Symposium
on Presenile Spongy
Encephalopathies
Venetia, June 4-9, 1965
Editors: G.L. Guazzi,
F. Seitelberger
65 figures. IV, 152 pages
(With contributions in
English, French and
German). 1967 (Acta
Neuropathologica, Sup-
plementum III)
DM 78,–; US $33.60
ISBN 3-540-03997-X

Symposium
on Neuroglia
Papers presented on the
12th annual meeting of
the Vereinigung Deutscher
Neuropathologen und
Neuroanatomen Berlin,
October 20-22, 1966
Editors: F. Erbslöh,
A. Oksche, F. Seitelberger
87 figures. IV, 166 pages
(In German with English
and German Summaries)
1968 (Acta Neuropatholo-
gica, Supplementum IV)
DM 86,–; US $37.00
ISBN 3-540-04355-1

F.W. Rieben
Zur Orthologie
und Pathologie der Arteria
vertebralis
(Vorgelegt in der Sitzung
vom 2. Juni 1973 von
W. Doerr)
12 Abbildungen
42 Seiten. 1973 (Sitzungs-
berichte der Heidelberger
Akademie der Wissen-
schaften, Mathematisch-
naturwissenschaftliche
Klasse, Jahrgang 1973,
3. Abhandlung)
DM 21,80; US $9.40

Symposium
on Pathology of Axons
and Axonal Flow
Organized by the
Österreichische Arbeits-
gemeinschaft für Neuro-
pathologie and the
Research Group of Neuro-
pathology of the World
Federation of Neurology
Wien, September 10 and
11, 1970
Editors: R.L. Friede,
F. Seitelberger
140 figures. IV, 266 pages
1971 (Acta Neuropatholo-
gica, Supplementum V)
DM 120,–; US $51.60
ISBN 3-540-05433-2

J. F. Kurtzke
Epidemiology of
Cerebrovascular Disease
42 figures. 212 pages. 1969
DM 74,–; US $31.90
ISBN 3-540-04591-0

H. Solcher
Zur Neuroanatomie
und Neuropathologie
der Frühfetalzeit
Untersuchungen an
Gehirnen menschlicher
Keimlinge einer Scheitel-
Fersen-Länge von 13 bis
38 cm. Mit einem Geleit-
wort von H. Jacob
39 Abbildungen
VII, 79 Seiten. 1968
(Monographien aus dem
Gesamtgebiete der Neu-
rologie und Psychiatrie,
Heft 127)
DM 54,–; US $23.30
ISBN 3-540-04283-0

Preisänderungen vorbehalten
Prices are subject to change
without notice

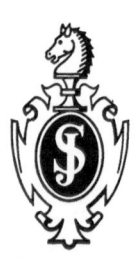

Springer-Verlag
Berlin
Heidelberg
New York

Acta Neuropathologica

Supplementum VI

Malignant Lymphomas
of the Nervous System

International Symposium

Organized by The Österreichische Arbeitsgemeinschaft
für Neuropathologie and the Research Group
of Neuropathology of the World Federation of Neurology

Wien, August 29–31, 1974

Edited by:

K. JELLINGER, Wien

F. SEITELBERGER, Wien

With 238 Figures

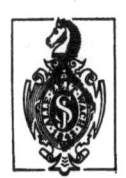 **Springer-Verlag Berlin Heidelberg GmbH**

Library of Congress Cataloging in Publication Data
Main entry under title:

Malignant lymphomas of the nervous system.

(Acta neuropathologica: supplementum; 6)
Bibliography: p.
Includes index.

1. Lymphoma-Congresses, 2. Nervous system—Tumors—Congresses. I. Jellinger, Kurt, ed.
II. Seitelberger, Franz, ed. III. Österreichische Arbeitsgemeinschaft für Neuropathologie.
IV. World Federation of Neurology. Commission für Neuropathology. V. Series. [DNLM
1. Lymphoma-Congresses. 2. Neoplasms, Nervous tissue-Congresses. W1 AC872NA
no. 6 / QZ380 M251 1974]

Library of Congress Cataloging in Publication Data

RC280.L9M34   616.9′94′8   75-2307

ISBN 978-3-540-07208-9

ISBN 978-3-540-07208-9   ISBN 978-3-662-08456-4 (eBook)
DOI 10.1007/978-3-662-08456-4

Contents

Contents

Introduction

More than 150 years have passed since involvement of the nervous system in
leukemia was first reported by BURNS, while the possibility of the primary
brain tumor derived from the lymphoreticular tissue was recognized much later.
BAILEY in 1929 described such neoplasms under the term perithelial sarcoma.
Later these tumors of the nervous system have been variously designated as
"Perivascular of perithelial sarcomas, reticulum cell sarcomas or microgliomas",
as controversy has evolved and still exists on the definition of this group of
neoplasms and on the nature of their cells of origin. Much of the unfortunate
confusion concerning the neoplastic lesions attributed to "microglia" and other
derivations of the RE system arose because their close relationship to extraneural cells has been ignored. On the other hand, communication in the field
of malignant lymphomas has become increasingly difficult because of the termino-
logic maze and conceptual diversities of traditional morphological classifications that have limited valid comparisons. Although at present we are still
far from a precise recognition of the basic features of lymphoproliferative
processes and from a fairly general agreement on the terminology of non-Hodgkin
lymphomas, there is encouraging evidence recently of some enlightment on the
nature of tumor cells that provides the basis for a reasonable and generally
acceptable lymphoma classification. It is now generally agreed upon that there
are no definite structural differences between ML arising in extraneural sites
and as a primary lesion in the CNS, but there are particular types of cytologic
reaction and growth pattern characteristic of CNS processes that add specific
dimensions to CNS lymphomas.

Those neoplasmas which may arise as a part of generalized disease or as
primary lesions confined to the CNS are not uncommon, but often escape recognition or identification as to their true nature. Limited epidemiological
experience suggests a relative rarity of metastatic CNS affection, occurring
in 10 to 23 percent of extraneural lymphomas and an almost equal incidence of
primary CNS lymphomas that constitute 0,3 to 1,8 percent of all intracranial
neoplasms. The increasing incidence of such tumors in immunologically suppressed
individuals, the rapid evolution of their clinical phenomena, the diagnostic
value of CSF examination, the remarkable response of CNS lymphomas to irradiation
and chemotherapy opposed by an increasing number of secundary and iatrogenic CNS
lesions are additional subjects of current interest.

In the last few years a series of conferences has been devoted to current
concepts in the classification and management of malignant lymphomas, which,
however, hardly considered the special problems related to the nervous system.
The present meeting which is organized by the "Österreichische Arbeitsgemeinschaft für Neuropathologie" under the auspices of the Research Group of Neuropathology of the WFN is therefore suggested to provide a timely review on the
many interrelated aspects of malignant lymphomas, with particular reference
to the nervous system including the still much debated problem of the nature
of microglia. This approach requires cooperation of experts which have been
invited to this meeting to shed some light on the large field of problems in
malignant lymphomas. Advances in general pathology, cytology and experimental
immunology are so rapid that this conference cannot reasonably be expected to
sufficiently answer the multitude of open questions. On the other hand, this
meeting may be considered to have been arranged too early as to provide new
concepts. Rather, its purpose must be to take stock of the available data and

to provide better communication on this field between general pathologists, neuropathologists, immunologists and clinical research workers, in order to provide impacts for future research.

It is hoped that publication of the papers will provide valuable information on the present state of knowledge. As the discussions cannot, unfortunately, be included in the printed text, a critical evaluation and suggestions for further work will be given in a concluding statement at the end of this volume.

We would like to express our gratitude to all participants of the symposium for contributing their efforts and for their co-operation in rapid publication of the Proceedings. We would like to thank Prof. H.M. ZIMMERMAN for his encouragement and infailing support in the organisation of the symposium.

We are indebted to Drs. HUME ADAMS, R.O. BARNARD, W. BLACKWOOD, W.G.P. MAIR and H. URICH for editorial support.

Our special thanks are due to all our collaborators and sponsors who have enabled the organisation ot his meeting. We are highly indepted to Springer-Verlag and to Mr. H. Rupprecht for providing publication of the symposium and for their appreciation of the editorial concerns.

K. JELLINGER   F. SEITELBERGER

Acta Neuropath. (Berlin), Suppl. VI, 1 - 16 (1975)
© by Springer-Verlag 1975

Morphology and Classification of Malignant Lymphomas and So-called Reticuloses [+)]

KARL LENNERT [++)]

Department of Pathology
University of Kiel, Germany

Summary: There is general agreement as to the definition and subclassification of Hodgkin lymphomas, which is acceptable for practical reasons. However, the nature of the different types of Hodgkin lymphomas needs further consideration.

On the other hand, today we are as far from agreement on non-Hodgkin lymphomas as ever before. Earlier European and American classifications have now to be reconsidered in the light of modern concepts of experimental immunology. It has become necessary to apply immunochemical and immunomorphological methods in addition to histological, histochemical, cytological, and ultrastructural techniques. Only such a complex approach has been able to provide new insight into the functional properties of the tumor cells.

The result was a new lymphoma classification, which conforms to LUKES' concept in many respects. It was fundamentally accepted by a group of European lymphoma experts and has been condensed and modified in order to be applicable by as many lymphoma centers as possible. It has received the name "Kiel Classification" 1974.

The main principles of the classification are as follows:
1. A distinction is made between malignant lymphomas of low-grade and those of high-grade malignancy; "-cytic", "-blastic" m.l.
2. The terms "sarcoma" and "leukemia" are avoided.

All types of malignant lymphoma can be leukemic, however with different frequencies. All B-cell lymphomas can also show a monoclonal immunoglobulin increase ("paraproteinemia") in the blood, mostly of IgM. So-called macroglobulinemia of Waldenström is therefore not itself an entity, but instead a clinical syndrome.

It has been shown that so-called reticulosarcoma is derived from immunoblasts, not from reticulum cells or histiocytes.

The group of reticuloses also needs reconsideration. The term "reticulosis" is cytologically incorrect in most cases. Otherwise it refers to a group of diseases which we do not yet understand.

Key words: Malignant lymphoma - malignant reticulosis - Hodgkin's disease - non-Hodgkin lymphoma - immunocytoma

An introductory survey of the classification and morphology of malignant lymphomas, including so-called reticulosis, will be given, and I have to talk about Hodgkin lymphomas, non-Hodgkin lymphomas, and reticuloses.

[+)] Supported by the Deutsche Forschungsgemeinschaft, SFB 111/C7.
[++)] E. KAISERLING and H. STEIN played important roles in the development of the non-Hodgkin lymphoma concept. H.-K. MÜLLER-HERMELINK contributed to the work on the normal cytology of the lymphatic tissue. L.-D. LEDER kindly allowed the use of his cytochemical techniques.

We can cover *Hodgkin lymphoma* in a few sentences. Today Hodgkin's disease is classified into four categories according to the conclusions drawn at the Rye conference (1):

1. lymphocytic predominance

2. nodular sclerosing

3. mixed

4. lymphocytic depletion.

This classification is based mainly on the studies of LUKES and co-workers, who distinguished six subgroups (2).

The Rye classification is clinically useful and reproducible. However, in some respects it is perhaps an oversimplification of the basic problems.

In addition to the above we have described an epithelioid cellular lympho-granulomatosis (3). This, however, is not a true type of Hodgkin's disease, but instead a lympho-epithelioid cell lymphoma which is composed primarily of lymphocytes (and functional variants) and epithelioid cells. The epithelioid cells are usually arranged in small clusters, not in the form of so-called tubercles. True Hodgkin or Sternberg cells are not found.

With so-called *reticulosis* there is great confusion in the terminology. If we exclude all non-neoplastic reticuloses, we find that there are a number of entities which have been thought to be reticuloses, but which have turned out in recent years to not be from reticulum cells or histiocytes (4).

We have distinguished three types of reticulosis based on the size of the cells (5), i.e. reticulosis with small, medium-sized, and large cells. According to recent cytological, cytochemical, and immunological data, however, these three types now have to be interpreted in a new way. The *small* cell variant, lymphoid reticulosis or leukemic reticuloendotheliosis (6), is now called hairy cell leukemia and is probably a B-cell lymphoma.

Medium-sized cellular reticulosis, histiomonocytic reticulosis, has been proven in cytochemical studies by LEDER (7) and others to be a variant of myeloid leukemia. They have shown that monocytes are not derived from the so-called RES, but instead from precursors in the bone marrow, which LEDER identified as promyelocytes. It is important for the pathologist to know that virtually all cases of monocytic leukemia reveal at least a small number of promyelocytes and myelocytes, as clearly demonstrated by the chloroacetate-esterase reaction in paraffin sections (8).

The group of *large* cellular reticuloses includes anaplastic monocytic leukemia, which is characterized by a strongly positive nonspecific esterase (alpha-naphthyl-acetate-esterase) reaction in cryostat sections or imprints, as is the case for monocytic leukemia. Unfortunately, this enzyme cannot be demonstrated in paraffin sections.

The other large cellular reticuloses are really leukemic variants of immuno-blastic sarcoma ("histioblastic leukemia" of MATHÉ et al. (9)). The esterase reaction is negative.

So we are left with what SCOTT and ROBB-SMITH (10) called *histiocytic medullary reticulosis*. We are in doubt as to the true nature of this disease. New facts, immunological ones in particular, are needed to prove that is a neo-plastic and not an immunological reaction like the graft-versus-host reaction. Together with NEZELOF we believe that *Farghuar's familial haemophagocytic reticulosis* is such a graft-versus-host reaction (11, 12).

I shall now consider *non-Hodgkin lymphomas* somewhat more extensively for several reasons.
1. Recent progress in the experimental research on lymphocytes and their significance in immunological reactions has been gigantic. The data indicate a correlation with malignant lymphomas, which are either equivalents of immunolo-

gical reactions or pure populations of lymphoid cells that are normally engaged in immunological reactions.

The most important result of modern immunological research has been the separation of lymphocytes into two lines: T- (thymus-derived) lymphocytes and B- (bursa or bone marrow-derived) lymphocytes.

2. By investigating malignant lymphomas with modern cytological, electron microscopic, cytochemical, and immunological methods (13) we have been able to show that they can be of both the B and T-lymphocyte lines. It has also become apparent that what have often been called reticulum cells or histiocytes are in fact transformed lymphocytes, which we now call immunoblasts.

Unfortunately, I do not have enough space to mention all of the interesting features of B and T-cells (14, 15, 16) and the methods we use to differentiate and identify the various types of lymphoma (17). I also regret that I cannot cite all of the important studies in this field which are in agreement with our own approach (18, 19).

However, I would like to present a very simple scheme demonstrating the basic cytological correlations of T and B-lymphocytes. It might also be useful to understand the different types of lymphoma, their interrelationships and variants.

Lymphocytes are derived from a type of hemopoietic stem cell which is certainly different from that of the three lines of the bone marrow.

These stem cells represent the origin of the T and B-lymphocyte series. *T-lymphocytes* are produced in the thymus and are then found in the thymus-dependent areas of peripheral lymphoid tissue, the paracortical area of lymph nodes for instance. Stimulation by an antigen induces the T-lymphocytes to transform into large pyroninophilic cells (blasts, T-immunoblasts). These cells either die or give rise to small T-lymphocytes, which react faster and with greater multiplication (through blast cells) to the same antigen. We call them T_2-lymphocytes, as opposed to the uncommitted T_1-lymphocytes. T-lymphocytes are responsible for cell-mediated immunity and not for immunoglobulin production. However, they are also engaged in most of the immunoglobulin responses as so-called helper cells: they help the B-cells to produce immunoglobulins.

B-lymphocytes, on the other hand, represent the precursors and effector cells (plasma cells) of immunoglobulin production, i.e. of humoral immunity. When a virgin B_1-lymphocyte is confronted with an antigen it can develop in either of two directions: a) It can transform into a large pyroninophilic cell (B-immunoblast). This is the precursor of either small lymphoplasmacytoid cells, which produce primarily IgM, or typical Marschalkó plasma cells, which produce chiefly IgG and IgA. b) Other B_1-lymphocytes aggregate to form a germinal center and at the same time transform into large blastic cells, which we used to call germinoblasts, but can now call centroblasts. These cells multiply very rapidly. They give rise to the polymorphous smaller forms, which used to be known as germinocytes and can now be called centrocytes, and then transform in B_2-lymphocytes. The germinal center is mainly engaged in providing active precursor cells of plasmacytopoiesis. However, it is not yet clear whether the centroblasts, their progeny, or both are the precursors for B-immunoblasts, which are then primarily engaged in the production of IgG and IgA, as is seen in the second response to a given antigen. B-lymphocytes bear surface immunoglobulin. After the switch to immunoglobulin production and, consequently, the development of plasma cells, they lose their surface immunoglobulin and produce it in their own cytoplasm (in the rough endoplasmic reticulum).

At the end of this presentation I shall try to correlate the different types of lymphoma with this cytological scheme.

However, I would first like to make some remarks on the terminology and the classification of non-Hodgkin lymphomas. This is an area of great confusion. I therefore prepared a comparison of several classifications (Table 1).

Table 1

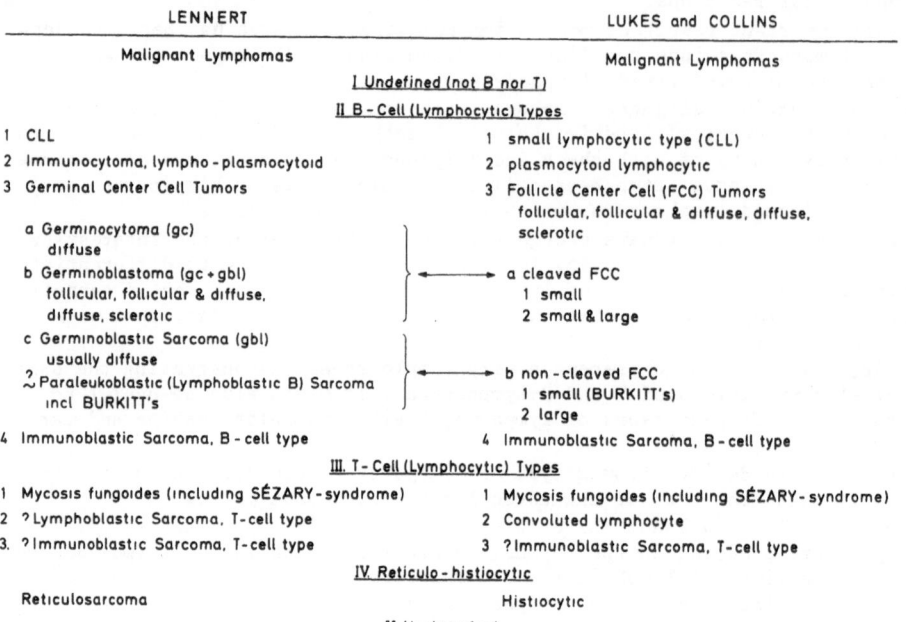

LENNERT	LUKES and COLLINS
Malignant Lymphomas	Malignant Lymphomas

I Undefined (not B nor T)

II B - Cell (Lymphocytic) Types

LENNERT	LUKES and COLLINS
1 CLL	1 small lymphocytic type (CLL)
2 Immunocytoma, lympho - plasmacytoid	2 plasmacytoid lymphocytic
3 Germinal Center Cell Tumors	3 Follicle Center Cell (FCC) Tumors follicular, follicular & diffuse, diffuse, sclerotic
a Germinocytoma (gc) diffuse	
b Germinoblastoma (gc + gbl) follicular, follicular & diffuse, diffuse, sclerotic	a cleaved FCC 1 small 2 small & large
c Germinoblastic Sarcoma (gbl) usually diffuse	
? Paraleukoblastic (Lymphoblastic B) Sarcoma incl BURKITT's	b non - cleaved FCC 1 small (BURKITT's) 2 large
4 Immunoblastic Sarcoma, B - cell type	4 Immunoblastic Sarcoma, B - cell type

III. T - Cell (Lymphocytic) Types

LENNERT	LUKES and COLLINS
1 Mycosis fungoides (including SÉZARY - syndrome)	1 Mycosis fungoides (including SÉZARY - syndrome)
2 ? Lymphoblastic Sarcoma, T-cell type	2 Convoluted lymphocyte
3. ? Immunoblastic Sarcoma, T-cell type	3 ? Immunoblastic Sarcoma, T-cell type

IV. Reticulo - histiocytic

LENNERT	LUKES and COLLINS
Reticulosarcoma	Histiocytic

V Unclassified

Here I shall have to restrict myself to the classification that we use now.
In May, 1974, the so-called European Lymphoma Club held a meeting in Kiel. We
agreed on a new classification based mainly on the one that I had presented
(cf. Table 1), but with a revised terminology. It is quite similar to the
classification of LUKES and COLLINS (20) which LUKES presented in a comparison
with my nomenclature at a meeting in London in October, 1973 (cf. Table 2).
The classification that had been agreed upon in Kiel was considered and discussed again in July, 1974, in Amsterdam, and finally accepted as the "Kiel
Classification". It has now been published by GERARD-MARCHANT *et al.* (21). I
shall use this classification in what follows as the basis for discussion
since it has been accepted by a group of experts in this field and because
other new classifications such as that of DORFMAN (22) or BENNETT *et al.* (23)
are only compromises and lack a definite cytological concept.

I shall begin with the essential points of the *Kiel Classification*.

1. We distinguish two main groups of malignant lymphomas, those of low-grade
and those of high-grade malignancy.
   The names of the low-grade malignant lymphomas end in the suffix "-cytic"
(or "-cytoid") and those of the high-grade ones in the suffix "-blastic". There
are four basic entities in the first group, three in the second group. Most of
the low-grade malignant lymphomas can transform into high-grade ones. However,
this occurs with different frequencies for the various types.

2. We omit the word lymphosarcoma completely because it has been used for so
long for so many different kinds of malignant lymphoma that it is most confusing. We also omit the word leukemia, at least from the main terms, since
in many cases it cannot be decided whether a leukemic blood picture exists or
not. All types of malignant lymphoma can be leukemic, although with different
frequencies for the different types.

Table 2

"Kiel Classification" 1974[1]	Rappaport's Classification[2]

Low-grade malignant lymphomas

lymphocytic

    CLL and others

                             m.l., well differentiated lymphocytic, diffuse

lympho-plasmacytoid

    (immunocytic)

                              m.l., lymphocytic with dysproteinemia

centrocytic

                              m.l., lymphocytic poorly differentiated? intermediate? diffuse(and nodular?)

centroblastic/centrocytic

    ⎧follicular
    ⎨follicular & diffuse
    ⎩diffuse

    with or without sclerosis

m.l. ⎰ well differentiated lymphocytic / poorly differentiated lymphocytic / lymphocytic-histiocytic / histiocytic ⎱ → nodular or diffuse

High-grade malignant lymphomas

centroblastic

                              m.l., histiocytic, nodular or diffuse undifferentiated

lymphoblastic

    Burkitt type

    convoluted cell type

    others

m.l., undifferentiated Burkitt's lymphoma

m.l. ⎰ poorly differentiated lymphocytic - diffuse? / undifferentiated - non-Burkitt ⎱

immunoblastic

                              m.l., histiocytic - diffuse

---

[1] Gérard-Marchant, Hamlin, Lennert, Rilke, Stansfeld, & van Unnik, 1974

[2] 1956, 1966

3. So-called reticulosarcoma turned out in most instances to be a tumor of B-immunoblasts. So we call it malignant lymphoma, immunoblastic. True reticulo-sarcoma and other apparently reticulocytic neoplasias such as reticulosis have been excluded from our classification.

4. Some of our American friends feel that the terms germinoblast and germino-cyte, which we have used for what LUKES calls non-cleaved and cleaved follicle center cells, are not acceptable because they could be confused with the ger-

minal cells of the gonads. Therefore we proposed the term centroblast instead
of germinoblast and the term centrocyte instead of germinocyte. The corresponding tumors are the centrocytic, the centroblastic-centrocytic, and the centroblastic.

In the following I would like to present all of the types of malignant lymphoma of the Kiel Classification. I shall mention some of the most familiar
synonyms in order to help you understand what is what in the different nomenclatures. For each type you will also find the percentage of cases with respect
to the total number of malignant lymphomas in our routine lymph node material.

I. LOW-GRADE MALIGNANCIES

1. *Malignant lymphoma, lymphocytic*

In the first group of low-grade malignancies I have added hairy cell leukemia
and mycosis fungoides together with Sézary syndrome, since I am now sure that
these are two further distinct entities of lymphocytic lymphoma.

The first subtype of lymphocytic lymphoma is the *CLL type*. It is the most
frequent in our routine material (12.5%).

The essential morphological feature of this type is the presence of so-called
lymphoblasts. These cells are often situated in lighter areas, which we call
proliferation centers. Here there are also many so-called prolymphocytes. Such
proliferation centers can be seen in most biopsy cases. They are difficult to
find in autopsy material because postmortal shrinking of the cells leads to a
monotonous lymphoid appearance.

Plasma cells or plasmacytoid cells are not found. There are also no PAS-positive globular inclusions in the lymphoid cells.

The second subtype of lymphocytic lymphoma is so-called *hairy cell leukemia*.
We prefer this term because it is a purely descriptive one and not wrong like
the term reticuloendotheliosis. This year the work of CATOVSKY et al. (24),
HAAK et al. (25), and STEIN et al. (26) has shown that hairy cells are a
special kind of B-lymphocyte.

We have studied 33 cases. The percentage of routine material was 0.2%. However, these were lymph node biopsies. The number of cases among bone marrow or
liver biopsies and removed spleens is much greater since the lymph nodes are
not regularly involved and, if so, they are not strongly infiltrated in most
cases. The meninges can be infiltrated in terminal cases (27).

The first infiltration takes place in the outer cortex, i.e. in the B-cell
region of the lymph node. The paracortical area (tertiary nodules) is not
affected until later and sometimes not until just before the death of the
patient.

The leukemic cells are somewhat larger than typical lymphocytes. The nucleus
is sometimes reniform and the chromatin pattern somewhat lighter than that of
lymphocytes. The distance between the nuclei is larger than in CLL. Mitotic
activity is generally not seen. Lymphoblasts or other blasts do not occur.
Hairy cells make up the whole cell population.

The term hairy cell was introduced by SCHREK and DONNELLY (28) since the
cells have long hair-like cytoplasmic projections. These are best seen under
the phase contrast or electron microscope and in enzyme stainings of blood
smears.

The most diagnostic feature of hairy cells is the existence of tartrate-
resistant acid phosphatase in smears, imprints or cryostat sections (29).

The third subtype of lymphocytic lymphoma is *mycosis fungoides (M.f.) including Sézary syndrome,* which we consider is a leukemic variant of mycosis
fungoides. We agree with LUTZNER et al. (30) and ZUCKER-FRANKLIN et al. (31)
that the main constituent of this lymphoma, the so-called Lutzner cell, is in

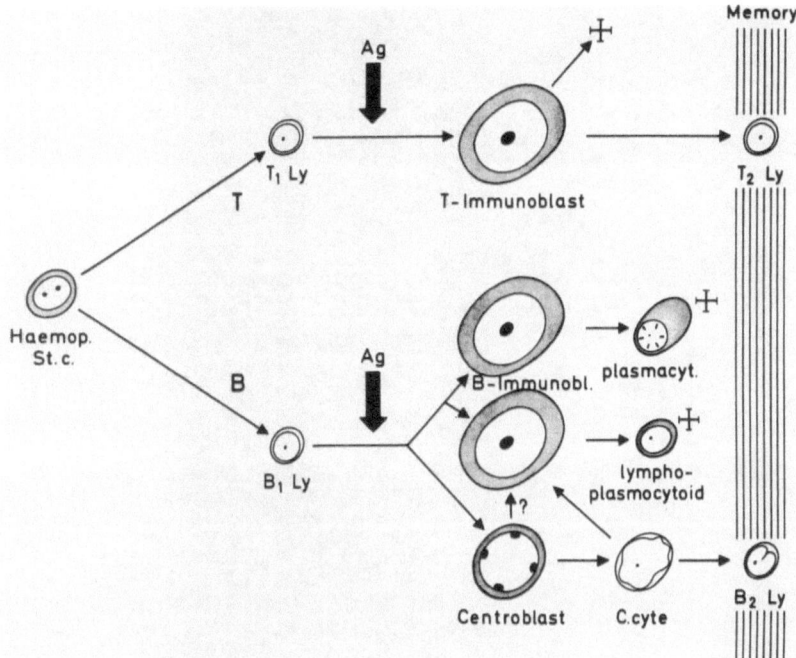

Fig. 1. The two lymphocyte systems in a simplified schema

fact a lymphocyte and not a histiocyte. This has been shown by many immunological and cytochemical studies.

M.f. and Sézary syndrome are relatively rare diseases (0.8% of our routine lymph node biopsies). VARJAKOJIS *et al.* (32) reported that in 14% of 45 autopsy cases there was meningeal infiltration.

Histologically the so-called infiltrative stage of M.f. and Sézary syndrome shows a somewhat polymorphous lymphocyte proliferation, which is seen at first in the so-called paracortical area of the lymph node. This agrees with the findings reported by LUTZNER *et al.* (30) and ZUCKER-FRANKLIN *et al.* (31) and speaks in favor of the T-lymphocyte nature of the proliferated cells.

In between the Lutzner cells there are always some larger cells with different morphological features (so-called M.f. cells). These cells are definitely of a different origin. Some of them represent polyploid Lutzner cells.

In the later stages of M.f., which clinicians call the tumor phase, a polymorphous of medium-sized to large cellular monomorphous appearance can develop.

Other lymphocytic lymphomas do exist. However, we still have to learn more about them. For instance, we have seen tumors whose cells fulfilled all of the immunocytological criteria of T-lymphocytes, but which were not identical with M.f.

2. Malignant lymphoma, lympho-plasmacytoid (immunocytic)

The second main group of low-grade malignancies, malignant lymphoma, lympho-plasmacytoid or immunocytic, is called "immunocytoma" for short. This is a frequent malignant lymphoma (9.5% of our routine node biopsies). The group includes macroglobulinemia Waldenström. On the whole, however, only 1/4 to 1/3 of the cases shows an increase of macroglobulins (IgM) in the blood!

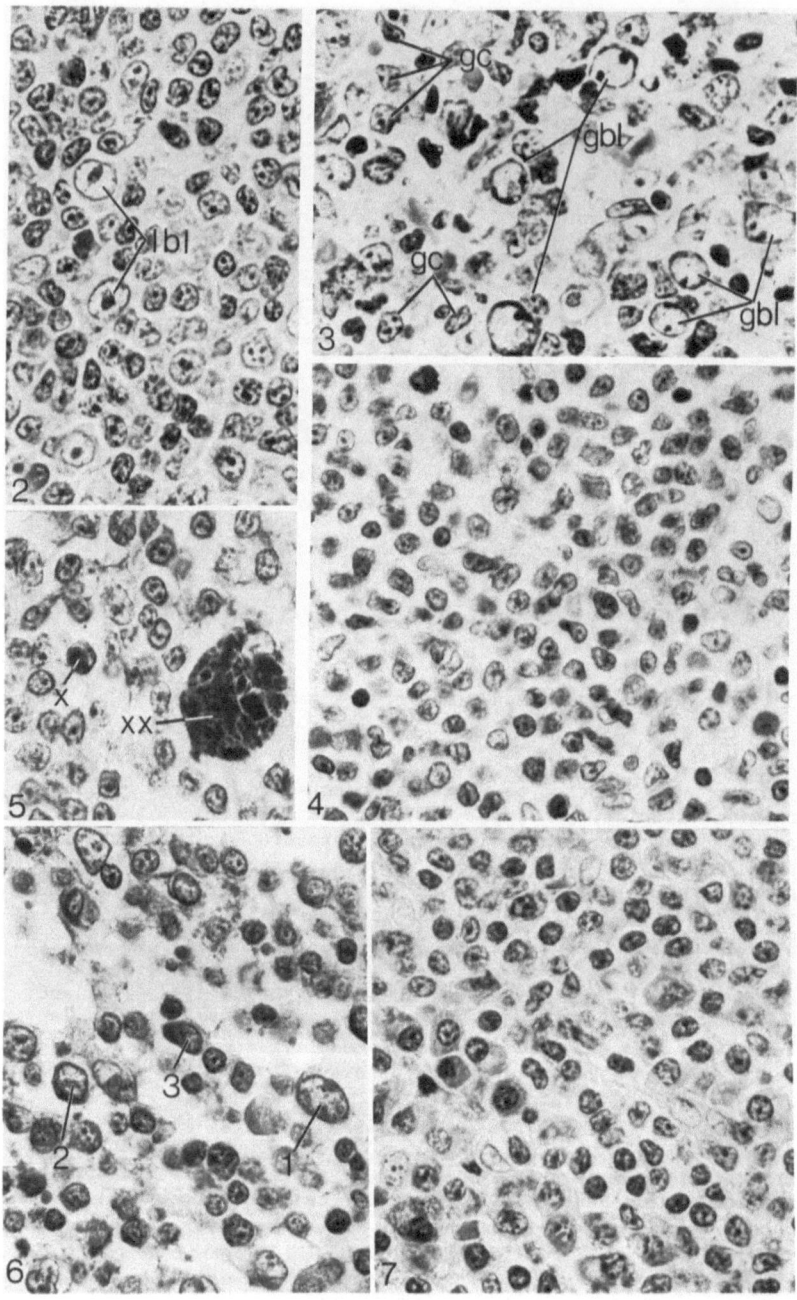

Plate 1:

Fig. 2. CLL. Note some lymphoblasts (lbl) with large central nucleoli. Giemsa

Fig. 3. Malignant lymphoma centroblastic/centrocytic. Note several centroblasts (gbl) with medium-sized nucleoli at the nuclear membrane. Some centrocytes (gc). Giemsa

We postulated this lymphoma entity on the basis of the following facts, which resulted from joint studies with STEIN and KAISERLING (13, 33)

There is a type of malignant lymphoma with diffuse proliferation which always contains a large number of lymphocytes and a smaller amount of plasma cells or plasmacytoid cells. These cells cannot be seen well enough in H & E slides and require special stains such as Giemsa or methyl green pyronine. In some cases we have also found centroblasts and centrocytes as well as plasmablasts and proplasmacytes. The number of mast cells is often relatively high.

We have investigated the tumor homogenates of such lymphomas (41 cases so far) and found an increase and sometimes an excessive amount of immunoglobulins, mostly IgM, occasionally IgA, IgG, or IgE, alone or in combination with IgM.

In nearly all of the cases which we studied immunochemically we also found globular PAS-positive inclusions in the nucleus and/or cytoplasm of the tumor cells. In most instances these inclusions represented retained immunoglobulins, which was also demonstrated in electron microscopic pictures.

An immunocytoma can also secrete immunoglobulins into the blood after producing them. This results in a monoclonal gammopathy.

Immunocytoma can be leukemic. It is then called CLL, lymphoplasmacytoid leukemia, or, in extreme cases, plasma cell leukemia. 30% of our material presented a leukemic blood picture.

About 8% of our cases showed a transformation into a blastic ("sarcomatous") variant, i.e. a high-grade malignancy.

3. *Malignant lymphoma, centrocytic* (synonyms: lymphocytic lymphosarcoma; malignant lymphoma, lymphocytic, well and/or poorly differentiated; germinocytoma)

Centrocytic malignant lymphoma is composed of small germinal center cells, which we used to call germinocytes and which LUKES and COLLINS (23) called follicle center cells with cleaved nuclei (cleaved FCC). This group made up 4.7% of our routine lymph node biopsies.

The lymphoma consists only of small polymorphous cells with irregular, often cleaved nuclei. They are somewhat larger than lymphocytes. The tumor can show rather high mitotic activity, but does not contain any lymphoblasts. The growth pattern is diffuse in most cases, although one sometimes finds nodular structures which are similar to primary lymph follicles. There are only a few, but very thick reticulin fibers.

No more than 10% of our cases showed a clear leukemic picture. However, we are not sure whether the number of cases would not be higher if an expert were to review the blood smears. This should be done the next time.

Fig. 4. Malignant lymphoma centrocytic. Only pleomorphous cells with cleaved nuclei are present. Giemsa

Fig. 5. Malignant lymphoma lymphoplasmacytoid with μ-chain disease. Intranuclear PAS-positive inclusions (x). PAS-positive deposits in a macrophage (xx). PAS

Fig. 6. Malignant lymphoma lymphoplasmacytoid with μ-chain disease. Polymorphous picture with an immunoblast (1), a plasmablast (2), and a proplasmacyte (3). The cytoplasm of the plasmablast and the proplasmacyte shows a diffuse PAS reaction. PAS

Fig. 7. Malignant lymphoma lymphoplasmacytic with macroglobulinemia. There are lymphocytes and Marschalkó plasma cells. Giemsa

Figs. 2 - 7: x 750

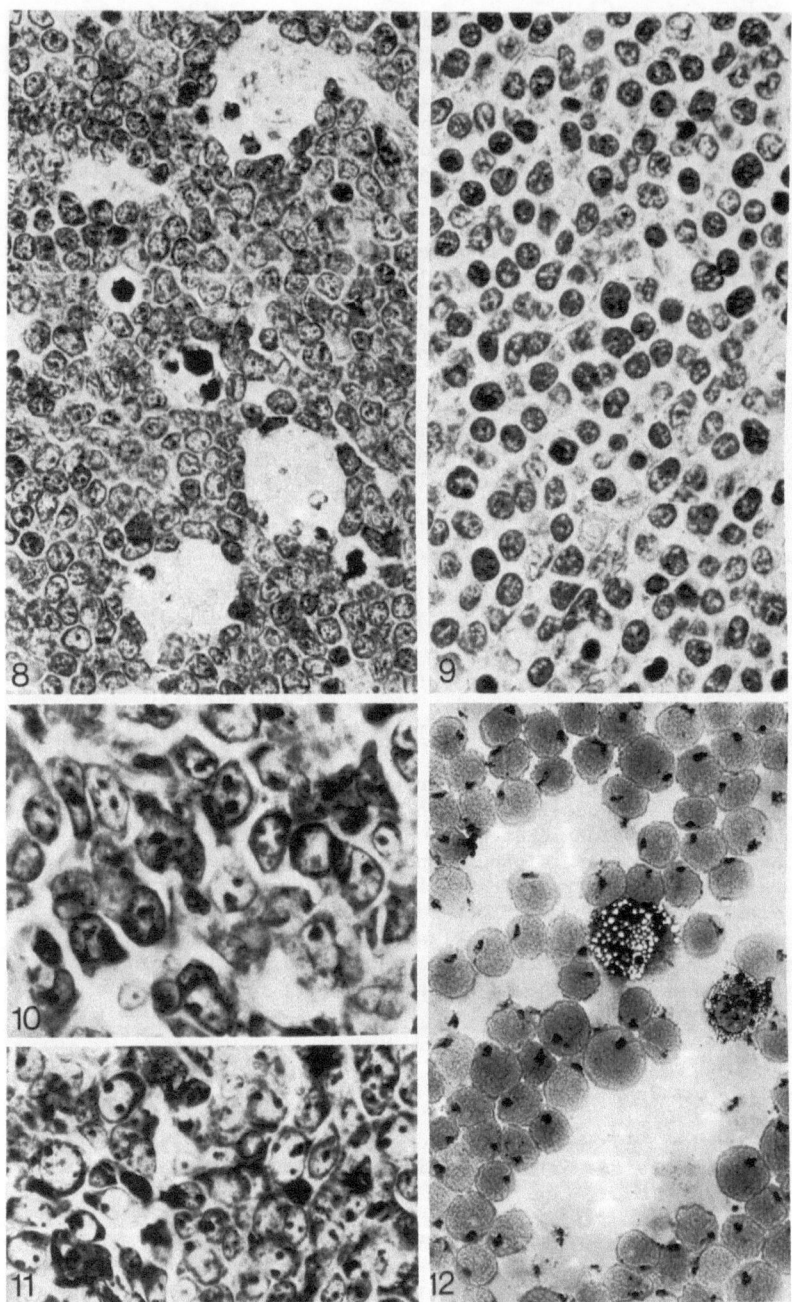

Plate 2:

Fig. 8. Malignant lymphoma, lymphoblastic, Burkitt type. Starry sky pattern. The cells are very close together. Giemsa

Fig. 9. Malignant lymphoma, convoluted type (acid phosphatase type). Note the "convoluted" nucleus (x). The cells lie separately. Giemsa

4. Malignant lymphoma, centroblastic/centrocytic (synonyms: Brill-Symmers' disease; follicular lymphoma; nodular lymphoma; germinoblastoma)

Malignant lymphoma, centroblastic/centrocytic is the most frequent type of non-Hodgkin lymphoma (12.1% of routine lymph node biopsies) beside the CLL type. It is now accepted by most hematopathologists that it is itself an entity (34, 35) and not a variant of the different types of lymphoma, as RAPPA-PORT (36) pointed out.

This tumor always consists of at least four types of cell: centroblasts, centrocytes, dendritic reticulum cells, and a few macrophages. The centroblasts are easily distinguishable from the lymphoblasts of CLL in Giemsa stained slides. They are transformed B-lymphocytes and by no means histiocytes or reticulum cells. Arguments in favor of this interpretation were reported in earlier papers (34, 35). It is not necessary to repeat them here because nearly all of the experts in this field now agree with this view. The dendritic reticulum cell is a specific cell of the normal follicle, in particular of the germinal center. This supports our opinion that follicular lymphoma is a special tumor entity, namely a tumor of the germinal centers.

Centroblastic-centrocytic lymphoma can also be leukemic at any stage of the disease. GALTON (37) reported that about 25% of his cases were leukemic.

The transformation into a blastic, i.e. a centroblastic variant, occurs often. We found it in about 40% of our autopsy material. The histological picture is then monomorphous and sometimes similar to that of Burkitt's tumor.

II. HIGH-GRADE MALIGNANCIES

1. Malignant lymphoma, centroblastic (synonyms: malignant lymphoma, histiocytic; reticulosarcoma in follicular lymphoma; germinoblastic sarcoma)

Centroblastic malignant lymphoma is the first lymphoma of high-grade malignancy. Until now we have made this diagnosis only when we found signs of a centroblastic-centrocytic lymphoma in the lymph nodes or other tissues, or when such a low-grade malignant lymphoma had already been established. However, it now seems that centroblastic lymphoma can also be primary.

It is very rare in routine lymph node biopsies (0.07%), in contrast to autopsy material.

The blastic variant of germinal center cell tumors can also be leukemic (37).

2. Malignant lymphoma, lymphoblastic

The second malignant lymphoma of high-grade malignancy is the lymphoblastic. We distinguish the Burkitt type, the convoluted cell type, and a large number of so-called "other" cases which are not yet fully understood. Together all of the lymphoblastic lymphomas make up 6.0% of our routine lymph node biopsies.

The *Burkitt type* is well known from many studies of the last 15 years (38, 39, 40, 41). It shows the typical starry sky pattern and a relatively monotonous proliferation of medium-sized, very basophilic (pyroninophilic) cells, which perhaps represent neoplastic centroblasts and/or centrocytes. The mitotic activity is high.

Fig. 10 and 11. Malignant lymphoma, immunoblastic. Basophilic cytoplasm. Large nucleoli. Giemsa

Fig. 12. Malignant lymphoma, convoluted type (acid phosphatase type). CSF. Two vacuolated strongly positive macrophages and tumor cells with a solitary positive reaction. Acid phosphatase reaction

Figs. 8 - 12: x 750

Since the tumor cells produce immunoglobulins in tissue cultures (42) we can be quite certain that this is a tumor of B-lymphocyte derivates.

Epstein-Barr viruses are always found in the tumor cells of African Burkitt's tumor. However, this is not true for most of the tumors of the same type in Europe, which are also called Burkitt's tumor outside of Africa and New Guinea. Only one of our 27 European cases (0.35% of our routine lymph node biopsies) showed evidence of Epstein-Barr viruses in the tumor (43). The basophilia of this tumor was much greater than that of all the other cases with the same general appearance.

Leukemic variants of this lymphoma are very rare (approx. 5%).

Lymphoblastic malignant lymphoma of the *convoluted cell type* was described by LUKES (44, 23) on the basis of the form of certain nuclei which are found with a low frequency in this lymphoma. The tumor is at least in part identical with what LEDER called extremely immature erythremia (45). The tumor cells possess a very distinctive marker: a focal accumulation of acid phosphatase activity. When this reaction is found in an imprint or cryostat section one can make the diagnosis immediately.

This tumor is most frequent in childhood and adolescence, although we have found cases in up to the sixth decade. The percentage of routine lymph node biopsies was 0.42%.

In most cases there is a large mediastinal mass, a thymic tumor in other words. The tumor cells form spontaneous rosettes (E-rosettes) with sheep erythrocytes. These features show that the tumor has a T-cell origin.

For neuropathologists it is important to know that this tumor can very extensively infiltrate the meninges. For instance, in one autopsy case we found a mediastinal mass and only a few bone marrow infiltrations, but widespread infiltration of the meninges of the brain.

What are called for the moment *"other"* lymphoblastic malignant lymphomas include all of the acute lymphocytic leukemias of childhood and the corresponding so-called sarcomas. However, we now avoid these terms. The synonyms most often used are: lymphoblastic sarcoma and leukemia; paraleukoblastic sarcoma and leukemia; acute lymphocytic leukemia (ALL); malignant lymphoma, poorly differentiated; malignant lymphoma, undifferentiated. 5.2% of our routine lymph node biopsies were of this type.

This group is still greatly in need of clarification. Therefore we shall mention only that the cells are a little or much larger than lymphocytes. They have a small, moderately basophilic cytoplasm and sometimes show a granular PAS reaction. This positivity does not represent immunoglobulin, but in most cases glycogen. All specific cytochemical marker enzymes are negative (for example peroxidase, chloroacetate-esterase, nonspecific esterase, etc.).

3. *Malignant lymphoma, immunoblastic* (synonyms: reticulosarcoma; malignant lymphoma, histiocytic)

The term immunoblastic lymphoma now covers most of the cases of reticulosarcoma of histiocytic lymphoma. At the meeting in Nagoya, 1971, we called it "immunoblastic sarcoma". It is a frequent lymphoma (8.1% of our routine lymph node biopsies).

As we have shown in immunochemical and electron microscopic studies together with STEIN and KAISERLING (46, 47), the reticulosarcoma of the former nomenclature is in fact a tumor which consists of immunoglobulin producing cells that are morphologically similar to B-immunoblasts or, if they have a lot of rough endoplasmic reticulum, plasmablasts. The immunoglobulin produced by the cells is usually IgM, sometimes IgA. "Macroglobulinemia" was found in some cases. Globular of diffuse PAS-positive inclusions are sometimes seen in the tumor cells.

Fiber production may be great or not. However, this does not mean that the tumor cells themselved produce fibers. On the contrary, we believe that the immunoglobulin producing and secreting tumor cells stimulate reticulum cells with fibroblastic ability to produce reticulin fibers (48). This would correlate with the enormous fiber production in multiple myeloma, which we found through quantitative fiber estimation in bone marrow (49).

The nonspecific esterase reaction, which is a marker of histiocytes, was negative in the tumor cells of all cases. There is often a large number of histiocytes, but *in addition to* the tumor cells! The histiocytes are not an essential part of the tumor itself, but are reactive like the fiber production. They can transform into epithelioid cells or Langhans' giant cells, as we have found in a number of immunoblastic lymphomas, especially those which produced very large amounts of IgM (48).

Nevertheless we are convinced that true reticulosarcoma does exist. So far we have had this suspicion in only 3 cases. However, we are not yet sure just what the exact criteria for true reticulosarcoma should be. We also have to take into consideration the fact that there are at least four types of reticulum cell in the lymphatic tissue: histiocytic, fibroblastic, dendritic, and interdigitating reticulum cells. So we can presume that each of these kinds of reticulum cell could also produce a special kind of reticulosarcoma.

If we correlate the different non-Hodgkin lymphomas with our cytological scheme we can make the following suppositions.

The *T-cell series* includes lymphoblastic lymphoma of the convoluted type and Sézary syndrome (which probably includes mycosis fungoides), which is a neoplasia of T-lymphocytes (T_1 or T_2 ?).

Most non-Hodgkin lymphomas are of *B-cell origin*. CLL is at least chiefly a B-lymphocytic lymphoma, in particular B_1-lymphocytic. In this type the transformation of the lymphocytes into immunoblasts seems to be blocked (18). Therefore "immunocytes" (plasma cells and plasmacytoid cells) are not produced. In contrast, lympho-plasmacytoid lymphoma is composed of a variable amount of (unblocked ?) lymphocytes (lympho-plasmacytoid cells, plasmacytes and precursors), sometimes together with germinal center cells (centroblasts, centrocytes), which are said to be precursors of the plasma cell series (16). Germinal centers are accumulations of B-cells, so tumors of germinal center cells (malignant lymphoma, centrocytic; malignant lymphoma, centroblastic-centrocytic) must be B-cell neoplasms. This has also been proven to be the case for Burkitt's tumor, which is a variant of lymphoblastic lymphoma. At least most cases of immunoblastic lymphoma are of B-immunoblastic origin. A T-immunoblastic lymphoma has yet to be found. For some lymphoblastic lymphomas the correlation is not yet clear. Either they are derived from B-cells or they can be undefined.

REFERENCES

1. LUKES, R.J., CRAVER, L.F., HALL, T.C., RAPPAPORT, H., RUBEN, P.: Report of the Nomenclature Committee. Cancer Res. *26*, 1311 (1966) a
2. LUKES, R.J., BUTLER, J.J., HICKS, E.B.: Natural history of Hodgkin's disease as related to its pathologic picture. Cancer (Philad.) *19*, 317 - 344 (1966) b
3. LENNERT, K., MESTDAGH, J.: Lymphogranulomatosen mit konstant hohem Epitheloidzellgehalt. Virchows Arch. Abt. A *344*, 1 - 20 (1968)
4. LENNERT, K.: Retikulosen und Retikulosarkom. Beitrag zum Rundtischgespräch. (Spanisch.) 6. Congr. Nacional de Anatomia Patológica, Murcia 1973. Patologia *7*, 35 - 38 (1974)
5. LENNERT, K.: Pathologische Anatomie der Retikulosen. Krebsforschung u. Krebsbekämpfung *5*, 48 - 67 (1964)

6. EWALD, O.: Die leukämische Reticuloendotheliose. Dtsch. Arch. klin. Med. *142*, 222 - 228 (1923)

7. LEDER, L.-D.: Der Blutmonocyt: Morphologie - Herkunft - Funktion und prospektive Potenz - Monocytenleukaemie. Exp. Med., Path. u. Klinik *23*. Berlin - Heidelberg - New York: Springer 1967

8. LEDER, L.-D.: Der Nachweis der Naphthol-AS-D-Chloracetat-Esterase und seine Bedeutung für die histologische Diagnostik. Verh. dtsch. Ges. Path. *48*, 317 320 (1964)

9. MATHÉ, G., GÉRARD-MARCHANT, R., TEXIER, J.L., SCHLUMBERGER, J.R., BERUMEN, L., PAINTRAND, M.: The two varieties of lymphoid tissue "reticulosarcomas", histiocytic and histioblastic types. Brit. J. Cancer *24*, 687 - 695 (1970)

10. SCOTT, R.B., ROBB-SMITH, A.H.T.: Histiocytic medullary reticulosis. Lancet 1939, II, pp. 194 - 198

11. LENNERT, K., MOHRI, N.: Histologische Klassifizierung und Vorkommen des M. Hodgkin. Internist *15*, 57 - 65 (1974)

12. NEZELOF, C., ELIACHAR, E.: La lymphohistiocytose familiale. Revue générale à propos de trois observations. Liens éventuels avec les syndromes secondaires. Nouv. Rev. franç. Hémat. *13*, 319 - 338 (1973)

13. LENNERT, K., STEIN, H., KAISERLING, E.: Cytological and functional criteria for the classification of malignant lymphomas. Symp. on Non-Hodgkin's Lymphomas, London 1973. Brit. J. Cancer, in press

14. GOOD, R.A.: Immunodeficiency in developmental perspective. Harvey Lect. Ser. *67*, 1 - 107 (1971-72)

15. VELDMAN, J.E.: Histophysiology and Electron Microscopy of the Immune Response. Diss. med., Groningen 1970. Groningen: N.V. Boekdrukkerij Dijkstra Niemeyer 1970

16. NIEUWENHUIS, P., KEUNING, F.J.: Germinal centres and the origin of the B-cell system. II. Germinal centres in the rabbit spleen and popliteal lymph nodes. Immunology *26*, 509 - 519 (1974)

17. LENNERT, K., STEIN, H., KAISERLING, E.: New criteria for the classification of malignant lymphomas. (Referat) 2. Meeting Europ. and Afr. Div. of Int. Soc. of Haemat., Prague 1973

18. PREUD'HOMME, J.L., SELIGMANN, M.: Surface bound immunoglobulins as a cell marker in human lymphoproliferative diseases. Blood *40*, 777 - 794 (1972)

19. JAFFE, E.S., SHEVACH, E.M., FRANK, M.M., BERARD, C.W., GREEN, I.: Nodular lymphoma - evidence for origin from follicular B lymphocytes. New Engl. J. Med. *290*, 813 - 819 (1974)

20. GERARD-MARCHANT, R., HAMLIN, I., LENNERT, K., RILKE, F., STANSFELD, A.G., VAN UNNIK, J.A.M.: Letter to the editor: Classification of non-Hodkin's lymphomas. Lancet 1974, II, pp. 406 - 408

21. DORFMAN, R.F.: Letter to the editor: Classification on non-Hodgkin's lymphomas. Lancet 1974, I, pp. 1295 - 1296

22. BENNETT, M.H., FARRER-BROWN, G., HENRY, K., JELLIFFE, A.M.: Letter to the editor: Classification of non-Hodgkin's lymphomas. Lancet 1974, II, pp. 405 - 406

23. LUKES, R.J., COLLINS, R.D.: New observations on follicular lymphoma. *In:* AKAZAKI, K., RAPPAPORT, H., BERARD, C.W., BENNETT, J.M., ISHIKAWA, E. (eds.): Malignant Diseases of the Hematopoietic System. GANN Monograph on Cancer Research No. 15, pp. 209 - 215. Baltimore-London-Tokyo: University Park Press 1973

24. CATOVSKY, D., PETTIT, J.E., GALETTO, J., OKOS, A., GALTON, D.A.G.: The B-lymphocyte nature of the hairy cell of leukaemic reticuloendotheliosis. Brit. J. Haemat. *26*, 29 - 37 (1974)

25. HAAK, H.L., DE MAN, J.C.H., HIJMANS, W., KNAPP, W., SPECK, B.: Further evidence for the lymphocytic nature of leukaemic reticuloendotheliosis (hairy-cell leukaemia). Brit. J. Haemat. *27*, 31 - 38 (1974)

26. STEIN, H., KAISERLING, E., STEIN, G.: Surface markers on hairy cells.
    Proc. of the Immunological Conf., Pavia 1974. Boll. Ist. sieroter. milan.
    53 Suppl., 305 (1974)
27. PLENDERLEITH, I.H.: Hairy cell leukemia. Canad. med. Ass. J. 102, 1056 -
    1060 (1970)
28. SCHREK, R., DONNELLY, W.J.: "Hairy" cells in blood in lymphoreticular
    neoplastic disease and "flagellated" cells of normal lymph nodes. Blood
    27, 199 - 211 (1966)
29. YAM, L.T., LI, C.Y., LAM, K.W.: Tartrate-resistant acid phosphatase
    isoenzyme in the reticulum cell of leukemic retikuloendotheliosis. New
    Engl. J. Med. 284, 357 - 360 (1971)
30. LUTZNER, M.A., EMERIT, I., DUREPAIRE, R., FLANDRIN, G., GRUPPER, C.,
    PRUNIERAS, M.: Cytogenetic, cytophotometric, and ultrastructural study
    of large cerebriform cells of the Sézary syndrome and description of a
    small-cell variant. J. nat. Cancer Inst. 50, 1145 - 1162 (1973)
31. ZUCKER-FRANKLIN, D., MELTON, J.W., III, QUAGLIATA, F.: Ultrastructural,
    Immunologic and Functional Studies on Sézary Cells: A Neoplastic Variant
    of Thymus-Derived (T) Lymphocytes. Proc. nat. Acad. Sci. Wash., 71,
    1877 - 1881 (1974)
32. VARIAKOJIS, D., ROSAS-URIBE, A., RAPPAPORT, H.: Mycosis fungoides: Pathologic
    findings in staging laparotomies. Cancer (Philad.) 33, 1589 - 1600 (1974)
33. STEIN, H., KAISERLING, E., LENNERT, K.: Lymphoplasmocytoid immunocytoma.
    A new entity of human non-Hodgkin's lymphoma. 10. Int. Congr. Int. Acad.
    of Path., Hamburg 1974
34. LENNERT, K.: Follicular lymphoma: A special entity of malignant lymphomas.
    1. Meet. Europ. Div. of the Int. Soc. of Haemat., Milano 1971
35. LENNERT, K.: Follicular lymphoma. A tumor of the germinal centers. In:
    AKAZAKI, K., RAPPAPORT, H., BERARD, C.W., BENNETT, J.M., ISHIKAWA, E.
    (eds.): Malignant Diseases of the Hematopoietic System. GANN Monograph on
    Cancer Research No. 15, pp. 217 - 231. Baltimore-London-Tokyo: University
    Park Press 1973
36. RAPPAPORT, H.: Tumors of the Hematopoietic System. Atlas of Tumor Pathology
    Sect. 3, Fasc. 8. Washington, D.C.: Armed Forces Institute of Pathology 1966
37. SPIRO, S., GALTON, D.A.G., WILTSHAW, E., LOHMANN, R.C.: Follicular lymphoma:
    A survey of 75 cases with special reference to the syndrome resembling
    chronic lymphocytic leukaemia. Brit. J. Cancer 1974, in press
38. BURKITT, D.: A sarcoma involving the jaws in African children. Brit. J.
    Surg. 46, 218 - 223 (1958/59)
39. O'CONOR, G.T.: Malignant lymphoma in African children. II. A pathological
    entity. Cancer (Philad.) 14, 270 - 283 (1961)
40. WRIGHT, D.H.: Cytology and histochemistry of the Burkitt lymphoma. Brit.
    J. Cancer 17, 50 - 55 (1963)
41. BERARD, C., O'CONOR, G.T., THOMAS, L.B., TORLONI, H.: Histopathological
    definition of Burkitt's tumour. Bull. Wld. Hlth. Org. 40, 601 - 607 (1969)
42. VAN FURTH, R., GORTER, H., NADKARNI, J.S., NADKARNI, J.J., KLEIN, E.,
    CLIFFORD, P.: Synthesis of immunoglobulins by biopsied tissues and cell
    lines from Burkitt's lymphoma. Immunology 22, 847 - 857 (1972)
43. GOETZ, O., LAMPERT, F., PELLER, P., PRECHTEL, K.: Histologisch und virolo-
    gisch gesicherter Burkitt-Tumor bei einem 10jährigen Knaben. Münch. med.
    Wschr. 112, 1373 - 1376 (1970)
44. LUKES, R.J.: Personal communication. Workshop Chicago 1973
45. LEDER, L.-D.: Fermenthistochemische Befunde bei chronischer Erythroblastose
    und akuter Erythrämie. Klin. Wschr. 43, 795 - 796 (1965)
46. STEIN, H., KAISERLING, E., LENNERT, K.: Neue Gesichtspunkte zur Systematik
    maligner Lymphome auf dem Boden immunchemischer Analysen. In: STACHER, A.
    (ed).: Leukämien und maligne Lymphome, pp. 195-201. München, Berlin,
    Wien: Urban & Schwarzenberg 1972

47. STEIN, H., KAISERLING, E., LENNERT, K.: Evidence for B-cell origin of reticulum cell sarcoma. Virchows Arch. Abt. A *364*, 51 - 67 (1974)
48. LENNERT, K.: Pathologisch-histologische Klassifizierung der malignen Lymphome. *In:* STACHER, A. (ed.): Leukämien und maligne Lymphome, pp. 181 - 194. München, Berlin, Wien: Urban & Schwarzenberg 1972
49. LENNERT, K., NAGAI, K., SCHWARZE, E.-W.: Pathoanatomical features of the bone marrow in polycythaemia vera and myelofibrosis. Clin. Haemat. *4*, (1975), in press

Prof. Dr. KARL LENNERT
Department of Pathology
University of Kiel
Postfach 4324
D - 2300 Kiel, Germany

Acta Neuropath. (Berlin), Suppl. VI, 17 - 20 (1975)

Ultrastructural Features of Human Lymphomas

F. MOLLO, G. MONGA, R. CODA and G. PALESTRO

Centro di Microscopia Elettronica, I e III Cattedra di Anatomia e Istologia
Patologica; Facoltà di Medicina di Torino, Italy

Summary: The diagnostic value of some ultrastructural details in a series of
73 lymphomas, 7 thymomas, 6 cases of Waldenström's disease,and 5 myelomas
has been critically reviewed. The light microscopical diagnoses of "reticulum
cell sarcoma" seems now inadvisable, since the majority of these cases, when
examined by electron microscopy, were found to be "blast cell sarcomas",
probably lymphoid in nature. Clear-cut relationships between cell ultrastructure and immunfluorescence data about surface Ig in lymphoid cell
populations have not been ascertained.

Key words: electron microscopy; lymphomas

INTRODUCTION

The reliability of traditional morphology for the classification of lymphomas
has been recently questioned (1, 2, 3, 4); on the other hand, any immunological approach has been considered as possibly venturesome at this time (5).
In our opinion, some information can be achieved by electron microscopy (EM),
when applied without strict light microscopical (LM) prejudice. In this note
we shall report a reconsideration of a series of previously studied human
lymphomas of lymph nodes (6), together with more recent observations about
new cases in lymph nodes, bone marrow, thymus, spleen, and stomach. Our aim
is mainly the presentation of EM features of some value from a diagnostic
point of view; preliminary observations concerning relationships between
EM and immunofluorescence (IF) characteristics of pathological lymphoid
populations are added.

MATERIAL AND METHODS

Ninety-three specimens (69 from lymph nodes, 9 from bone marrow, 7 from
thymus, 5 from spleen, and 3 from stomach) were examined in EM, in 91 patients.
The pathological diagnoses before EM examination could be provisionally
grouped as follows: 39 Hodgkin's lymphomas (HL); 5 debatable HL; 29 non-
Hodgkin's lymphomas (nHL), that is 11 large cell lymphomas (LCL), 1 acute
and 4 chronic lymphatic leukaemias (CLL), 13 small cell lymphomas (SCL);
5 lymphoepithelial and 2 granulomatous thymomas; 6 Waldenström's diseases;
5 myelomas. EM study of peripheral blood was also performed in 5 of these
patients, and IF data about surface Ig in peripheral blood and/or tissue
lymphoid cells were available in 12 patients.

RESULTS

The most characteristic EM feature in HL (beside Sternberg cells) was the
presence in the connective tissue of peculiar banded structures (Fig. 1).

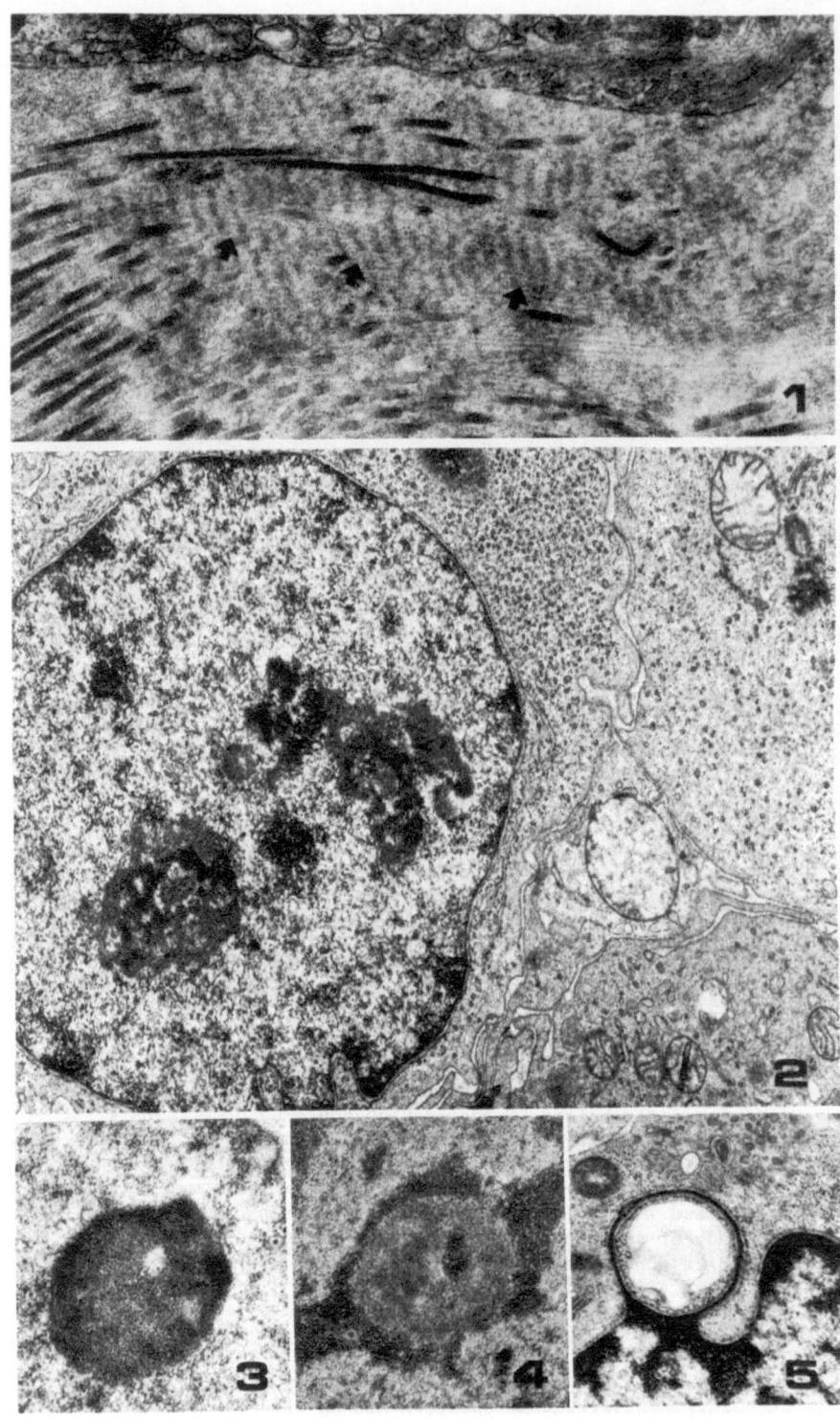

They were always present and usually abundant in HL, and in granulomatous
thymomas; their finding was occasional (and not significant) in some cases
of nHL, but characteristically abundant in 3 out of 5 cases previously considered as debatable HL.

Among nHL, accurate EM examination of many sections from several blocks
revealed that, in 10 cases out of 11 LCL, the predominant elements were
"blast cells", characterized by many polyribosomes, swollen mitochondria,
nucleus with scarce peripheral clumping of chromatin, and nucleoli with
rather prominent nucleolonema (Fig. 2). In one case only, most cells showed
rather abundant endoplasmic reticulum, vesicles and lysosomes, that is an
"histiocytic" or "reticulum cell" pattern; similar aspects were also present
in 2 cases out of those previously considered as debatable HL. In SCL, lymphoid cells were clearly predominant. Compact and/or sponge-like nucleoli
(Fig. 3) were characteristic of the cases without hematological data
suggesting leukaemias, and then considered as lymphosarcomas (LS); nucleoli
with a prominent shell of nucleolus-associated chromatin (Fig. 4) were
particularly abundant in CLL. Polyribosomal patterns appeared more frequent
in LS, whereas monoribosomal ones in CLL.

In the present series, nuclear pockets (Fig. 5) were observed in cells of
lymphoid and blastic type (besides the Sternberg cells and occasionally
in granulocytes); on the contrary they were not found in cells with histiocytic or "reticular" patterns.

Preliminary observations about relationships between EM and IF data may
be synthesized as follows. In cases of HL, and in blood specimens in which
Ig-unstained cells (T lymphocytes) were clearly predominant, a major (but
not strictly proportional) part of lymphocytes were small to medium in size;
they showed a nucleus with rather condensed chromatin, and scanty cytoplasm
with prevalent monoribosomal pattern. In cases of SCL, and in blood specimens in which Ig-stained cells (B lymphocytes) by far predominated, EM
examination could show medium to large lymphocytes with less condensed
nuclear chromatin, and more abundant cytoplasm rich in polyribosomes; however, numerous lymphocytes of the above described type (mainly in CLL), and
intermediate forms were also present.

COMMENTS

Banded structures in the stroma, nucleolar features, and nuclear pockets
have been discussed in previous works from this laboratory (6); our present
observations confirm previous results, also in different tissues.

Further information has been achieved by reconsideration of our cases of
LCL. A major part of them could well correspond to features described by

---

Fig. 1. Hodgkin's lymphoma: banded structures (arrows) in the connective
tissue (x 13.600)

Fig. 2. Blast cell sarcoma: blast cells showing clear nucleus, nucleoli with
prominent nucleolonema, many polyribosomes, and swollen mitochondria
(x 27.600)

Fig. 3. Lymphosarcoma: a lymphoid cell with compact nucleolonema (x 22.000)

Fig. 4. Chronic lymphatic leukaemia: a lymphoid cell with prominent shell
of nucleolus-associated chromatin (x 22.000)

Fig. 5. Lymphosarcoma: lymphoid cell with a nuclear pocket, circumscribing
a cytoplasmic vacuole (x 18.000)

others as "undifferentiated reticulosarcomas", or "lymphoreticulosarcomas"
(7), "reticulum cell sarcomas virtually without endoplasmic reticulum" or
"with smooth endoplasmic reticulum" (8), "reticulosarcomas, histioblastic
type" (9). Our present opinion is that EM features of the predominant cells
in these cases correspond with a lymphoid (rather than a "reticular") nature;
the present suggestion seems in agreement with the immunological approaches
to the classification of lymphomas (1, 2, 3, 4). Our inability to differentiate in tumour proliferations the patterns described as characteristic of
"lymphoblasts" and "hemocytoblasts" (7), "germinoblasts" and "basophilic
stem cells" (8), and so on, leads us to simply denominate these cases, from
a cytological point of view, as "blast cell sarcomas". The existence of
true "reticulum cell sarcomas" can not be denied, but this is anyway not
reliable diagnosis when proposed solely by LM.

Our preliminary observations on pathological populations of lymphocytes
do not support, nor do the results of others (10, 11), clear-cut relationships between cell ultrastructure and IF data about surface Ig.

REFERENCES

1. STEIN, H., LENNERT, K., PARWAKESCH, M.R.: Malignant lymphomas of B-cell
   type. Lancet II, 855-857 (1972)
2. JAFFE, E.S., SHEVACH, E.M., FRANK, M.M., BERARD, C.W., GREEN, I.:
   Nodular lymphoma - Evidence for origin from follicular B lymphocytes.
   New Engl. J. Med. *290*, 813-819 (1974)
3. DORFMAN, R.F.: Classification of non-Hodgkin's lymphomas. Lancet I,
   1295-1296 (1974)
4. LUKES, R.J.: *In:* REBUCK, J.W., BERARD, C.W. (eds.): Monograph, International Academy of Pathology (in press)
5. MATHÉ, G., BELPOMME, D.: T and B lymphocytic nature of leukaemias and
   lymphosarcomas: a new but still uncertain parameter for their classification. Biomedicine *20*, 81-85 (1974)
6. MOLLO, F., MONGA, G., STRAMIGNONI, A.: Electron microscopy in morphological classification of human lymphomas. J. Submicr. Cytol. *3*, 105-
   120 (1971)
7. BERNHARD, W., LEPLUS, R.: Fine structure of the normal and malignant
   human lymph node. Oxford: Pergamon Press, Paris: Gauthier-Villars,
   New York: McMillan 1964
8. MORI, Y., LENNERT, K.: Electron microscopic atlas of lymph node cytology
   and pathology. Berlin-Heidelberg-New York: Springer 1969
9. MATHÉ, G., GÉRARD-MARCHANT, R., TEXIER, J.L., SCHUMBERGER, J.R.,
   BERUMEN, L., PAITRAND, M.: The two varieties of lymphoid tissue "reticulosarcomas", histiocytic and histioblastic type. Br. J. Cancer
   24, 687-695 (1970)
10. PERKINS, W.D., KARNOVSKI, M.J., UNANUE, E.: An ultrastructural study
    of lymphocytes with surface-bound immunoglobulin. J. Exptl. Med. *135*,
    267-276 (1972)
11. ZUCKER-FRANKLIN, D., BERNEY, S.: Electron microscope study of surface
    immunoglobulin-bearing human tonsil cells. J. Exptl. Med. *135*, 533-
    548 (1972)

Prof. Franco MOLLO
Istituto Anatomia Patologica - via Santena 7
I-10126 Torino, Italy

Acta Neuropath. (Berlin), Suppl. VI, 21 - 29 (1975)

Morphological Classification of Malignant Lymphomas: Ultrastructural, Cytochemical and Immunological Results [+])

H. E. SCHAEFER, G.R.F. KRÜGER, R. FISCHER

Pathologisches Institut der Universität Köln, Germany

Summary: Except for tumors clearly producing immunoglobulin (e.g. plasma-cytoma), the different classes of malignant lymphomas do not correlate with a constant surface immunoglobulin pattern. Beside a prevailing IgM-surface type in a high number of different lymphoma classes even T-like or O-cells occur in most tumor types provided they are studied in a sufficient number. The possibility of dedifferentiation of immunologic cell qualities has to be envisaged. In this context intracellular lambda-chain crystals occurring in chronic lymphocytic leukaemia may provide a morphological hallmark of anaplastic deterioration of immunoglobulin synthesis. - The ambiguous significance of PAS-positive inclusions and virus-like micro-tubular complexes in lymphoma cells is discussed. - In conclusion the recent discovery of hairy cell leukaemia provides a good example of the value of nomenclatures based on empiricism rather than on short-lived theories.

Key words: surface immunofluorescence - cytoplasmic crystals - PAS-reaction - microtubular (virus-like) inclusions - hairy cell leukaemia

INTRODUCTION

After the presentation of the "Kiel Classification 1974", there does not seem to be much that can be added now. At least, instead of unfolding an additional own concept of classification, we shall elaborate on several immunological and morphological features that may throw some light on the biology of peculiar lymphomas and the evolving problems of their classifi-cation.

The present-day discussion on typing of lymphomas is widely stimulated by the discovery of B- and T-lymphocytes in experimental immunology. No wonder, that many efforts have been made to transfer the principles of the T- and B-system from its physiological origin to the field of oncology.

Surface immunoglobulins

The presence of membrane-bound surface immunoglobulins (Ig) is a convenient marker for B-cells as shown in animals (1 - 3). Our determination of such Ig on the surface of lymphoma cells from blood, spleen or lymphnode suspen-sions using a fluorescence method (4), as well as compiled data from literature (9 - 13) show the following (Tab. 1).

[+]) Supported by Deutsche Forschungsgemeinschaft

Table 1. *Immunologic Characteristics of Lymphoma Cells*
Surface Immunofluorescence and Rosette Formation

Types of malignant lymphomas (ML)	Number of cases	B-cells monoclonal	B-cells bi- and polyclonal	T-cells	0-cells
ML, lymphocytic well differentiated (chronic lymph. leuk.)	121 -13-	68% IgM (5-13)-10-	8% IgM, A,G (10, 11)	6% (5,12,13)	12% (10)-3-
ML, lymphocytic poorly differentiated	43 -4-	16% IgM (5-13)-3-	12% IgM, A,G (10,11)	20% (13)	45% (10)-1-
ML, "histiocytic" (former reticulum cell sarcoma)	-4-	-3- IgM			-1-
Hairy cell leukaemia (leukaemic reticulo-endotheliosis)	-3-	-2- IgM -1- IgA			

( ) references, -- our own cases

The percentages given in this table have been obtained from collective results of 184 patients including 32 of our own. A tumour was classified as belonging to a monoclonal immunological type, when more than 75% of lymphoid cells carried specific surface receptors of an equal type. As this table shows, certain immunological types of cells appear to predominate in some of the histological types of lymphomas, such as for instance IgM-cells in chronic lymphocytic leukaemia. However, any clear-cut correlation between the immunological cell type and a given histological type of the tumour is lacking.

Moreover polyclonal populations have been observed. They are characterized by cell lines of divergent Ig-surface types belonging to one cytomorphological type participating in a lymphoma, and their sum must approach 100%. Besides there is evidence, that a few malignant lymphomas are made up by cells carrying more than one immunoglobulin receptor on their surface (10), thus complicating further the correlation between histological and immunological classification of lymphomas. It should be added that more recent results from TERNYNCK and collaborators (14) lay stress on an obligate monoclonal light chain pattern of chronic lymphocytic leukaemia.

Besides the bulk of B-cell lymphomas, there is a smaller number of T-cell and so-called null-cell lymphomas. T-cells are characterized by spontaneous rosette formation with sheep erythrocytes, and by the absence of surface immunoglobulins. Null-cells contain neither a surface marker, nor do they show rosette formation. But one should keep in mind, that the indicated available markers for human T-cells are very feeble. On one hand the quantitation of rosette-forming T-cells is subject to a number of variables, and the fundamental nature of this phenomenon remains to be solved (15). On the other hand a lack of surface immunoglobulins may be caused by neoplastic dedifferentiation of former B-cells, or may be a relative one. A positive immunofluorescence in part is a matter of quantity rather than quality, for 50 000 to 150 000 Ig-molecules must be present on a cell to give detectable surface Ig-fluorescence (16), and in chronic lymphocytic leukaemia it has been shown, that at least the number of light chain sites on the cell surface becomes considerably reduced (14).

Crystals in anaplastic lymphocytes

Indeed ultrastructural investigations may indicate, that the neoplastic anaplasia leads to considerable deterioration of certain cell functions. In 2 out of 14 cases of chronic lymphocytic leukaemia we detected conspicous crystalline inclusions in the blood lymphocytes. Those crystals are almost invisible in routine PAPPENHEIM-stained smears. In one case they were faintly contrasting as colourless needles against the surrounding cytoplasm, due to some background staining resulting from a histochemical acid phosphatase reaction. Electron microscopically these inclusions show geometrical shapes with quadrangular or trapeziform profiles. On higher magnification and at suitable section angles a lattice with periodic distances of 8 nm becomes visible. In part these crystals are surrounded by a somewhat whrinkled membrane without evident connection to the endoplasmic reticulum.

Besides this type of crystalline inclusions, in another case we observed smaller but more numerous crystalline profiles composed of denser stripes in an parallel arrangement. In contrast to the type mentioned before the subunits of those crystals had a periodicity of 21 nm, and they appeared not quadrangular but hexagonal in their outlines. In this case the growth of those crystals could be traced, beginning with an accumulation of dense strands of material in the perinuclear space and in cisternae of the endoplasmic reticulum and finishing with densely packed stripes (Fig. 1).

In the first case the inclusions exhibited a vivid λ-, but only a faint μ-chain fluorescence. The majority of lymphocytes with and without crystals belonged to the IgM-surface type. Obviously those inclusions are not rare in chronic lymphocytic leukaemia (11), and they are indicative of a deteriorated immunoglobulin synthesis. It seems likely, that the crystals are not composed of complete Ig-molecules, since in our cases there is a constant λ-chain fluorescence whereas heavy chains are hardly detectable. In our cases and in those from the literature, where crystals contained

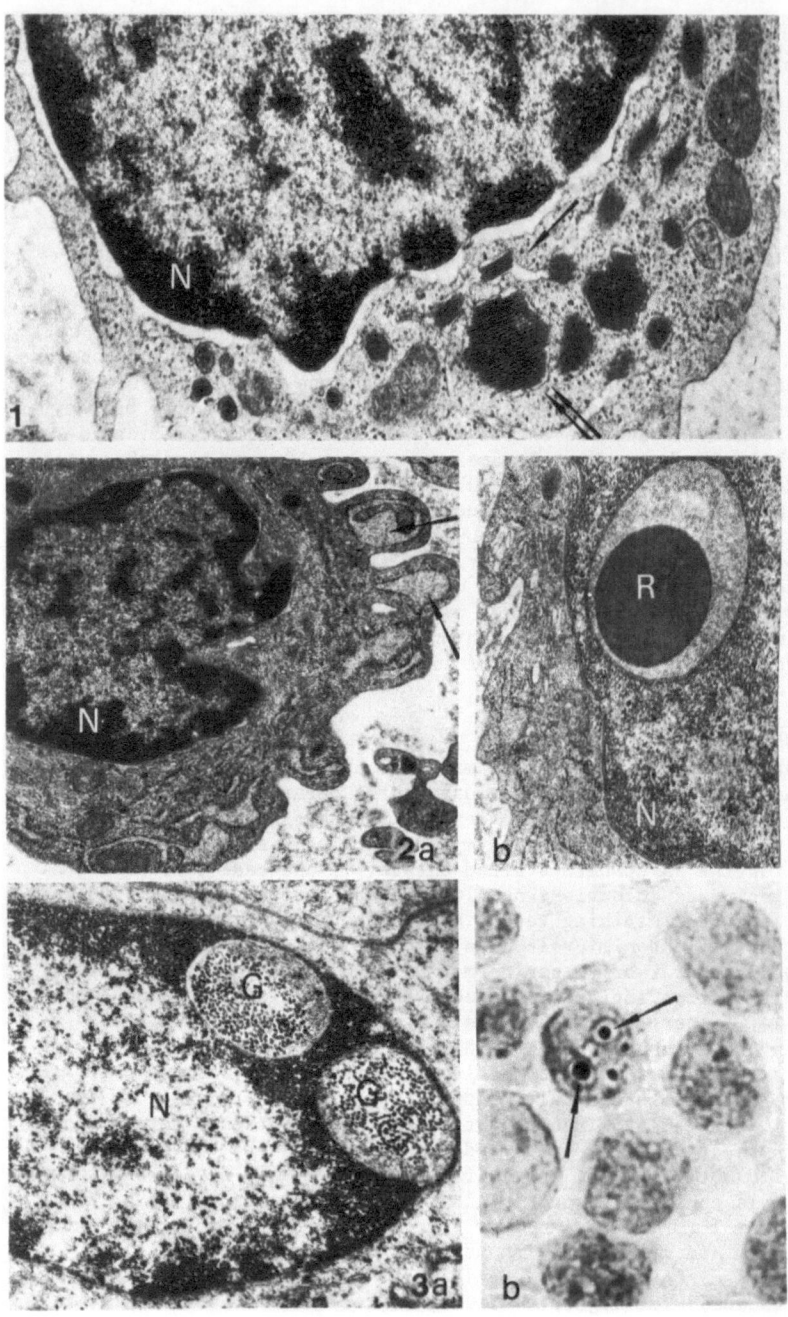

Fig. 1. Chronic lymphocytic leukaemia. Blood lymphocyte. Accumulation of dense material (arrow) in endoplasmic cisternae and development of hexagonal crystals (double arrow) composed of dense stripes (periodicity about 21 nm). N = nucleus. x 22 500

IgM (17) or µ-chains respectively (18), the PAS-reaction was negative, in-
spite of the well known carbohydrate content of IgM. This fact indicates
that no complete glycoprotein is formed. Either the synthesis or the binding
of protein to carbohydrate is blocked off in the leukaemia lymphocytes. In
sum, there is a double kind of underlying disturbance: incomplete synthesis
of Ig and hampered release. One might speculate that more severe anaplasia
could disturb the Ig-synthesis more thoroughly with resulting null-cells.

Different types of PAS-reaction

As mentioned before, immunoglobulins are glycoproteins (19), and therefore
they may show a positive PAS-reaction. But this reaction is visibly positive
only if immunoglobulins with high hexose contents are accumulated, such as
IgM (20, 21), and IgA, whereas the reaction of IgG is virtually negative
(22). Accumulations with a sufficient density are well known from WALDEN-
STRÖM's macroglobulinaemia (20, 21). But they may also be present in multiple
myeloma (22).

   This may be demonstrated in a case of IgA-plasma cell leukaemia. Ultrastructurally the leukaemia cells show densely arranged circular cisternae
of endoplasmic reticulum. More mature cells develop considerable clasmatocytic activity of the peripheral cytoplasm, which contains distended
cisternae with a flocculent content in its interior (Fig. 2a). This may
represent accumulated immunoglobulins on the way to be secreted. Moreover
there occur some nuclear pockets with invaginated perinuclear cisternae
containing the same flocculent material that tends to condensate like
RUSSEL bodies (Fig. 2b). In light microscopy at corresponding sites the
PAS-reaction shows perinuclear or seemingly intranuclear positive bodies.
Faintly stained granules in the peripheral cytoplasm obviously represent
the more flocculent IgA of the distended ergastoplasmic cisternae occurring
there.

   The PAS-reaction may be used as a screening method for the detection of
Ig-producing lymphomas as recently recommended (23). But correlating our
cytochemical and ultrastructural results we have found, that many cytoplasmic PAS-positive inclusions represent merely glycogen or glycogen-
like carbohydrates.

   This may be demonstrated in a case of giant follicular lymphoma (germinoblastoma) exhibiting typical follicular lymph node infiltration, with its
characteristic circular arrangement of argyrophilic fibres. On PAS-stained
smears one can see few cells containing red globular bodies in peri- or
intranuclear sites (Fig. 3b) These sites appear to be identical with some
of those numerous nuclear pockets that are in some way characteristic for
germinoblastoma cells (24). But unlike in the case of plasma cell leukaemia,
those pockets contain variable cytoplasmic constituents, but no intra-
cisternal material suggestive of Ig-nature. On further examination, a
minority of nuclear pockets are encountered that are stuffed with typical

---

Fig. 2 a and b. IgA plasma leukaemia with PAS-positive inclusions corresponding to *a)* distended endoplasmic cisternae within clasmatocytic protuberances (arrows), and to *b)* aggregated material like RUSSEL bodies (R)
in a nuclear pocket with supposed immunoglobulin content. N = nucleus.
a) x 9 500, *b)* x 10 500

Fig. 3 a and b. Germinoblastoma (giant follicular lymphoma). Lymph node.
a) Nuclear pockets containing clusters of glycogen (G) corresponding to
b) intranuclear PAS-granules (arrows) in lymph node smears from the same
case. *a)* x 9 500

glycogen granules obviously responsible for the positive PAS-reaction
(Fig. 3a).

It seems to us that this glycogen conditioned type of PAS-reaction is
far more frequent in lymphoma cells than the Ig-type. It may occur in normal
lymphocytes, and is increased in certain lymphocytic proliferations (25).
As pointed out by BESSIS (17), the broad PAS granules as seen in light
microscopy have no corresponding ultrastructural bodies of equivalent shape
or dimension. They result apparently from coalescence of cytoplasmic glycogen
when cell smears are made. The largest amount of glycogen conditioned PAS-
inclusions may be found in lymphoma cells derived from CSF.

On the whole, PAS-positive inclusions are heterogenuous in nature. They
may indicate Ig-accumulations without providing evidence for malignancy,
since RUSSEL bodies of non malignant plasma cells are PAS-reactive as well,
if a hexose-rich Ig is present, The glycogen type, too, is not indicative
of malignancy, but its enormous increase sometimes correlates with neoplastic
proliferation, thus indicating metabolic distress of anaplastic cells.

Microtubular (virus-like) complexes in lymphocytes

A rarely encountered cytoplasmic inclusion with unresolved significance
should be mentioned briefly. In 3 out of 14 cases of chronic lymphocytic
leukaemia studied electron microscopically, up to 10% of the blood lymphocytes
contained bizarr polygonal or roundish inclusion bodies composed of densely
fasciculated tubules with equal diameters of about 20 nm. In part the tubules
are loosely meshed and interwoven. The resulting microtubular complexes as
we call them are in part membrane bound and range from 200 to 400 nm (Fig. 4).

They resemble similar structures found in lymphocytes from normal and
antibody deficient persons (27). Originally they have been described by
HOVIG and associates (28) in a more vacuolar variant in lymphocytes from
a lymphopenic female suffering from chronic rheumatoid arthritis. On the
other hand similar inclusions occur in glomerular endothelial cells in lupus
erythematosus (30, 31, 32) and elsewhere, for instance in nuclei of nerve
cells in subacute inclusion-body encephalitis (33) and in polymyositis (34).
They have been regarded by several authors as nucleoprotein strands of an
unidentified myxovirus (30, 31, 33, 34, for criticism see 32). To the best
of our knowledge there is no evidence up to now whether those supposed
subviral structures are real representatives of viral infection of lymphoma
cells or not. Nevertheless it is our impression, that those inclusion bodies
are remarkably increased in some cases of chronic lymphocytic leukaemia.

Remarks on hairy cell leukaemia

So far our data presented here intend to underline the inadequacy of solitary parameters for purposes of classification. But the recent terminologi-
cal evolution of the so-called hairy cell leukaemia (35, 36) demonstrates,
that a seemingly inconspicous cytological marker may define an entity of
lymphoma without any theoretical background. Because of its uniform clinical
picture it is useful to separate this type of leukaemia.

The essential marker in this condition consists of hair-like protrusions
stretching out from the periphery of large lymphoid cells usually appearing
in the blood in moderate numbers (Fig. 5b). The neoplastic proliferation
causes slight enlargement of lymph nodes and an early splenie tumour with
diffuse or nodular infiltration. Later on infiltrates appear in the bone
marrow exhibiting a reticular arrangement of cells best visible with HEIDEN-
HAIN's haematoxylin stain or with india ink negative staining. Moreover
a slight diffuse argyrophilic fibrosis develops accounting for the former
classification of this disease as "lymphoid myelofibrosis" (37, 38). One of
our 4 cases showed terminal meningeal infiltrates, especially along the

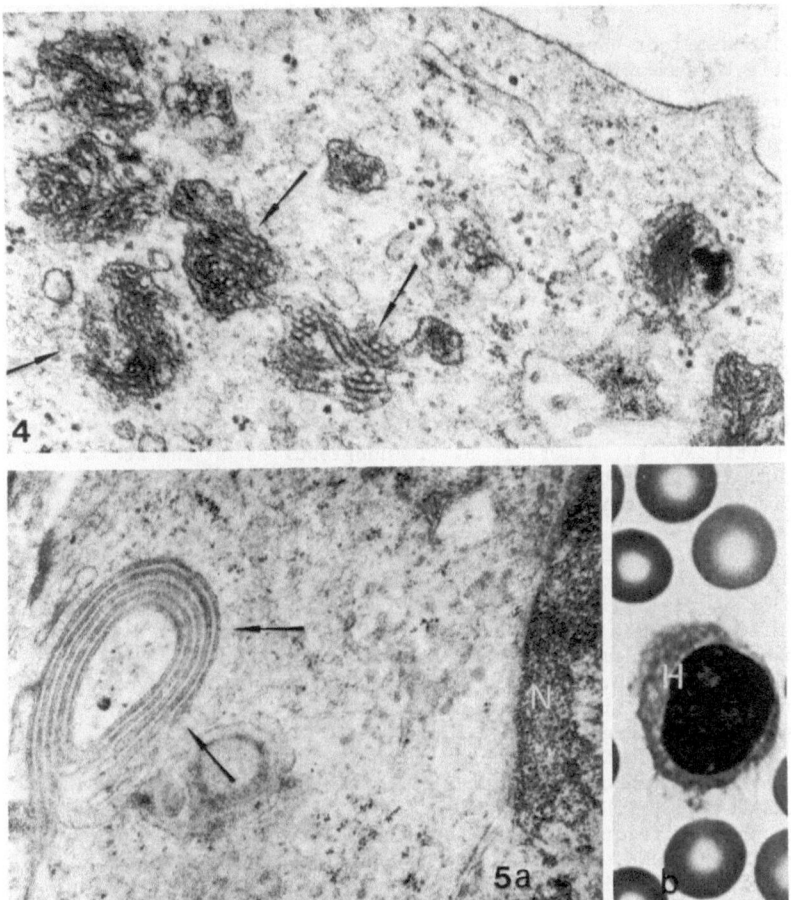

Fig. 4. Chronic lymphocytic leukaemia. Blood lymphocyte. Cytoplasmic inclusions of myxovirus-like microtubular complexes. x 48 000

Fig. 5. Hairy cell leukaemia. *a)* Spleen. Curled up cytoplasmic protuberances ("hairs") (arrow). N = nucleus. x 22 500. *b)* Same case. Hairy cell (H) in a blood smear

cauda equina. Interestingly enough hairy cells exhibit their cytoplasmatic protuberances not only while present in the blood stream. Within spleen infiltrates they are preformed, and curled up or tightly crammed into narrow spaces (Fig. 5a).

Regardless of current discussions whether these cells are of reticulo-endothelial, lymphatic (39) or other origin, the term "hairy cell leukaemia" is widely accepted, and due to its originality it has triggered world wide efforts to investigate this very type of haemoblastosis (for review see 40). In view of this phenomenon we advocate a pragmatic type of nomenclature enjoying general consent and understanding rather than one fitting in to short lived streams of theory.

REFERENCES

1. RAFF, M.C.: Two distinct populations of peripheral lymphocytes in mice
   distinguishable by immunofluorescence. Immunology *19*, 637-650 (1970)
2. RABELLINO, E., GREY, H.M.: Immunoglobulins on the surface of lymphocytes.
   III. Bursal origin of surface immunoglobulins on chicken lymphocytes.
   J. Immunol. *106*, 1418-1420 (1971)
3. KINCADE, P.W., LAWTON, A.R., COOPER, M.D.: Restriction of surface immunoglobulin determinants to lymphocytes of the plasma cell line. J. Immunol.
   106, 1421-1423 (1971)
4. PAPAMICHAIL, M., HOLBOROW, E.J., KEITH, H.I., CURREY, H.L.F.: Subpopulations of human peripheral blood lymphocytes distinguished by combined
   rosette forming and membrane immunofluorescence. Lancet *II*, 64-66 (1972)
5. SANDILANDS, G.P., GRAY, K., COONEY, A., BROWNING, J.D., GRANT, R.M.,
   ANDERSON, J.R., DAGG, J.H., LUCIE, N.: Lymphocytes with T and B cell
   properties in a lymphoproliferative disorder. Lancet *I*, 903-904 (1974)
6. DAGUILLARD, F., FONTAINE, L., TARDIEU, M.: B and T lymphocytes in chronic
   lymphatic leukaemia. Lancet *I*, 308-309 (1974)
7. GREY, H.M., RABELLINO, E., PIROFSKY, B.: Immunoglobulins on the surface
   of lymphocytes. IV. Distribution in hypogammaglobulinemia, cellular
   immune deficiency, and chronic lymphatic leukaemia. J. Clin. Invest.
   50, 2368-2375 (1971)
8. CATOVSKY, D., OKOS, A., WILTSHAW, E., GALETTO, J., GALTON, D.A.G.,
   STATHOPOULOS, G.: Prolymphocytic leukaemia of B and T cell type.
   Lancet *II*, 232-234 (1973)
9. SUMIYA, M., MIZOGUCHI, H., KOSAKA, K., MIURA, Y., TAKAKU, F., YATA, J.:
   Chronic lymphocytic leukaemia of T-cell origin? Lancet *II*, 910 (1973)
10. PIESSENS, W.F., SCHUR, P.H., MOLONEY, W.C., CHURCHILL, W.H.: Lymphocyte
    surface immunoglobulins. Distribution and frequency in lymphoproli-
    ferative diseases. New. Engl. J. Med. *288*, 176-180 (1973)
11. PREUD'HOMME, J.L., SELIGMAN, M.: Surface bound immunoglobulins as a
    cell marker in human lymphoproliferative diseases. Blood *40*, 777-794 (1972)
12. AIUTI, F., LACAVA, V., FIORILLI, M., CIARLA, M.V.: Lymphocyte surface
    markers in lymphoproliferative disorders. Acta Haemat. *50*, 275-283 (1973)
13. SHEVACH, E.M., HERBERMANN, R., FRANK, M.M., GREEN, I.: Receptors for
    complement and immunoglobulin on human leukaemic cells and human lympho-
    blastoid cell lines. J. Clin. Invest. *51*, 1933-1938 (1972)
14. TERNYNCK, T., DIGHIERO, G., FOLLEZOU, J., BINET, J.-L.: Comparison
    of normal and CLL lymphocyte surface determinants using peroxidase-
    labeled antibodies. I. Detection and quantitation of light chain
    determinants. Blood *43*, 789-795 (1974)
15. SELIGMAN, M.: B-cell and T-cell markers in lymphoid proliferation. New
    Engl. J. Med. *290*, 1483-1484 (1974)
16. MARCHALONIS, J.J., ATWELL, J.L., CONE, R.E.: Isolation of surface
    immunoglobulin from lymphocytes from human and murine thymus. Nature
    235, 240-242 (1972)
17. BESSIS, M.: Cellules du sang normal et pathologiques. l.c.p. 721-723
    Paris: Masson et Cie. 1972
18. HUREZ, D., FLANDRIN, G., PREUD'HOMME, J.L., SELIGMAN, A.: Unreleased
    intracellular monoclonal macroglobulin in chronic lymphocytic leukaemia.
    Clin. exp. Immunol. *10*, 223-234 (1972)
19. WALDMANN, R.H., HENNEG, CH.S.: Die Struktur der Antikörper. Verhandl.
    dtsch. Ges. Path. *54*, 28-37 (1970)
20. DUTCHER, T.F., FAHEY, J.L.: The histopathology of the macroglobulinemia
    of WALDENSTRÖM. J. nat. Cancer Inst. *22*, 887-918 (1953)
21. DUTCHER, T.F., FAHEY, J.L.: Immunocytochemical demonstration of intra-
    nuclear localization of 18 S gamma macroglobulin in macroglobulinemia
    of WALDENSTRÖM. Proc. Soc. Exper. Biol. Med. *103*, 452-455 (1960)

22. BRITTIN, G.M., TANAKA, Y., BRECHER, G.: Intranuclear inclusions in multiple myeloma and macroglobulinemia. Blood *21*, 335-351 (1963)
23. STEIN, H., LENNERT, K., PARWARESCH, M.R.: Malignant lymphomas of B-cell type. Lancet *II*, 855-857 (1972)
24. MORI, Y., LENNERT, K.: Electron microscopic atlas of lymph node cytology and pathology. Berlin, Heidelberg, New York: Springer 1969
25. MITUS, W.J., BERGNA, L.J., MEDNICOFF, J.B., DAMESHEK, W.: Cytochemical studies of glycogen content of lymphocytes in lymphocytic proliferations. Blood *13*, 748-756 (1958)
26. HUHN, D.: Neue Organelle im peripheren Lymphozyten? Dtsch. med. Wschr. *93*, 2099-2100 (1968)
27. HUHN, D., TYMPNER, K.D.: Elektronenmikroskopische Untersuchungen der Lymphozyten bei verschiedenen Formen von Antikörpermangel im Kindesalter. Blut *20*, 169-177 (1970)
28. HOVIG, T., JEREMIC, M., STAVEM, P.: A new type of inclusion bodies in lymphocytes. Scand. J. Haemat. *5*, 81-96 (1968)
29. GYÖRKEY, F., MIN, K.-W., SINCOVICS, J.G., GYÖRKEY, P.: Systemic lupus erythematosus and myxovirus. New Engl. J. Med. *280*, 333 (1969)
30. GYORKEY, F., MIN, K.-W., GYÖRKEY, P.: Submicroscopic structures resembling myxovirus in 5 cases of human systemic lupus erythematosus (SLE). Amer. J. Path. *55*, 13a (1963)
31. KAWANO, K., MILLER, L., KIMMELSTIEL, P.: Virus-like structures in lupus erythematosus. New Engl. J. Med. *281*, 1228-1229 (1969)
32. HAAS, J.E., YUNIS, E.J.: Tubular inclusions of systemic lupus erythematosus. Ultrastructural observations regarding their possible viral nature. Exp. mol. Path. *12*, 257-263 (1970)
33. SHAW, C.-M., BUCHAN, G.C., CARLSON, C.B.: Myxovirus as possible etiologic agent in subacute inclusion-body encephalitis. New Engl. J. Med. *277*, 511-515 (1967)
34. CHOU, S.M.: Myxovirus-like structures in case of human chronic polymyositis. Science *158*, 1453-1455 (1967)
35. SCHRECK, R., DONNELLY, W.J.: Hairy cells in blood in lymphoreticular neoplatic disease and "flagellated" cells of normal lymph nodes. Blood *27*, 199-211 (1966)
36. PLENDERLEITH, J.H.: Hairy cell leukaemia. Canad. med. Ass. J. *102*, 1056-1060 (1970)
37. DUHAMEL, G., LEVY, V.G., OUAHNICH, M.: Un cas de myélofibrose lymphoide. Etude anatomo-clinique et critique. Sem. Hôp. (Paris) *43*, 3450 - 3455 (1967)
38. DUHAMEL, G.: Lymphoid myelofibrosis. Acta haemat. (Basel) *45*, 89-96 (1971)
39. STEIN, H., KAISERLING, E., STEIN, G., KLEIN, U.E.: Leukaemic reticuloendothelioses (hairy cell leukaemia). Evidence for the lymphatic origin of hairy cells from the detection of lymphocyte-specific surface antigen and surface immunoglobulins. Blood, submitted for publication.
40. DÜLLMANN, J., WULFHEKEL, M., DRESCHER, S., HAUSMANN, K.: Die Haarzellenhämoblastome ("hairy cell leukaemia"). Klinische licht- und elektronenmikroskopische Befunde. Dtsch. med. Wschr. *99*, 859 - 863 (1974)

Prof. Dr. H.E. SCHAEFER
Pathologisches Institut der Universität zu Köln
Abteilung für Feinstrukturelle Pathologie
5 Köln 41 /Deutschland
Josef-Stelzmannstr. 9

Acta Neuropath. (Berlin), Suppl. VI, 31 - 36 (1975)

Classification of Malignant Lymphomas by Means of Membrane Markers

H. HUBER, G. MICHLMAYR, CH. HUBER

Medizinische Universitätsklinik Innsbruck, Austria

Summary: In the majority of patients with lympho- and reticulum cell sarcomas, high numbers of B-lymphocytes were found in affected lymph nodes, but were rarely observed in the peripheral blood. In chronic lymphocytic leukaemia receptor properties of B-lymphocytes were defective in several aspects. In patients with Hodgkin's disease the relative number of both lymphocyte populations in the blood were within the normal range and in lymph node suspensions marked alterations were unusual. A preferential proliferation of T-lymphocytes, perhaps accompanied by a reduced life span, was however suggested by double labelling experiments.

Key words: Lymphocyte subpopulations - Membrane markers - Malignant lymphomas Immunopathology of lymphomas

INTRODUCTION

The concept of a functional heterogeneity of lymphoid cells (1) has been applied to various lymphoproliferation disorders. By the use of membrane markers specific for T-or for B-lymphocytes a better understanding of the immunopathological features of lymphoproliferative disorders has been obtained, which also facilitates the differential diagnosis of these diseases. Employing several markers blood lymphocytes as well as those obtained from affected lymph nodes from a larger group of patients have been investigated. In some studies the proliferating lymphocytes (lymphocytes in DNA synthesis) were characterized by the combined use of ^{3}H-thymidine labelling and a representative membrane marker.

METHODS

B-lymphocytes were evaluated autoradiographically using ^{125}I-labelled anti-immunoglobulin (Ig) antisera and ^{125}I-labelled heat-aggregated gammaglobulin (2). T-lymphocytes were assessed by their capacity to form rosettes with unsensitized neuraminidase-treated sheep red blood cells (E_N) (3). Techniques employed in the double labelling experiments have been described (4), at least 5×10^3 lymphocytes were evaluated.

RESULTS AND DISCUSSION

1. Specificity of the markers

The specificity of the markers used in our experiments was tested in double labelling experiments. After reaction with aggregated IgG (AGG) the lymphocyte

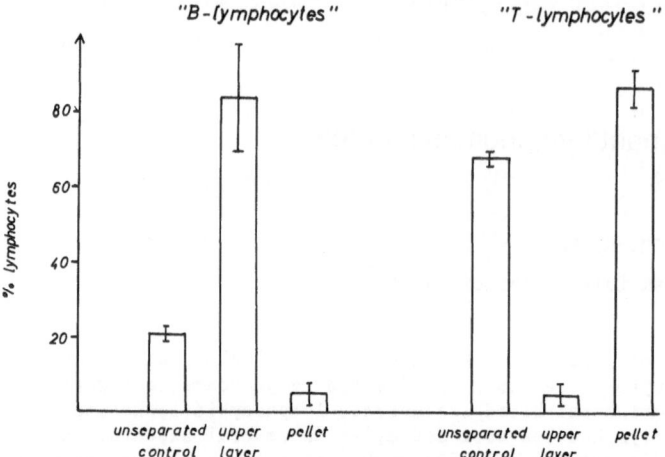

Fig. 1. Specifity of the membrane markers: Centrifugation experiments. Suspensions of blood lymphocytes were reacted with E_N and centrifuged using a FICOLL density gradient. The percentage of "B" - and " T " - lymphocytes in the pellet and in the supernatant were evaluated by standard techniques (see methods)

suspension was incubated with E_N. Only about 3 % of the lymphocytes reacted with both markers. In further experiments lymphocytes were incubated with E_N. After centrifugation using a FICOLL density gradient, the cells in the pellet and in the supernatant were tested with a B-cell marker (Fig. 1). In the fraction enriched with rosette-forming cells few cells bound aggregated IgG (AGG), whereas the majority of the lymphocytes in the supernatant were positive in this respect. Under normal as well as pathological conditions a closely comperable percentage of lymphocytes stained with atisera as with AGG (2).

2. Chronic lymphocytic leukaemia

In most matients with chronic lymphocytic leukaemia (CLL) the leukaemia lymphocytes behave as B-cells (5). This finding has been amply documented in recent years. Of 18 patients studied in detail 17 showed the typical pattern: very high percentages of blood lymphocytes reacting with AGG as well as with anti-Ig antisera (Fig. 2). The percentage of T-lymphocytes was inversely related to the lymphocyte count; patients with high numbers of leukaemic cells had few rosette-forming cells. In contrast, patients with reactive lymphocytosis suffering from virus-diseases showed high numbers of T and a relative depletion of B-lymphocytes (Fig. 2).

A further characterization of membrane-bound Ig was achieved by the use of deaggregated monospecific antisera. In 7 of 9 patients investigated evidence for a monoclonal proliferation of the neoplastic cells was obtained. A further difference compared with normal B-lymphocytes was observed when the density of the membrane receptors was evaluated.

A semiquantitative estimation of the silver grain counts after labelling with AGG or anti-immunoglobulin antisera suggested that the average number of receptor sites was lower in the majority of these leukaemic cells (2). A recirculation defect, as suggested by a comparison of the percentage of leukaemic lymphocytes in blood and thoracic duct as well as by labelling experiments apparently provides further evidence for a membrane defect of these pathological cells (6).

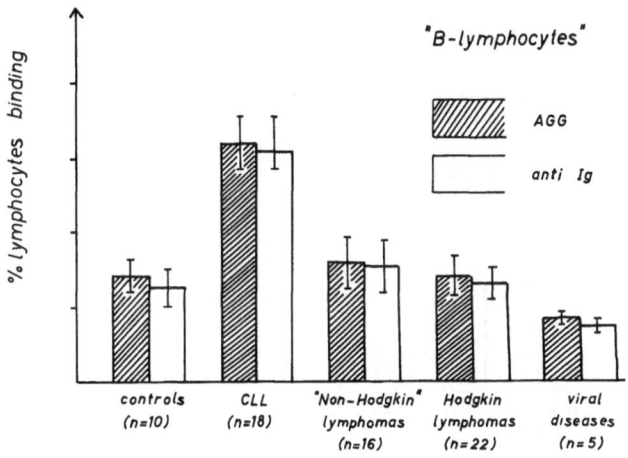

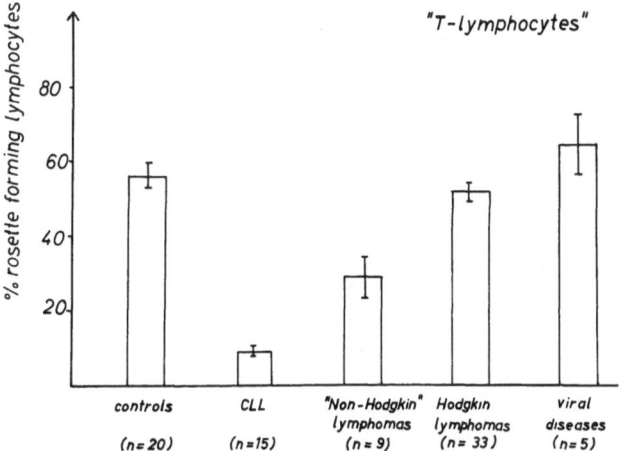

Fig. 2. Results with membrane markers on blood lymphocytes in various lymphoproliferative disorders

3. Non-Hodgkin lymphomas

A marked increase of blood lymphocytes with membrane-bound Ig and receptors for AGG was observed in only 4 out of 16 patients with non-Hodgkin lymphomas. These patients showed increased white cell counts and atypical mononuclear cells in their blood. The average percentage of rosette-forming lymphocytes was lower than in the controls, the lowest percentage being observed in patients with increased white cell counts (Fig. 2). In contrast, cell suspensions of affected lymph nodes showed high numbers of lymphocytes reacting with AGG as well as with anti-Ig-antisera in 10 of 12 patients investigated. In comparison with the controls, rosette-forming lymphocytes were markedly reduced (Fig. 3). Results comparable to the controls were observed in one lymph node with nodular involvement. Only in one case of histiocytic lymphoma were the cells neither reactive with our B nor the T-cell marker. When the cells were tested with monospecific antisera, a monoclonal nature of the cells in terms of their Ig coat was suggested. In contrast to the CLL-lymphocytes, however, the density of the membrane receptors was apparently not reduced (2).

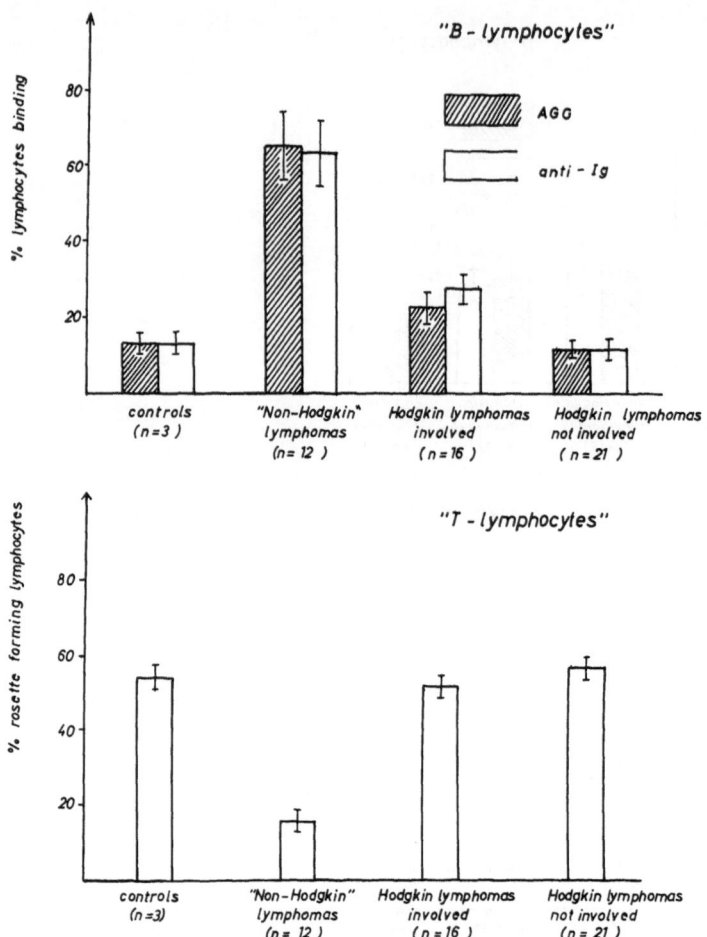

Fig. 3. Results with membrane markers on lymph node lymphocytes in various lymphoproliferative disorders

4. *Hodgkin's-disease*

The B/T cell ratio of blood lymphocytes in patients with Hodgkin's disease was comparable to the normal controls (Fig. 2). In absolute counts a slightly reduced number of T-lymphocytes was observed in patients after intensive (cytotoxic or radiation) therapy (3). The diminished transformation rate in the presence of phytohaemagglutinine, mainly found in patients in advanced stages of the disease, was apparently not related to reduced relative numbers of T-lymphocytes.

In further experiments we studied a number of lymph node biopsies obtained from staging laparotomies. Even in suspensions from histologically affected lymph nodes REED-STERNBERG cells were rarely observed in the cell suspension tested. Because of the variety of cells present in these preparations only typical small and medium sized lymphocytes were evaluated. The percentages of B-lymphocytes was slightly higher in affected in comparison to histologically uninvolved lymph nodes (Fig. 3). Particularly in the spleen relative

Table 1. *Proliferation of rosette-forming and non-rosette forming lymphocytes in Hodgkin's disease and infectious mononucleosis*

	controls	Hodgkin's disease (untreated)	infect. mononucleosis
number of patients	10	11	5
I: DNA-synthesizing blood lymphocytes (%)	1.7 ± 0.4	5.4 ± 0.9 [+)	43.8 ± 15.6 [+)
II: E_N-binding lymphocytes % in DNA-synthesis	1.4 ± 0.4	7.6 ± 2.4 [+)	65.3 ± 27.7 [+)
III: non-E_N-binding lymphocytes % in DNA-synthesis	1.9 ± 0.3	3.5 ± 1.0	17.7 ± 6.8 [+)
ratio II : III	0.7	2.2	3.7

[+) p values versus normal controls < 0.05

high percentages of lymphocytes positive with anti-Ig antisera or aggregated IgG were counted. These differences were, however, not significant.

When tested with monospecific anti-Ig antisera, the "polyclonal" nature of these cells became evident.

According to these experiments a predominant involvement of one of the lymphocyte subpopulations was not evident in our Hodgkin's-patients. These studies did not exclude, however, that one of the subpopulations proliferates preferentially, but also turns over more rapidly. A maked shortening of the life span of some lymphocytes in patients with advanced Hodgkin's disease has indeed been reported (7).

In order to gain some information on the proliferating cell itself in terms of its membrane reactivity, rosette-forming lymphocytes were evaluated after incubation with ^{3}H-thymidine. In this way the proliferative capacity of T-lymphocytes was estimated. The percentage of lymphocytes in DNA-synthesis, which did or did not bind E_N was counted.

The frequency of rosette-forming cells in blood lymphocytes labelled with ^{3}H-thymidine was twice as high in patients with Hodgkin's disease as that observed in normal controls. These differences were even more pronounced in untreated patients with Hodgkin's disease, where approximately 7 of 10 lymphocytes in DNA synthesis were rosette-forming lymphocytes (Table 1). A preferential proliferation of T-lymphocytes was also observed in patients with infectious mononucleosis. A T-lymphocyte response to a yet unknown stimulus together with a reduced life span of some lymphocytes may well play an important role in the pathogenesis of Hodgkin's disease.

REFERENCES

1. PETERSON, R.D.A., COOPER, M.D., GOOD, R.A.: The pathogenesis of immunologic deficiency diseases. Amer. J. Med. *38*, 578-604 (1965)
2. HUBER, CH., DWORZAK, E., FINK, U., MICHLMAYR, G., BRAUNSTEINER, H., HUBER, H.: Receptor sites for aggregated gammaglobulin (AGG) on lymphocytes in lymphoproliferative diseases. Brit. J. Haemat. (in press)
3. MICHLMAYR, G., HUBER, CH., FINK, U., FALKENSAMMER, M., HUBER, H.: T-Lymphozyten in peripherem Blut und Lymphknoten bei lymphatischen Systemerkrankungen. Schweiz. Med. Wschr. *104*, 815-820 (1974)
4. HUBER, CH., MICHLMAYR, G., FALKENSAMMER, M., FINK, U., NEDDEN, G., zur, BRAUNSTEINER, H., HUBER, H.: Increased proliferation of T-lymphocytes in the blood of patients with Hodgkin's disease. Clin. exp. Immun. (submitted for publication)
5. SELIGMANN, M., PREUD'HOMME, J.L., BROUET, J.C.: B and T cell markers in human proliferative blood diseases and primary immunodeficiences, with special reference to membrane bound immunoglobulins. Transplant. Rev. *16*, 85-113 (1973)
6. FLAD, H.D., HUBER, CH., BREMER, K., MENNE, H.D., HUBER, H.: Impaired recirculation of B lymphocytes in chronic lymphocytic leukaemia. Eur. J. Immun. *3*, 688-693 (1973)
7. SCHICK, P., TREPEL, H., THEML, H., BENEDEK, S., TRUMPP, P., KABOTH, W., BEGEMANN, H., FLIEDNER, T.M.: Kinetics of lymphocytes in Hodgkin's disease. Blut *37*, 223 (1973)

Prof. Dr. H. HUBER
Medizinische Univ.-Klinik
Anichstraße 35
A - 6020 INNSBRUCK - Austria

Acta Neuropath. (Berlin), Suppl. VI, 37 - 40 (1975)

Differentiation of Lymphoid Cells of the B Cell Series According to Membrane and Cytoplasmic Determinants

W. KNAPP, G. BAUMGARTNER and J. HOLOWIECKI

Institut für Immunologie der Universität Wien and 1. Medizinische Abteilung and Ludwig Boltzmann-Institut für Hämatologie und Leukämieforschung im Hanusch-Krankenhaus, Wien, Austria

Summary: Previous investigations have shown that a large proportion of normal human lymphocytes bearing membrane-bound IgM have also independently moving IgD molecules on their surface. Since it is known that in the majority of chronic lymphatic leukaemias (CLL) high numbers of lymphocytes with easily detectable membrane IgM can be found, we investigated CLL cells for the presence of membrane-bound IgD. In all 18 cases studied, high proportions of cells bearing surface IgD and IgM could be found. In none of the 18 cases crystalline Ig inclusions could be detected.

Key words: Surface Ig in CLL - Membrane Immunoglobulins - IgD and IgM - Lymphocytes

INTRODUCTION

Previous investigations have shown that a large proportion of normal human lymphocytes having M-IgM are found also to bear IgD on their membranes (1, 2). In this paper, data will be presented which show that this is also the case for the lymphocytes in a group of patients with chronic lymphatic leukaemia (CLL).

MATERIALS AND METHODS

The fluorescence staining technique was essentially performed as described previously (1, 3). Fluorescein isothiocyanate labelled conjugates against human IgM and human IgD and a tetramethylrhodamine isothiocyanate labelled anti-human IgG (F(ab)$_2$)) conjugate were used. The reactivity of the anti-IgG (F(ab$_2$)) conjugate with the three main Ig classes IgG, IgM and IgA and the class specificity of the anti IgM and the anti IgD conjugates was checked with the monoclonal bone marrow system (4) and the DASS system (5).

RESULTS

In Table 1 the results of the membrane fluorescence studies are listed. The number of lymphocytes ranged between 5 and 90 x 13^3/µl with a mean of 25.49. In the differential white blood cell count, the lymphocytes made up 59 - 99% (mean of 86%). The percentage of lymphocytes with detectable surface Ig (total Ig) ranged between 72 and 100% (mean 91.1%). The percentage

Table 1. *Membrane bound IgM and IgD on peripheral Lymphocytes in chronic lymphatic leukaemia*

Patients	No. Leuco-cytes x 10^3	% Lympho-cytes	% Membrane		
			Ig tot.	IgD	IgM
Do	9,5	91	99	96	95
Ho	52	83	99	98	98
Bi	6,8	59	75	46	68
Zi	55	93	95	90	95
Ha	28	87	95	63	95
Kr	16	93	93	96	99
Na	35	90	88	99	85
Br	26	84	95	94	95
Ko	N.T.	N.T.	96	92	94
Br	21	76	100	100	99
Pf	20	85	96	99	97
Fu	90	99	80	61	76
Wa	5	62	72	50	71
Ma	10	94	92	91	94
Ra	72	95	93	91	94
Ha	30	90	100	89	100
Ge	20	88	84	77	83
Ce	27	93	88	73	83

with detectable surface IgM ranged between 68 and 100% (mean 90.06%), with surface IgD between 46 and 100% (mean 83.6%). It is evident from these data that in all cases the sum of the percentages of IgM and IgD positive cells exceeds the percentage of cells stained for total Ig. It seems to be justified therefore to conclude that all or a high proportion of these cells carry both IgM and IgD molecules on their surface.

Cytocentrifuge preparations of the same cell preparations were also stained for detection of crystalline Ig inclusions in the cytoplasm of these cells. In none of the investigated cell preparations, however, such inclusions could be found.

DISCUSSION

In previous investigations of cord blood lymphocytes of healthy babies and peripheral lymphocytes from healthy adults, we could show that IgD and IgM are present on the same cells and move independently from each other (1). Comparable findings have also been reported by ROWE *et al.* (2).

The finding that both IgD and IgM are simultaneously present in a relatively high proportion of normal lymphocytes is remarkable in two respects.

Firstly it is in contrast to the distribution pattern of the other Ig classes, where restriction to one class is the general rule, secondly it is surprising that a high proportion of lymphocytes bear Ig of a class on their membranes, which is present in sera only in very small amounts.

The special function of IgD on the surface of lymphocytes which carry also IgM is not as yet clear. ROWE *et al.* (2) speculated that both IgD and IgM should have the same combining site, whereby a) the class of the receptor determines the signal-tolerance of induction, or b) IgD constitutes the first antigen receptor in the shift of the Ig synthesis form $\delta \rightarrow \mu \rightarrow \gamma$ with δ and μ showing overlap. Thus the appearance of IgM as a receptor would indicate a step in differentiation towards a plasma cell.

The absence of cells bearing exclusively IgD on the surface in the presence of lymphocytes bearing either only IgM or both IgD and IgM in spleen-, liver- and bone marrow-lymphocytes of 13 to 18 weeks old fetuses (6) seems to be in contrast to the latter assumption.

The observation of high numbers of IgD bearing lymphocytes, some of which carried simultaneously μ-chains in the absence of lymphocytes carrying IgM without IgD and of IgG or IgA bearing cells in two immunodeficient children (7) would be in agreement with the latter assumption.

This would be of special interest in regard to observations in CLL (3), where a monoclonal proliferation of cells with surface Ig was found, while the percentage of cells with cytoplasmic fluorescence was decreased. Obviously, there is a block in the further differentiation to Ig secreting cells. Crystalline Ig inclusions in the lymphocytes of two patients with CLL and the three cases in literature (3, 8, 9) may represent a side step from the normal differentiation into Ig secreting plasma cells: there is already a cytoplasmic localization but not yet an adequately functioning secretory apparatus.

The finding of crystalline Ig inclusions in some but not in all cases of CLL indicates that the block in the differentiation is not a fixed one, it can accur somewhat earlier or later. If the assumption holds true that IgD is the first step in the shift of the Ig production of one cell line from one class to another, one should expect therefore to find some cases of CLL which bear only IgD, some with IgD and IgM and some with IgM exclusively. In our group of 18 patients with CLL, a different pattern was observed. All 18 cases showed a high proportion of lymphocytes carrying IgM as well as IgD on the surface. This would mean that the differentiation of these cells is blocked right at the step where IgD and IgM overlap. One might expect that IgD disappears as soon as the cells start to secrete IgM. We therefore also investigated the lymphocytes of these patients for the presence of crystalline Ig inclusions. In none of the 18 cases, however, could inclusions be found.

The number of patients so far studied is too small to draw any definitive conclusions. It seems to be worthwhile however to follow these lines, since the simultaneous presence of two Ig receptors on the same cell indicates a remarkable genetic event and the investigation of these markers in malignant lymphocyte proliferations might give a better understanding of the under- lying mechanisms.

REFERENCES

1. KNAPP, W., BOLHUIS, R.L.H., RADL, J., HIJMANS, W.: Independent movement of IgD and IgM molecules on the surface of individual lymphocytes. J. Immunol. *111*, 1295 (1973)
2. ROWE, D.S., HUG, K., FORNI, L., PERNIS, B.: Immunoglobulin D as lymphocyte receptor. J. exp. Med. *138*, 965 (1973)

3. KNAPP, W., SCHUIT, H.R.E., BOLHUIS, R.L.H., HIJMANS, W.: Surface immunoglobulins in chronic lymphatic leukaemia, macroglobulinaemia and myeloma-
   tosis. Clin. exp. Immunol. *16*, 541 (1974)
4. HIJMANS, W., SCHUIT, H.R.E., KLEIN, F.: An immunofluorescent procedure
   for the detection of intracellular immunoglobulins. Clin. exp. Immunol.
   4, 457 (1969)
5. KNAPP, W., HAAIJMAN, J.J., SCHUIT, H.R.E., RADL, J., BERG, P., v.d.,
   PLOEM, J.S., HIJMANS, W.: Conjugate specificity in immunofluorescence.
   Microfluorometric evaluation of the specificity of conjugates with the
   defined antigen substrate spheres (DASS) system. Ann. N.Y. Acad. Sci.
   (in press)
6. VOSSEN, J.M., HIJMANS, W.: Membrane associated immunoglobulin determinants
   on bone marrow- and blood lymphocytes in the pediatric age group and on
   foetal tissues. Ann. N.Y. acad. Sci. (in press)
7. PREUD'HOMME, J.L., CLAUVEL, J.P., SELIGMAN, M.: Immunoglobulin D bearing
   lymphocytes in primary immunodeficiencies. (In preparation)
8. HUREZ, D., FLANDRIN, G., PREUD'HOMME, J.L., SELIGMAN, M.: Unreleased
   intracellular monoclonal macroglobulin in chronic lymphatic leukaemia.
   Clin. exp. Immunol. *1o*, 223 (1972)
9. CAWLEY, I.C., BARKER, C.R., BRITCHFORD, R.D., SMITH, J.L.: Intracellular
   IgA immunoglobulin crystals in chronic lymphocytic leukaemia. Clin.
   exp. Immunol. *13*, 407 (1973)

Dr. W. KNAPP
Institut für Immunologie der Universität Wien
Borschkegasse 8 a
Austria

Acta Neuropath. (Berlin), Suppl. VI, 41 - 45 (1975)
© by Springer-Verlag 1975

Studies of the Mechanism of Growth Promotion
of Lymphoma Cells by 2-Mercaptoethanol *in vitro*

J.D. BROOME and H.N. JAYARAM

Department of Pathology
State University of New York - Downstate Medical Center
Brooklyn, N.Y., U.S.A.

Summary: Rates of incorporation of thymidine and uridine, but not leucine,
decrease markedly in L1210(V) cells within 1 hour of incubation in DULBECCO's
medium containing 10% serum. 2-Mercaptoethanol (2-ME) after a latent period
of more than 5 hours causes an increase in nucleotide incorporation. Bovine
serum albumin can substitute for serum in the medium, but a higher concentration of 2-ME is required for growth. After charcoal treatment of the
albumin less 2-ME is required. These experiments suggest that inhibition of
the tumor cells is caused by a serum factor whose effect is antagonized by
the thiol.

Key word: Lymphoma Cells - Growth Promotion - Thiols - 2-Mercaptoethanol -
Nucleotide Incorporation

INTRODUCTION

There is fundamental and practical value in the study of growth control mechanisms in lymphocytes and knowledge of the extent to which they are retained
or lost in the neoplastic state. Evidence for one such mechanism found in
lymphocytes and in 13 of 22 lines of mouse lymphoma cells tested, is the
dependence for growth *in vitro* on certain specific thiols or their corresponding disulfides (1). Since these agents are not naturally occurring, it is
clear that they are compensating for substances of conditions found *in vivo*.
Experiments to understand the mechanism of this effect form the subject of the
present paper. They have been performed with cells of the thiol-disulfide
dependent mouse lymphoma L1210(V) and a variant L1210(A) obtained from it,
which grows independently of such substances.

MATERIALS AND METHODS

Media: DULBECCO's modification of EAGLE's medium was used with air and 5% CO_2
atmosphere (1); unless otherwise stated, 10% horse serum and 5μM 2-mercapto-
ethanol (2-ME) were added. Albumin preparations were purchased from Sigma
Chemical Co., St. Louis, Mo.

Lymphoma cells: The cells used, L1210(V) have been described in previous
publications (1, 2). They were maintained as ascites tumors in B6D2F1 mice.
A variant line L1210(A) was obtained by culturing these cells in the medium
just described for 4 weeks and subsequently changing to medium lacking 2-ME.
A small number of cells survived, and proliferated. They maintained the

character of thiol-disulfide independence on prolonged culture and animal passage.

Assays for tumor growth in vitro: These were performed on the basis of increase of cell count in a 48 hour period as described (1).

Incorporation of thymidine, uridine and L-leucine: Cells obtained from ascites tumors were washed twice and incubated in DULBECCO's medium containing 10% horse serum and 25mM Hepes. Labelled ^3H or ^{14}C-thymidine, uridine or L-leucine were added and aliquots of cell suspension exposed for 10-60 minutes pulses at the times indicated in the figures. Cells were collected and incorporated radioactivity measured as described (1, 3).

RESULTS

Although cells of V and A did not differ significantly in the amount of thymidine incorporated when they were exposed to the labelled compound in heparinized ascitic fluid, a marked difference was observed when they were washed and suspended in DULBECCO's medium with 10% serum. It can be seen in Fig. 1 that in the first hour approximately 5 times more thymidine was incorporated by A as by V. The level fell off further in V, and after 5-6 hours was barely detectable, contrasting again with the rising rate of incorporation by A cells. 2-Mercaptoethanol (2-ME) which earlier experiments showed to support the continued proliferation of V cells, did not have an immediate stimulating effect on thymidine incorporation. At 5 hrs. the rate of incorporation in V cells was three times greater in the thiol containing medium than in the non-thiol and was only similar to that seen in the first hour. By 24 hours, however, the former culture was proliferating vigorously, and the rate of thymidine incorporation was comparable to that of A cells.

The diminishing rate of uptake of thymidine was accompanied by a similar change in uridine incorporation (Fig. 2). In this experiment, 2-ME caused a definite increase in the thymidine incorporation at 12 hours, whereas uridine incorporation did not increase comparably till 24 hours. In marked contrast, the rate of leucine incorporation decreased only slowly in the absence of thiol and at 24 hours was still 65% of that in the first hour. Thiol produced only a moderate increase in incorporation in this early period. Thus the principal metabolic changes observed in V cells after suspension in culture medium were a rapid decrease in thymidine and uridine incorporation, without a concommitant reduction in protein synthesis.

The results which have just been described using cells freshly explanted into culture, are similar to those obtained with cells growing in culture with 2-ME for 2 weeks and then resuspended in fresh medium lacking thiol (Fig. 3). Within 3-4 hours thymidine incorporation showed a 20% decrease and by 5-6 hours was half that seen in the initial period. The rate of uridine incorporation decreased rather more slowly, but by 24 hours had reached 25% of its initial figure. Protein synthesis, measured by leucine incorporation continued virtually unchanged through this period.

A major question raised by these findings is whether the lymphoma cells are affected by lack of a substance present *in vivo* which is not provided by the medium, or alternatively whether there is a growth inhibitory substance in the medium, particularly in its serum compenent. To examine this problem experiments were undertaken to grow cells in medium which lacked serum. Neither A nor V cells proliferated in protein free medium. However, A cells were found to proliferate at the same rate in DULBECCO's medium containing 5g/L bovine serum albumin as in medium containing 10% serum. COHN's fraction V, or x3 crystallized albumin were equally effective. V cells

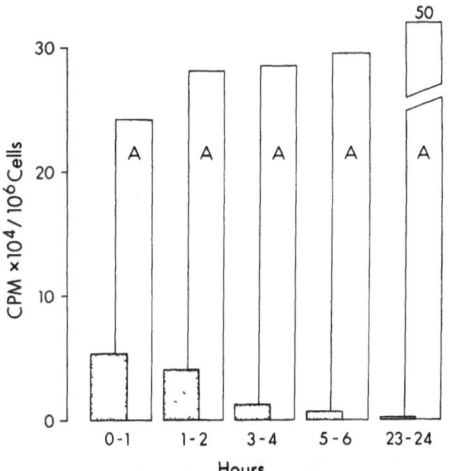

Fig. 1. Uptake of H³-Thymidine by L1210 Cells in Dulbecco's Medium

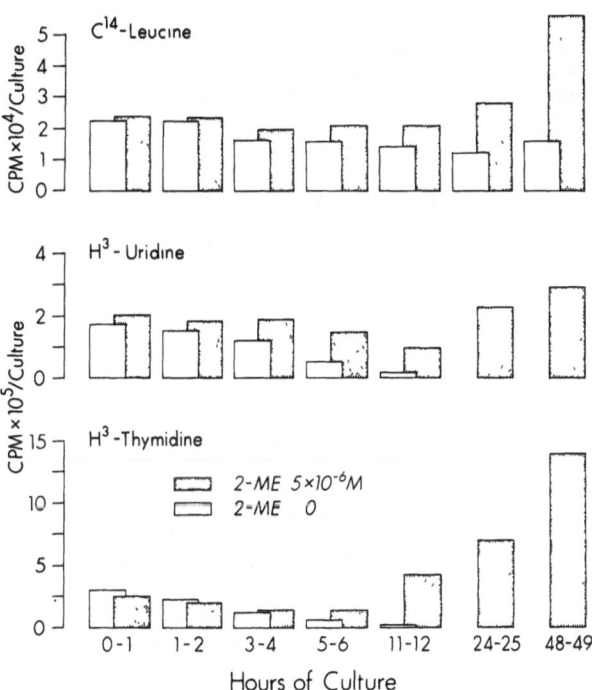

Fig. 2. Effect of 2-ME on Incorporation of Protein, RNA and DNA Precursors by L1210(V) Cells *in vitro*

grew optimally in medium containing 10% horse serum with 5 μM 2-ME but when horse serum was substituted by albumin no growth occurred (Table 1). However, when the 2-ME was increased to 50 μM, vigorous proliferation was seen. The suggestion from this experiment that the albumin preparation may contain a

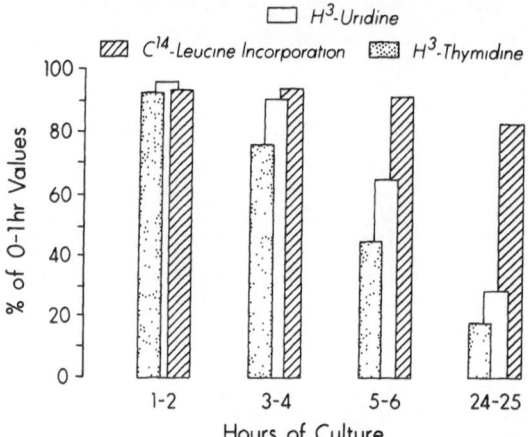

Fig. 3. Rates of Synthetic Processes after Removal of 2-ME from L1210(V)
Cells *in vitro*

Table 1. *Effects of bovine serum albumin (BSA). Supplements on the ability
of L1210 cells to proliferate in Dulbecco's medium*

BSA Preparation	Albumin Concentration (g/L)	2-ME Concentration (μM)	Cell Proliferation	
			L1210(V)	L1210(A)
Crystalline	0	0-5	0	0
	5	5	0	+
	5	50	+	+
Crystalline Charcoal- treated	5	5	+	+
	10	5	0	+

factor or factors inhibitory to the growth of V cells whose effect is count-
eracted by 2-ME, is reinforced by experiments using crystalline bovine albumin
absorbed with charcoal at pH3.0 by the method of CHEN (4). Protein, after
this treatment was considerably less inhibitory, and V cells proliferated
with 5 μM 2-ME, at an albumin concentration of 5g/L. At 10 g/L however, this
2-ME concentration was inadequate for growth, although cell viability was
maintained in the test period.

DISCUSSION

The experiments described show a growth control mechanism in L1210(V) cells
mediated by culture medium containing serum which causes the rapid decrease
in exogenous thymidine and uridine incorporation. That this is specific and
not part of a general depression of cell metabolism is demonstrated by the
maintenance of protein synthesis at scarcely diminished rate for a period

of at least 24 hours. The decrease in thymidine and uridine incorporation
is most conveniently explained by inhibition of DNA and RNA synthesis. Further
experiments (not reported) have not thus far provided evidence for inhibition
of uptake of these bases nor for significant changes in intracellular pool
size.

The experiments substituting purified albumin for whole serum in the presence of 2-ME suggest that growth control is mediated through a protein bound
substance in serum, which may be concentrated on albumin and partially freed
from it by charcoal absorption. This process removes fatty acids but it is
to be expected that other substances are also affected. The action of 2-ME
and presumably other thiols and disulfides is then to antagonize this inhibitory effect. It should be noted that serum is not the physiological fluid
to which cells are exposed, except under unusual circumstances of tissue
trauma, and several modifying effects on cell growth have been attributed
to it in other systems (5). Mouse splenic lymphocytes survive better in
culture, and lectin-induced mitosis is enhanced by thiols and disulfides
which are required for the growth of L1210(V) cells (1). It is therefore
possible that the mechanism of action of thiols on L1210(V) cells will elu-
cidate a growth control mechanism of normal lymphocytes which is retained
in this and other lymphoma cell lines.

REFERENCES

1. BROOME, J.D., JENG, MW.: Promotion of replication in lymphoid cells by
   specific thiols and disulfides *in vitro*. J. Exp. Med. *138*, 574-592 (1973)
2. HUTCHISON, D.J., HERSOHN, O.L., BJERREGARD, M.R.: Growth of L1210 mouse
   leukaemia cells *in vitro*. Exp. Cell Res. *42*, 157-170 (1966)
3. BROOME, J.D.: Studies on the mechanism of tumor inhibition by L-asparagi-
   nase. J. Exp. Med. *127*, 1055-1072 (1968)
4. CHEN, R.F.: Removal of fatty acids from serum albumin by charcoal treatment. J. Biol. Chem. *242*, 173-181 (1967)
5. BALK, S.D.: Stimulation of the proliferation of chicken fibroblasts by
   folic acid or a serum factor (s) in a plasma-containing medium. Proc.
   Natl. Acad. Sci. U.S.A. *68*, 1689-1692 (1971)

BROOME, J.D., M.D.
Dept. of Pathology, Downstate Medical Center
(State University of New York)
Brooklyn, N.Y. 11203
U.S.A.

Acta Neuropath. (Berlin), Suppl. VI, 47 - 52 (1975)

Myxovirus-Like Particles in Cells of American Burkitt's-Type Lymphoma

NINA A. POPOFF and THEODORE I. MALININ

Department of Pathology (Neuropathology)
University of Miami School of Medicine and
Veterans Administration Hospital
Miami, Florida, U.S.A.

Summary: Distinct tubular arrays associated with cisternae of endoplasmic reticulum were observed in neoplastic lymphoid cells in a primary American Burkitt's-type lymphoma. A late relapse of the disease was complicated by severe CNS involvement. The pathogenesis of CNS involvement and the significance of the tubular arrays are discussed.

Key words: Tubular Arrays - Burkitt's Lymphoma - Viral Particles - Ultrastructure

INTRODUCTION

The occurrence of Burkitt's type lymphoma outside Africa is now well established (1). The American Burkitt's Lymphoma Registry to date documented nearly 100 cases of the disease (2). The tumors in these cases showed a characteristic anatomic distribution and were morphologically similar to those reported from Africa (3). The mean age of onset was reported at 10.2 years in American patients and 8 years for patients studied in Uganda (1). Lymphadenopathy due to the tumor is rare and extranodal neoplastic growth, as a rule, is not accompanied by significant leukemic changes in the peripheral blood (14). CNS involvement is common and presents a serious complication of relapse in patients with Burkitt's lymphoma. Distinct histologic and cytologic features of the tumor permit its differentiation from other types of lymphomas of the histiocytic or lymphocytic variety (5).

The present report deals with the occurrence of tubular arrays in neoplastic and endothelial cells in the primary American Burkitt's type lymphoma. The significance of these structures and the pathogenesis of CNS involvement are discussed.

CLINICAL HISTORY

A 16-month-old white female was admitted to the hospital with an enlarging mass in the right labia, noted at 12 months of age. Physical examination was otherwise negative. One month prior to the onset of the tumor, the child received measles vaccination. A biopsy of the lesion revealed an undifferentiated lymphoma, Burkitt's type. No lymphadenopathy or bone involvement was present. Following local radiotherapy and administration of Vincristine and Azathioprine, the tumor disappeared and the child was well for five months. At 21 month's of age she was noted to stumble to the left, and her right

eye turned inward. She became unable to walk, irritable and lethargic. The
head circumference was larger than the 97th percentile for her age. Hct. was
48%, Hgb. 13,3 gm/100 ml; WBC 2900 per cu. mm. with 48% lymphocytes. Serum
immunoglobulin levels were: IA 105 mg%; IgM 40 mg% and IgC 700 mg%. Neurological examination showed marked ataxia on reaching and in gait. The optic
fundi were poorly visualized and there was a bilateral VI nerve paresis. The
reflexes were hypoactive and there were bilateral Babinski signs. Skull
x-rays revealed diffuse widening of sutures. Cerebral angiography showed
mild hydrocephalus and no mass lesions. The patient developed persistent
seizures and became comatose on the third hospital day. The child was placed
on continuous ventricular drainage. The CSF pressure was 220 mm H_2O, the
protein 161 mg.% and the cell count 1500 WBC per ml. with 97% mononuclear
cells. Radiotherapy was initiated. The seizures and the coma, however, persisted and the child expired 18 days following the onset of neurological
symptoms.

MATERIALS AND METHODS

Small blocks of tumor obtained from a biopsy of the labial lesion were fixed
in 3.5% glutaraldehyde (pH 7.3), postfixed in 1% osmium tetroxide, dehydrated
and embedded in Epon. Sections were double stained with uranyl and lead salts,
and examined in a Phillip's EM-300 electron microscope. Paraffin-embedded-
formalin-fixed tissues were stained with hematoxylin and eosin, methyl green-
pyronine, Giemsa, periodic acid-Schiff's and Gordon-Sweet reticulum stains.
Tissues from autopsy materials were studied in an identical manner.

RESULTS

The original subcutaneous tumor consisted of poorly differentiated lymphoid
cells, with scanty cytoplasm and round-to-oval nuclei. Reticulated chromatin
enclosed one or two nucleoli. The tumor cell cytoplasm exhibited marked
pyroninophilia. Interspered throughout the tumor were large pale histiocytes
forming a "starry-sky" pattern. Their clear cytoplasm often contained ingested
cellular debris (Fig. 1). Necropsy revealed lymphomatous tumor infiltrates in
both kidneys, liver, thymus, and subepicardial tissue. The markedly edematous
brain showed clouding of the leptomeninges which was especially prominent
over the brain stem and superior surface of the cerebellum. On section, a
0.5 cm hemorrhagic area was seen in the right anterior basal ganglia. Some
dilatation of the temporal and occipital horns was present with compression
of the lateral ventricles rostrally.
  Microscopically, lymphomatous infiltration of the meninges was present
throughout the cerebrum, brain stem and cerebellum. The infiltrates extended
along the peripheral portion of the cranial nerves and obliterated most of the
perivascular spaces. The cell population within meningeal infiltrates showed
generally a greater degree of distintegration as compared to other affected
organs of the body. Invariably present were large mulberry-like phagocytic
reticulo-endothelial cells, measuring up to 250 μ (Fig. 2). Their cytoplasm
contained numerous ingested neoplastic lymphoid cells, cellular debris and
karyorrhectic nuclei.

ULTRASTRUCTURAL STUDIES

The appearance of neoplastic cells in the primary tumor was rather uniform.
The spread of the tumor occurred throughout the dermis and was arrested at
the limiting membrane of the stratum Malpighii. Nuclei of numerous tumor

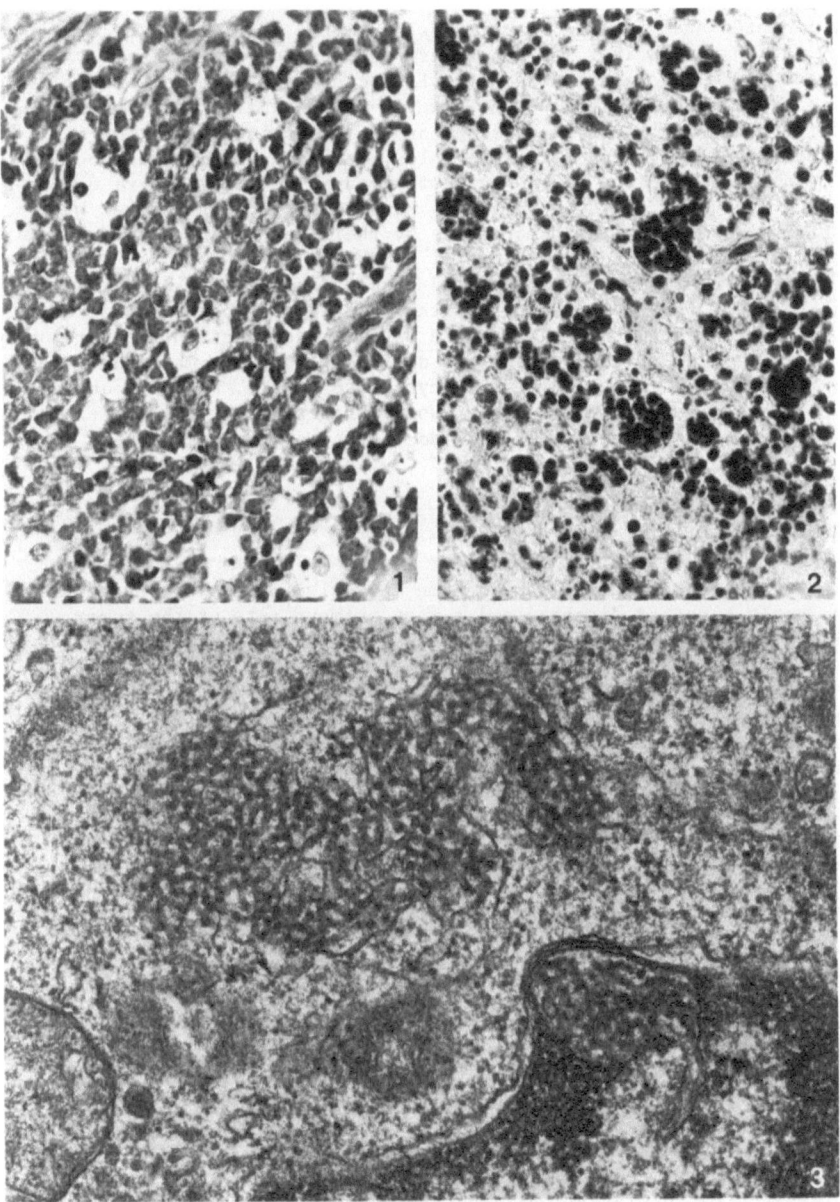

Fig. 1. Subcutaneous tumor. Large pale histocytes form a prominent "starry sky" pattern. x 425

Fig. 2. Lymphomatous infiltrate, right basal ganglia. Phagocytic reticulo-endothelial cells contain ingested neoplastic lymphoid cells and cellular debris. x 400

Fig. 3. Aggregates of tubular structures are associated with highly distorted systernae of ER. An indented intranuclear cytoplasmic process contains similar particles. x 57,500

cells were indented and showed a conspicuous chromatin margination. Occasionally extensions of nuclear membranes were seen to be indented by a cytoplasmic process. The moderately dense cytoplasm contained abundant free RNP granules frequently grouped in rosettes. Many cells exhibited additional signs of differentiation, such as development of membranous ER and Golgi apparatus. Some cells contained lipid vacuoles, membrane-bound dense bodies, and short cytoplasmic bundles of 120A wide filaments. Desmosomes were not observed among the tumor cells. Intervening non-neoplastic histiocytes were easily distinguishable from the tumor cells by their more abundant cytoplasm, which contained well developed cysternae of rough E.R.

A striking feature of many well preserved neoplastic lymphoid cells, the endothelial cells of some capillaries and the cytoplasm of occasional granulocytes was the presence of tubular arrays in intimate association with granular E.R. (Fig. 3). The tubular aggregates were delineated by unit membranes derived form the wall of highly distorted cysternae of E.R. Not infrequently the particles were also seen between the two membranes of the nuclear envelope. The tubular arrays were not identified in the postmortem tissues.

DISCUSSION

The patient in the present study showed some unusual findings with respect to the very early onset of disease, and a rare primary site of the tumor. A late relapse with CNS involvement occurred 5 month's following the initial onset and treatment of the disease.

In view of the absence of lymphatics within the CNS and an infrequent finding of tumor cells in the peripheral blood, the pathogenesis of meningeal and parenchymal invasion remains obscure. CNS manifestation of the disease during a late relapse may be the result of tumor reinduction impelled by the same agent which induced the primary tumor. The evidence that late relapse tumors originate from a different clone of tumor cells than the initial tumor is in support of this theory (6).

A common etiologic agent for Burkitt's lymphoma has not been documented to date. The widespread occurrence of the Epstein-Barr virus (EBV) indicate that it may be an important but inadequate causative agent. Recent epidemiologic studies suggest that malaria may be one such co-factor in the pathogenesis of African Burkitt's tumor, since the incidence of epidemicity of this neoplasm frequently parallels that of malaria (7, 8). Despite clinical and histopathologic similarities between African and American forms of Burkitt's lymphoma, the EBV genomes could not be detected in association with American Burkitt's lymphoma (9). Thus the apparent absence of the viral DNA in the American tumor tissue provides evidence against the etiologic role of the EBV in American Burkitt's lymphoma. However, biologic action of oncogenic agents may be complex and virus variation as well as host factors can both play a role in its determination.

The significance of tubular arrays and the mechanisms by which they are formed remains unclear. Since these structures occur in a variety of tissues and conditions, they cannot be considered unique for any particular cell type or pathologic process. On the other hand, the predilection of these structures for lymphoid and reticulo-endothelial cells and their frequent association with either viral or suspected viral conditions cannot be overlooked (10). Despite the fact that cytochemical analysis of the tubular arrays (10, 11) did not demonstrate nucleic acids, their viral origin cannot be entirely ruled out. The tubular arrays may possibly represent incomplete forms of a latent virus, and thus stimuli responsible for cell proliferation may also

lead to an increased production of the particles. Experimental production
of tubular arrays by treating lymphoid cell cultures with halogenated-
pyrimidine 5-bromo-2-deoxyuridine (BUDR) (12) tends to support this contention,
since BUDR is also known to activate latent virus infection in mammalian cells
(13, 14).

Another possibility is that the tubular structures may reflect production
of antibody protein. The finding of tubular arrays in umbilical cord lymphocytes from infants born to mothers with autoimmune disease (15) suggests
placental transmission of a maternal agent capable of inducing these structures. If the tubular arrays are related to the production of immunoglobulins,
especially the IgG, the release of such materials and their interaction with
the complement systems may markedly enhance phagocytosis (16). Such increased
ingestive capacity of histiocytic cells was observed within meningeal and
parenchymal infiltrates in our material. Finally, if the tubular arrays are,
in fact, related to immunoglobulin production, a possibility must be entertained of a response to the rubeola virus by the lymphoid cells in a host
with altered immunologic state.

REFERENCES

1. COHEN, M.H., BENNETT, J.M., BERNARD, C.W., ZIEGLER, J.L., VOGEL, C.L.,
   SHEAGREN, J.N., CARBONE, P.P.: Burkitt's Tumor in the United States.
   Cancer *23*, 1259-1272 (1969)
2. LEVINE, P.H., CHO, B.R.: Burkitt's lymphoma: Clinical features of North
   American Cases. Cancer Res. *34*, 1219-1212 (1974)
3. O'CONNOR, G.T., RAPPAPORT, H., SMITH, E.B.: Childhood lymphoma resembling
   "Burkitt's Tumor" in the United States. Cancer *18*, 411-417 (1965)
4. CARBONE, P.P., BERNARD, C.W., BENNET, J.M., ZIEGLER, J.L., COHEN, M.H.,
   GERPER, P.: Burkitt's tumor. Ann. Inst. Med. *70*, 817-832 (1969)
5. BERARD, C., O'CONNOR, G.T., THOMAS, L.B., TORLONI, H.: Histopathological
   definition of Burkitt's tumor. Bulletin of the World Health Organization
   40, 601-607 (1969)
6. FIALKOW, P.L., KLEIN, G., CLIFFORD, P.: Second malignant clone underlying
   a Burkitt tumor exacerbation. Lancet *2*, 629 (1972)
7. BURKITT, D.P.: Etiology of Burkitt's lymphoma - an alternative hypothesis
   to a vectored virus. J. Nat. Cancer inst. *42*, 19 (1969)
8. MORROW, R.H.: Burkitt's lymphoma in Africa. Cancer Res. *34*, 1211-1215
   (1974)
9. PAGANO, J.S., HUANG, C.H., LEVINE, P.: Absence of Epstein-Barr viral DNA
   in American Burkitt's lymphoma. New Eng. J. Med. *289*, 1395-1399 (1974)
10. SCHAFF, Z., HEINE, U., DALTON, A.J.: Ultramorphological and ultracyto-
    chemical studies on tuboreticular structures in lymphoid cells. Cancer
    Res. *32*, 2696-2706 (1972)
11. SCHAFF, Z., BARRY, D.W., GRIMLEY, P.M.: Cytochemistry of tuboreticular
    structures in lymphocytes from patients with systemic lupus erythematosus
    and in cultured human lymphoid cells: Comparison to a paramyxovirus. Lab.
    Invest. *29*, 577-586 (1973)
12. GRIMLEY, P.M., BARRY, D.W., SCHAFF, Z.: Induction of tubular structures
    in the endoplasmic reticulum of human lymphoid cells by treatment with
    5-Bromo-2-Deoxyuridine. J. Nat. Cancer Inst. *51*, 1751-1755 (1973)
13. GERBER, P.: Activation of Epstein-Barr virus by 5-bromodeoxyuridine in
    "virus free" human cells. Proc. Nat. Acad. Sci. U.S.A. *69*, 83-85 (1972)
14. ROWE, W.P., LOWRY, D.R., TEIGH, N., *et al*.: Some implication of the
    activation of murine leukaemia virus by halogenated pyrimidines. Proc.
    Nat. Acad. Sci. U.S.A. *69*, 1033-1035 (1972)

15. KLIPPEL, J.H., GRIMLEY, P.M., DECKER, J.L.: Lymphocyte inclusions in new-
    borns of mothers with systemic lupus erythematosus. New Eng. J. Med. *290*,
    95-97 (1974)
16. STOSSEL, T.P.: Phagocytosis (First of three parts). New Eng. J. Med. *290*,
    717-723 (1974)

Nina A. POPOFF, M.D.
Department of Pathology
Jackson Memorial Hospital
1700 N.W. Tenth Avenue
Miami, Florida 33152
U.S.A.

Acta Neuropath. (Berlin), Suppl. VI, 53 - 56 (1975)

Acid Phosphatase of Azurophilic Granules of C3HST4 Lymphoma

A. COPPOLA

Department of Pathology, S.U.N.Y. Downstate Medical Center
Brooklyn, New York, U.S.A.

Summary: A transplantable mouse lymphoblastic tumor with unusual azurophilic
granules has been recently reported.
   The present tumor has been studied with Gomori and Novikoff methods for
lysosomal marker, acid phosphatase. By electron microscopy enzyme was found
in granules surrounded by single or double membrane, which displayed a wide
morphologic range appearing as 1. vesicular, 2. multivesicular, 3. compound,
4. granular and 5. tubular bodies.
   The occurrence and the amount of enzyme activity in the granules appeared
dependent on their morphology. It was least in vesicular bodies and most in
granular organelles, characteristically at their periphery. Since the present
tumor, labelled C3HST4, is an unusual rich source of azurophilic granules,
it might be useful for further studies of lysosomal bodies. Their functions
are poorly understood. Similar structures have been observed in normal human
lymphocytes and those from chronic lymphocytic leukemia.

Key words: Transplantable Lymphoma - Azurophilic Granules - Electron Microscopy - Acid Phosphatase - Lysosomes

INTRODUCTION

A spontaneous transplantable murine lymphoma labelled C3HST4 has been recently reported (1). This tumor arose as spontaneous lymphoma in a 20 month old
C3H/HeJax mouse and it was converted readily into an ascitic form. The main
features of this tumor are represented by a tendency to metastasize to
numerous organs and by the presence of a large number of cytoplasmic azurophilic granules in 79.3% $\pm$ 16.6 of malignant lymphocytes. (2).
   The object of the present study was to demonstrate
1. the various morphology of these organelles and
2. the localization of a hydrolitic enzyme, acid phosphatase, within these
granules supporting the hypothesis as to their lysosomal nature.

MATERIAL AND METHODS

10 C3H/HeJax mice were implanted intraperitoneally with 500.000 C3HST4 tumor
cells. On the 11th post-implantation day, when approximately 50 to 80 million
cells were present in the peritoneal cavity, the mice were killed by cervical
dislocation. The tumor cells were harvested from the peritoneal cavity and
treated for routine electron microscopy and cytochemical demonstration of
acid phosphatase (3).

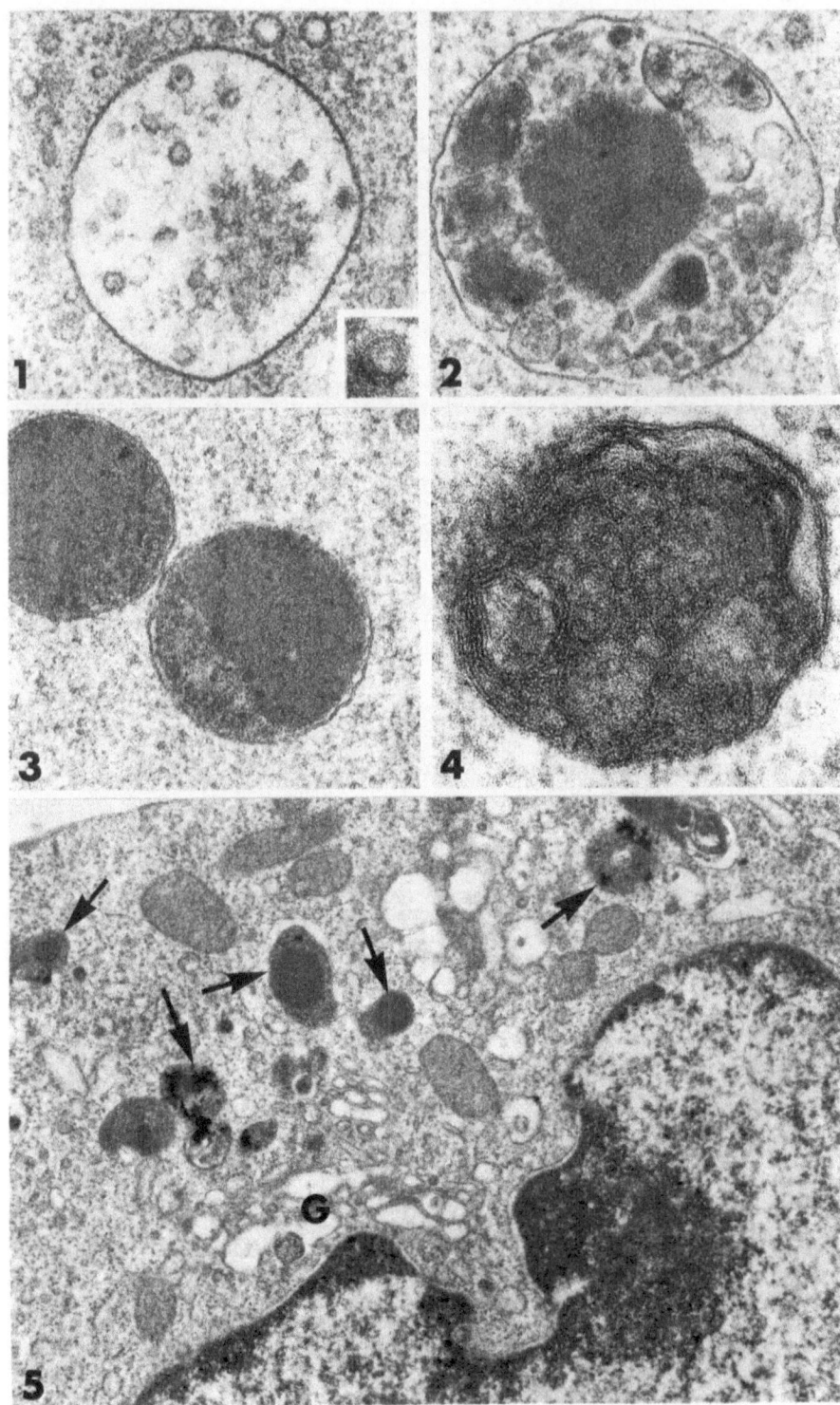

RESULTS

The cells treated for routine electron microscopy had the general features
of immature lymphoblasts. Most of the cells revealed the presence of a variable number of inclusion bodies presumed to correspond to the azurophilic
granules seen by light microscopy. All these were seen adjacent to the nuclear
indentation and often in close association with the Golgi apparatus. Only
occasionally were they seen in distant areas.
   These granules displayed a wide morphologic range appearing as
1. Vesicles which were electron translucent or frequently containing a small
amount of granular material.
2. Other granules similar to the previously described vesicles but containing
several internal smaller vesicles. The matrix among the vesicles was composed
of fine granular material. They were invariably limited by a double membrane.
(Fig. 1.).
3. Another variety of cytoplasmic granules containing several smaller vesicles
in close association with the inner aspect of the double layered limiting
membrane and displaying a dense granular material in the center. (Fig. 2).
4. Some cytoplasmic granules having a homogeneous granular appearance (3).
5. Occasionally cytoplasmic bodies with a laminated appearance (Fig. 4).

Localization of Acid Phosphatase

Specimens prepared for the cytochemical demonstration of acid phospatase
revealed localized lead deposits in several granules of C3HST4 lymphoma cells
suggesting the lysosomal nature of these cytoplasmic bodies.
   The lead deposit seemed to be characteristically located at the periphery
of the granules rather than in association with the central dense core.
(Fig. 5). Not all the granules appeared acid phophatase positive. Enzyme
activity was least in the vesicular bodies and most in the granular organelles.
Perhaps such variation reflects the stages of development of these organelles.

DISCUSSION

In the last decade there have been numerous reports concerning azurophilic
granules of all white blood cells (5, 6, 7, 8, 9). The granules of lymphocytes particularly have been extensively studied. These granules are seen
more numerous in large lymphocytes (10, 11, 12), and occasionally they have
been reported in cases of chronic lymphocytic leukemia (12). They are generally
considered to be lysosomes containing numerous enzymes, but their exact function is poorly understood.

Fig. 1. Multivesicular body containing granular material and smaller vesicles
which have limiting membrane and contain amorphous substance. Uranyl acetate
x 54,000. Insert x 110,000

Fig. 2. Compound body with condensed material in the center. Uranyl acetate
x 54,000

Fig. 3. Membrane limited inclusion body entirely filled by granular material.
Uranyl acetate x 54,000

Fig. 4. Tubular body with laminated or "fingerprint" appearance. Uranyl
acetate x 54,000

Fig. 5. This electron micrograph reveals the localization of acid phosphatase
around granules which are frequently seen gathered near the Golgi zone (G).
Uranyl acetate x 19,500

The C3HST4 murine lymphoma represents a good animal model for the study of azurophilic granules of lymphocytes, because the majority of cells contain a large number of such organelles. Azurophilic granules, as already reported, were seen in close association with the Golgi apparatus suggesting this as the site of origin. The variable morphology may be related to different stages of maturation. The occurrence and the amount of acid phosphatase in the granules appears dependent on their morphology: it is least in vesicular bodies and most in granular inclusions.

In conclusion, we would like to emphasize that the C3HST4 lymphoma may be useful for further studies of azurophilic granules of lymphoid cells and eventually we hope to be able to explain their role in benign and malignant lymphocytes.

REFERENCES

1. COPPOLA, A.: A spontaneous transplantable malignant lymphoma in C3H/Hejax mice (abstract). Fed. Proc., *31*, 614 Abs. March-April (1972)
2. COPPOLA, A.: A transplantable mouse lymphoma with unusual azurophilic granules. Amer. J. Path. *73*, 233-246 (1973)
3. GOMORI, G.: Microscopic Histochemistry: Principle and practice, p. 273. Chicago: 1952 University of Chicago Press
4. BAINTON, D.F., FARQUHAR, M.G.: Difference in enzyme content of azurophil and specific granules of polymorphonuclear leucocytes. I. Histochemical staining of bone marrow. J. Cell Biol. *39*, 286-298 (1968)
5. BAINTON, D.F., FARQUHAR, M.G.: Differences in enzyme content of azurophil and specific granules of polymorphonuclear leucocytes. II. Cytochemistry and electron microscopy of bone marrow cells. Cell Biol. *39*, 299-317 (1968)
6. NICHOLS, B.A., BAINTON, D.F., FARQUHAR, M.G.: Differentiation of monocytes. Origin, nature and fate of their azurophil granules. Cell Biol. *50*, 498-515 (1971)
7. WETZEL, B.K., SPICER, S.S., HORN, R.G.: Fine structural localization of acid and alkaline phosphatase in cells of rabbit blood and bone marrow. J. Histochem. Cytochem. *15*, 311-334 (1967)
8. ANDERSON, D.R.: Ultrastructure of normal and leukemic leukocytes in human peripheral blood. J. Ultrastruct. Res. *16*, Suppl. 9, 5-42 (1966)
9. MIALE, J.B.: Laboratory Medicine: Hematology, 4th edition. St. Louis: The C.V. Mosby Co. 1972
10. HUHN, D.: Fine structure of blood and blood marrow. New York: Ed. Hafner Publishing Company Inc., 1969
11. BESSIS, M.: Living blood cells and their Ultrastructure. New York-Heidelberg-Berlin: Springer 1973

A. COPPOLA, M.D.
Department of Pathology, S.U.N.Y. Downstate Medical Center
Brooklyn, New York 11203
U.S.A.

Acta Neuropath. (Berlin), Suppl. VI, 57 - 63 (1975)

The Fine Structure of the Lymphocyte Nucleus Under Conditions of Phytohaemagglutinin Stimulation

IVAN VALKOV

Department of Anatomical Pathology[+)]
Faculty of Medicine of Sofia, Bulgaria

Summary: The nucleus of PHA (phytohaemagglutinin) cultured lymphocytes is studied by EDTA, Thalium-Schiff and uranyl-lead techniques. Scattering of the dense chromatin, increase in the number of NB (nuclear bodies) and nucleolar modifications are established. Transportation is seen of granules similar to perichromatin ones from the nucleus into the cytoplasm. Morphometric investigation reveals a decrease between 7,7 and 26,3% of the dense chromatin and also thatthe number of PCG (perichromatin granules) to be the greatest in the untransformed PHA lymphocytes, e.g. B lymphocytes. It is established in new born chickens that the lymphocytes of the bourse of Fabricius are richer in PCG than these of the thymus.

Key words: T and B lymphocytes - morphometry - perichromatin granules - chromatin

Blast transformation in the phytohaemagglutinin (PHA) cultures is subject of many studies on the metabolic modifications connected with cell division preparation. Quantitative peculiarities of the process are studied by biochemical methods. Early structural modifications cannot be undertaken by routine electron microscopic technique.

MATERIAL AND METHODS

For the study of structural nuclear modifications including the early ones we used the EDTA technique of W. BERNHARD (1) for the RNP structures visualization, the Thalium-Schiff technique of G. MOYNE (2) for the DNA demonstration and uranyl-lead staining of guinea pigs lymph node lymphocytes, cultivated for 1, 2, 3, 4, 5, 6, 24 and 48 hours in the presence of PHA. The morphometric study was performed on electron micrographs of EDTA treated material. The nuclear surface, dense chromatin surface and the number of perichromatin granules (PCG) per cell profile were measured. Specimens of the thymus and of the bourse of Fabricius taken from new born chickens in the moment of the hatch out were treated by EDTA technique and put to morphometric study in the same manner.[++)]

[+)]   The article is from the Cancer Research Institute, Electron Microscopy Service, directed by Dr. W. BERNHARD, Villejuif (France)
[++)] For details of the techniques see Nr. 1 and 2 in References and also:
VALKOV, I., MOYNE, G., ROBINEAUX, R.: Eur. J. Immunol. 1974 (in press)
VALKOV, I., MOYNE, G.: J. Microsc. (Paris) 1974 (in press)

RESULTS

In uncultivated cell suspension the predominant cell type is the small lymphocyte. Clumps of dense chromatin, situated mainly under the nuclear membrane
are compact and their borderlines are sharply outlined (Fig. 1 a,b). Very
often a large central dense chromatin mass is seen. By the Thalium-Schiff
technique it is well demonstrated the internal layer of the nuclear envelope
(Fig. 1 c). Perinucleolar chromatin clumps are abundant and usually they
surround more than 2/3 of the nucleolar profile (Fig. 1 a). Intranucleolar
chromatin clumps are small and scanty.

The nucleolus is very often ring shaped or with a homogeneous structure
(Fig. 1 a). In rare cases when the nucleolus is found in the nuclear periphery a thin layer stained like dense chromatin (200 - 300 Å in width) is
observed separating it from the nuclear membrane. This layer is better
demonstrated by the Thalium-Schiff technique and by the EDTA technique also
in the later stages of the specimens [+] (Fig. 2 a).

The EDTA technique visualizes the RNP structures after dense chromatin
bleaching. Perichromatin and interchromatin granules are clearly seen (Fig.
1 b). The nucleolus is well preserved, but usually the central area of the
ring shaped nucleolus is bleached (Fig. 2 d).

In 1 hour PHA culture specimens, certain lymphocytes showed a slight tendency of augmentation of the fibrillar branches arising from the heterochromatin clumps. In three hour culture specimens, using the Thalium-Schiff
technique, certain nuclei showed initial fragmentation of the dense chromatin
clumps, accompined by borderline clouding (Fig. 2 a). An initial decrease in
the quantity of perinucleolar chromatin and augmentation of the nucleolar
size with features of transformation towards reticular tipe is observed. In
4-6 hour cultures these modifications are better demonstrated. In 24 and 48
hour cultures the majority of the lymphocytes are transformed. Their nuclei
are bigger with an increased number of pores and nuclear pockets (Fig. 2 c).
Fragmentation of the dense chromatin clumps is advanced. The inner borderline of the marginal chromatin clumps is rough, rich in thin branches which
gradually merges into the euchromatin. Sometimes the central dense chromatin
block is little modified (Fig. 2 b). The amount of perinucleolar chromatin
is reduced but the intranucleolar chromatin appears greater than in untransformed lymphocytes. The nucleolus is bigger with a reticular structure (Fig.
2 c), sometimes spotted and very often attached in one or two places to the
nuclear envelope.

Nuclear bodies (NB) are more numerous in the PHA cultures (8,03% of the
cell profiles) than in the controls (3,55%). Regarding the morphological
type, the so called simple NB (3) are predominant (Fig. 2 d). The complex
type and the compartmental ones are seen as a rule in the stimulated cells.

The morphometric study on the evolution of the dense chromatin surface,
compared with the nuclear surface (per cell profile) reveals a difference
even in the cells of one hour cultures (decrease of 7,7%). In the later
stages this difference is greater (26,0% in 24 h and 26,3% in 48 h). Regarding
the PCG number per unit area of the nuclear surface it is found that they are
most numerous in the untransformed lymphocytes of the PHA cultures (Fig. 3).

It is observed that the PCG are disposed at the periphery of the dense
chromatin clumps and sometimes in the channels near the pores. In single
cases of stimulated lymphocytes they can be seen just in the pores as elongated or deformed like "dumb bells". Granules with identical morphology are
rarely observed in the cytoplasm or in the perinuclear space.

[+] It coincides with the so called Internal dense lamella which is obviously
rich in DNA.

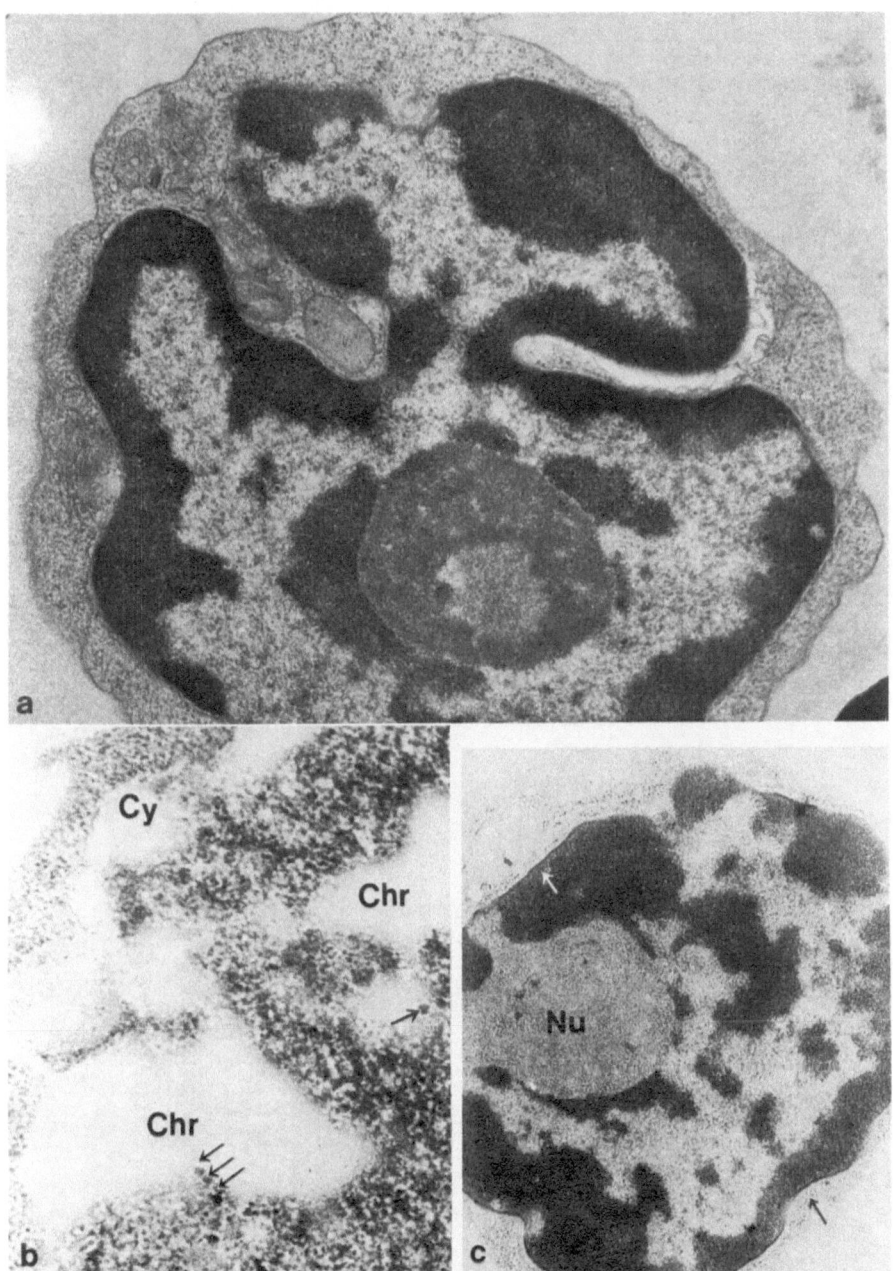

Fig. 1 a - c. Zero culture lymphocytes.
a) Uranyl-lead staining. Dense chromatin clumps are sharply outlined. Abundant perinucleolar chromatin. Ring shaped nucleolus (x 22 000). b) EDTA technique. Part of one untransformed lymphocyte. Chr-bleached chromatin clumps. Cy - cytoplasm. Arrows - perichromatin granules (x 33 000). c) Thalium-Schiff technique. Only DNA is stained. Nu - nucleolus. Arrows - inner nuclear membrane layer (x 12 000)

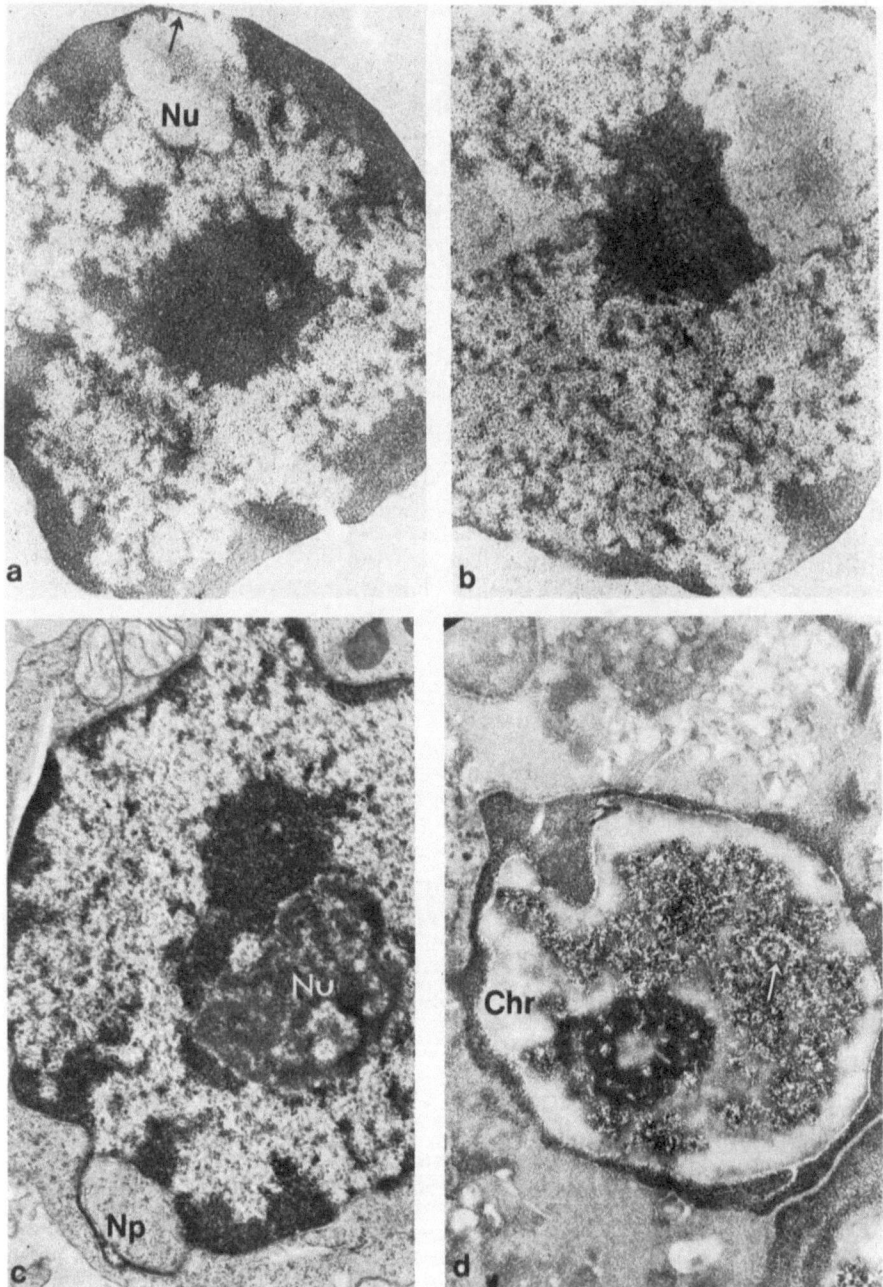

Fig. 2 a - d. PHA stimulated lymphocytes.
a) Three hour PHA culture, Thalium-Schiff technique. Initial fragmentation of
the dense chromatin clumps. Arrow - DNA containing layer separating the
nucleolus (Nu) from the nuclear envelope (x 15 000). b) 24 hour PHA culture.
Schiff-thalium technique. Advanced fragmentation of dense chromatin clumps.
The central chromatin clump is not modified (x 15 000). c) 24 hour culture.

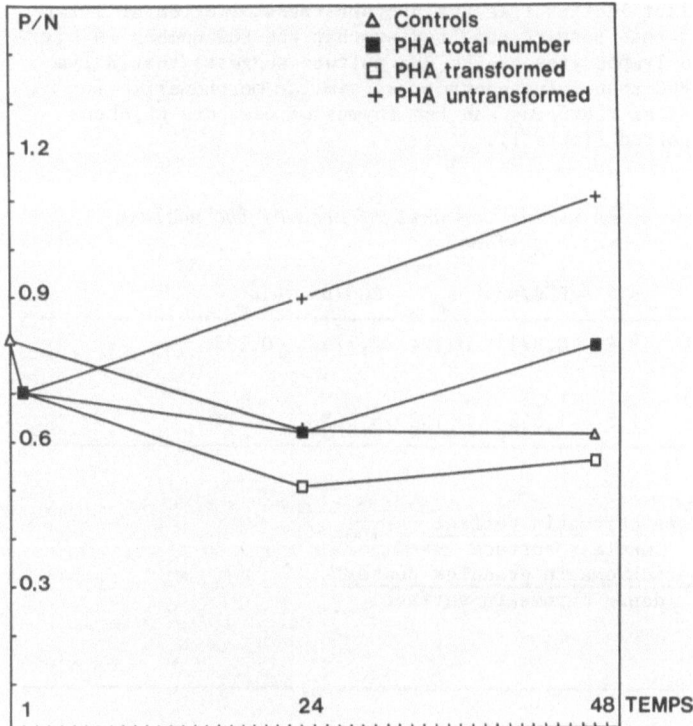

Fig. 3. Evolution of the perichromatin granules number per unit of area of the nuclear surface in the course of the PHA stimulation.

DISCUSSION

The present study reveals early chromatin modifications, provoked by PHA action, even in 1 hour culture specimens. Chromatin changes mark the transition of the inactive DNA into the active one, e.g. a morphological expression of the DNA derepression, which makes the RNA transcription possible (4). This finding corresponds to the data concerning the early start of nonhistone proteins and RNA synthesis (5, 6). Peripherally disposed dense chromatin clumps are observed to be more sensitive to the PHA action than the central chromatin clumps. Perinucleolar chromatin is found to be reduced and the intranucleolar chromatin to be increased in the course of blast transformation. In parallel with that, transformation of the ring shaped of homogeneous nucleolus into reticular form occurs. These modification are probably an expression of an increase in the rate of nucleic acid and protein synthesis (7). Augmentation of the NB number in different cell systems is also refered to as an expression of the increased protein synthesis (3).

Uranyl-lead staining. Marginal dense chromatin is obviously decreased.
Np - nuclear pocked. Nu - reticular nucleolus (x 16 000). d) 24 hour culture.
EDTA technique. Chr - bleached dense chromatin. Scanty perinucleolar chromatin.
One ring shaped nucleolus in transforming towards a reticular one. Arrow -
nuclear body of simple type (x 14 000)

It is admitted that plant lectins like PHA provoke transformation of T lymphocytes only (8, 9). In this respect our finding that the PCG number is bigger in the untransformed lymphocytes of the PHA culture suggests that B lymphocytes are richer in PCG than T lymphocytes. By similar morphometric investigation on the bourse of Fabricius and the thymus of new born chickens this hypothesis was supported (Table 1).

Table 1. *Perichromatin granules number per unit of area of the nuclear surface and of the dense chromatin surface*

	NC	DC/N	s_m	PCG/N	s_m	PCG/DC	s_m
Thymus	28	58,4	3,4	0,883	0,124	1,725	0,332
Burse of Fabricius	25	35,5	1,8	1,848	0,158	5,465	0,517

NC: number of the cells

DC/N: average ratio: $\dfrac{\text{dense chromatin surface}}{\text{nuclear surface}} \times 100$

PCG/N: average ratio: $\dfrac{\text{perichromatin granules number}}{\text{dense chromatin surface}}$

s_m: standard deviation

The present observation suggests the ability of whole PCG passing into the cytoplasm. It corresponds to the data obtained by LE GOASCOGNE *et al.* (10) in testosterone stimulated prostata cells. According to MONNERON *et al.* (11) the PCG, probably carriers of messenger RNA, could leave the nucleus after despirilization only. It seems that the passage of whole granules is possible only in rare cases under conditions of strong cell stimulation.

REFERENCES

1. BERNHARD, W.: A new staining procedure for electron microscopical cytology. J. Ultrastruct. Res. *27*, 250-265 (1969)
2. MOYNE, G.: Feulgen-derived technique for electron microscopical cytochemistry of DNA. J. Ultrastruct. Res. *45*, 102-123 (1973)
3. DUPUY-COIN, A.M., KALIFAT, S.R., BOUTEILLE, M.: Nuclear bodies as proteinaceous structures containing ribonucleoproteins. J. Ultrastruct. Res. *38*, 174-187 (1972)
4. FRENSTER, J.H.: Biochemistry and molecular biophysics of heterochromatin and euchromatin. In: Lima de Faria, A. (ed.) Handbook of molecular Cytology, 252-276. Amsterdam-London: North Holland P.C. 1969
5. LEVY, R., SHOSHANA, L., ROSENBERG, S.A., SIMPSON, R.T.: Selective stimulation of nonhistone chromatin protein synthesis in lymphoid cells by Phytohemagglutinin. Biochemistry *12*, 224-228 (1973)
6. RUBIN, A.D., COOPER, H.L.: Evolving patterns of RNA metabolism during transition from resting state to active growth in lymphocytes stimulated by phytohemagglutinin. Proc. Natl. Acad. Sci. U.S.A. *54*, 469-476 (1965)
7. SMETANA, K., FREIREICH, E.J., BUSCH, H.: Chromatin structures in ring - shaped nucleoli of human lymphocytes. Exp. Cell Res. *52*, 112-128 (1968)

8. JANOSSY, G., SHOHAT, M., GREAVES, M.F., DOURMASHKIN, R.R.: Lymphocyte
   activation. IV. The ultrastructural pattern of the response of mouse T
   and B cells to mitogenic stimulation *in vitro*. Immunology *24*, 211-227 (1972)
9. SHORTMAN, K., BYRD, W.J., CEROTTINI, J.-C., BRUNNER, K.T.: Characterisation
   and separation of mouse lymphocytes subpopulations responding to phytohemagglutinin and pokweed mitogens. Cell Immunol. *6*, 25-40 (1973)
10. LE GOASCOGNE, C., BAULIEU, E., ROBER, P. Discussion in: Gene Transcription
    in Reproductive Tissue, 30-32, Diszfalsy, E. (ed.) Stockholm: Karolinska
    Institutet 1972
11. MONNERON, A., BERNHARD, W.: Fine structural organisation of the interphase
    nucleus in some mammalian cells. J. Ultrastruct. Res. *27*, 266-268 (1969)

Dr. Ivan VALKOV
Department of Anatomical Pathology
Academy of Medicine
1, Georgi Sofiiski Str.
SOFIA 31 / Bulgaria

Acta Neuropath. (Berlin), Suppl. VI, 65 - 68 (1975)

Studies on Lymphocyte Sensitization to Encephalitogenic Protein in Tumor Patients

CH. CERNI und M. MICKSCHE

Institut für Krebsforschung der
Universität Wien, Austria

Summary: The specific lymphocyte sensitization of patients with malignant
diseases against a basic protein, isolated from human brain, was studied by
the lymphocyte migration inhibition technique. A sensitization of lymphocytes
of cancer patients against this encephalitogenic factor (EF) was first reported by FIELD and CASPARY in 1970. Their test system was the Macrophage-
Electrophoretic-Mobility-Test (MEMT). In 17 out of 18 patients with malignant
disease we found a specific inhibition or enhancement of the migration area
of lymphocytes of more than 15%.

Key words: cancer patients - encephalitogenic factor - sensitization of
lymphocytes - migration inhibition test

INTRODUCTION

Immunological methods for early detection of cancer have attracted attention
during the last decade. Recent investigations on the carcinoembryonic antigen,
first isolated by GOLD *et al.* (1), have shown that this glycoprotein is of no
diagnostic significance. Other tests like the T-globulin-test, which was
thought to demonstrate a tumor specific circulating globulin, have proved to
be non-specific (2). There still exists the demand for a reliable in-vitro
test for cancer detection.

In 1970 FIELD and CASPARY (3) reported that lymphocytes of cancer patients
are generally sensitized against a basic protein isolated from human brain.
Peripheral lymphocytes of these patients, incubated with this encephalitogenic factor (EF) release a mediator (Macrophage-Slowing-Factor = MSF) which
lowers the electrophoretic mobility of guinea pig macrophages. By this very
sophisticated MEMT they could also demonstrate a lymphocyte sensitization
against EF in patients with degenerative diseases of the CNS. This cross-
reactivity is still confusing and needs further investigations (4).

Recently a more cancer specific protein was isolated from different tumors.
It is surprising that most of the malignant tumors contain that common cancer
basic protein (CBP) (5). Till now there are only two confirmations of the
results of this group (6, 7).

Because of the demand for a diagnostic cancer test and in the course of a
search for tumor specific antigens, with emphasis on the immunreactivity of
lung cancer patients (8) we investigated the sensitization of lymphocytes
in cancer patients against this basic protein.

The test system we applied is the lymphocyte-migration-inhibition-technique
because of its specifity and sensitivity.

MATERIALS AND METHODS

The lymphocyte sensitization of 18 male patients with different malignant
diseases of different stages, and 7 healthy male controls were examined.

10 patients had inoperable bronchogenic carcinomas, 2 patients had gastric carcinomas, 2 bowel carcinomas, 1 had a melanoma and 3 had lymphomas.

As the sensitization of lymphocytes in cancer patients occurs in the very early stage of disease, persists for years after successful surgery and is independent of metastasis and stage of tumor (3) we did not discuss the clinical data in detail.

Healthy male blood donors of about the same age as the patients served as controls.

Isolation of lymphocytes

50 ml heparinized blood was diluted 1:4 with saline. The diluted blood was carefully pipetted on a Ficoll-Ronpacon-gradient and centrifuged for 15 minutes at 3000 rpm. The lymphocyte layers were harvested and washed in Hanks with 5% FCS. The cell concentration was adjusted to 5×10^6 lymphocytes per ml. The suspension consisted of about 95% pure lymphocytes.

Migration inhibition test

The migration inhibition technique as described by FALK and ZABRISKIE (9) was applied with some modifications. Aliquot amounts of the cell suspension were incubated with different concentrations of the EF (25µg, 50µg and 100µg). Afterwards the suspensions were aspirated into capillary tubes and centrifuged at low speed. The capillary tubes were cut on the cell-medium interface and put immediately into Sylke-Moore-Tissue-Chambers, which were filled with MEM with 5% FCS, pretested for non-toxicity. The incubation period was 16 hours. The size of migration area was determined with a planimeter. Inhibition was calculated by $\dfrac{\text{Area with AG}}{\text{Area without AG}}$.

Each test was done in duplicates or triplicates.

Isolation of Encephalitogenic Factor (EF)

EF was isolated according the original method of FIELD and CASPARY (10). Human brain was obtained maximal 8 hours postmortem, homogenized in cold saline and lyophilized. The lyophilisate was defatted and alcaline extraction was performed with 5% NaCl. The pellet obtained by centrifugation was further extracted by N/100 HCl. Extracts above pH 3,0 were discarded. Those which were more acid were pooled. Protein was precipitated by saturated ammoniumsulfate at 4°C. The redissolved precipitate was dialyzed against N/100 HCl.

Further purification was achieved by column chromatography on Sephadex G 100. Material was millipore filtered and stored a + 4°C.

The encephalitogenic activity of the isolated material was demonstrated in guinea pigs Hartley II strain.

Table 1 summarizes the characterization and the biological activities of the EF.

RESULTS

The sensitization of lymphocytes of 18 patients with different malignant diseases against EF was examined in the migration-inhibition-test (Fig. 1). The lymphocytes of 7 patients with inoperable bronchogenic carcinomas showed a specific inhibition of the migration with at least one concentration of EF. One patient had a borderline value of 14%, two patients had a stimulation of the migration area, that means the migration area with antigen was larger than the control. We defined an inhibition, or respectively stimulation of more than 15% as specific. Two patients with gastric carcinomas showed an inhibition, two patients with bowel carcinomas a stimulation, and one patient

Table 1. *Encephalitogenic Factor (EF)*

Characterization

1. Source is myelin of CNS of different species
2. Basic protein obtained by acid extraction (pH 3,5)
3. Molecular weight: 30 000 to 40 000 Dalton
4. Electrophoretic mobility almost kathodically
5. Localization on plasma membranes

Biological Activities

1. Induction of EAE in experimental animals
2. Animals with EAE show DHR against EF
3. Sensitization of lymphocytes of cancer patients
4. Sensitization of lymphocytes of patients with
   degenerative disease of the CNS
5. Release of Macrophage-Slowing-Factor (MSF)
6. Release of Migration-Inhibition-Factor (MIF)

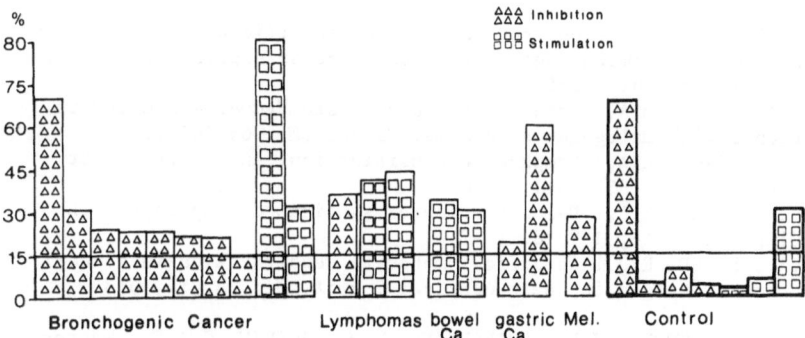

Fig. 1. Lymphocyte sensitization against EF of 7 controls and 18 patients with
different malignant diseases assayed by the LMIT

with melanoma an inhibition. One patient with lymphoma had an inhibition, the
other two showed an enhancement of the migration areas.

Five of 7 healthy controls showed no sensitization of their lymphocytes
against EF, neither inhibition nor stimulation. The inhibition of one of the
controls and the probably specific stimulation of another one is hard to explain as no clinical details or previous diseases have been available. Such
unknown diseases could account for these results. This clearly demonstrates
that controls have to be chosen carefully and pretested by routine laboratory
tests.

DISCUSSION

Our aim was to repeat some of the experiments of FIELD and CASPARY in a more
convenient test system as the MEMT. Our results demonstrate that sensitized
lymphocytes of patients with malignant disease do react specifically with EF
in the MIT. Till now there is no evidence whether there are two different
mediators of cell-mediated immunity, one which lowers the electrophoretic
mobility of guinea pig macrophages and one which inhibits the lymphocyte
migration, or whether there is just one mediator produced by sensitized lym-

phocytes expressing two different biological activities depending on the indicator cell and the test system.

There is also evidence that in some of our tests an additional factor is released by sensitized lymphocytes which induces a stimulation of the migration area. This Migration-Enhancement-Factor (MEF) was recently described by WEISBAR (11). After addition of antigen the maximal production of MEF varies individually between hours and days and the MEF reacts naturally as antagonist of MIF. As the incubation period in our testsystem is always 16 hours, the enlarged areas of migration may be due to an early production of MEF by the lymphocytes of some of our patients.

At present the migration-inhibition-technique is sensitive and specific for the demonstration of a sensitization of lymphocytes to EF but still too troublesome to be applied as a routine test or even as a screening method for early detection of cancer.

Our further investigations will be concentrated on the isolation and testing of the probably more specific cancer basic protein (12).

REFERENCES

1. GOLD, P., FREDMAN, S.O.: Demonstration of tumor-specific antigen in human colonic carcinomata by immunological tolerance and absorption technique. J. Exp. Med. *121*, 439-462 (1965)
2. ZAWADSKI, Z.A., KRAJ, M.A.: Attempts to demonstrate "tumor-globulin" in sera of patients with malignant neoplasms. Cancer *33*, 965-969 (1974)
3. FIELD, E.J., CASPARY, E.A.: Lymphocyte sensitization: An in vitro test for cancer? Lancet II, 1337-1341 (1970)
4. FIELD, E.J., CASPARY, E.A.: Demonstration of sensitized lymphocytes in blood. J. Clin. Path. *24*, 179.181 (1971)
5. CASPARY, E.A., FIELD, E.J.: Specific lymphocyte sensitization in cancer: Is there a common antigen in human neoplasia? Brit. Med. J. II, 613 - 617 (1971)
6. PRITCHARD, J.A.V., MOORE, J.L., SUTHERLAND, W.H., JOSLIN, C.A.F.: Macrophage-electrophoretic-mobility (MEM) test for malignant disease - an independant confirmation. Lancet II, 627-629 (1972)
7. GOLDSTONE, A.H., KERR, L., IRVINE, W.J.: The macrophage electrophoretic migration test in cancer. Clin. Exp. Immunol. *14*, 469-472 (1973)
8. CERNI, C., KOKRON, O., MICKSCHE, M.: Kombination von in vitro und in vivo-Methoden zur Bestimmung des Immunstatus von Krebspatienten - "Immunprofil". Wr. Klin. Wochensch. *86/9*, 258-259 (1974)
9. FALK, R.E., ZABRISKIE, A.: The capillary technique for measurement of inhibition of leucocyte migration - an assessement of cell. mediated immunity. In: BLOOM, B.R., GLADE, P.R. (eds.): In Vitro Methods in Cell-Mediated Immunity, p. 301-307. New York: Acad. Press 1971
10. CASPARY, E.A., FIELD, E.J.: An encephalitogenic protein of human origin: some chemical and biological properties. Ann. N.Y. Acad. Sci. *122*, 182 - 198 (1965)
11. WEISBART, R.H., BLUESTONE, R., GOLDBERG, L.S., PEARSON, C.M.: Migration enhancement factor: A new lymphokine. Proc. Nat. Acad. Sci. *71/3*, 875 - 879 (1974)
12. CARNEGIE, P.R., CASPARY, E.A., FIELD, E.J.: Isolation of an "Antigen" from malignant tumors. Brit. J. Cancer *28*, Suppl. I 219-223 (1973

Dr. C. CERNI
Institut für Krebsforschung d. Univ. Wien
Borschkegasse 8 a
A - 1090 WIEN/Austria

Acta Neuropath. (Berlin), Suppl. VI, 69 - 74 (1975)

Malignant Lymphomas of the Nervous System

H. M. ZIMMERMAN

Department of Pathology
Montefiore Hospital and Medical Center,
and Albert Einstein College of Medicine
Bronx, New York, U. S. A.

Summary: In a series of some 7,000 patients with tumors of the central nervous
system, 208 patients (about 3%) had some form of a malignant lymphoma. Slightly less than half of these tumors were primary in the brain; the remainder
had cranial involvement as part of a generalized process. The tumors consisted
of Hodgkin's disease, lymphosarcomas, reticulosarcomas and plasmacytomas. The
brain was involved in one of two ways: either as localized tumor masses resembling certain gliomas, or as diffusely invasive neoplasms resembling exudative
cellular inflammatory processes. They had a peculiar predilection for the septum pellucidum but occurred also in the cerebral lobes, basal ganglia, brain
stem and cerebellum. They all produced a fibrillary stroma of reticulin fibers
and they spread along the perivascular spaces, in the cerebrospinal subarachnoid space, or intraventricularly on and beneath the ependymal lining. One
type of lymphoma often fused into another - thus a single tumor often consisted of Hodgkin's sarcoma, lymphosarcoma and reticulosarcoma.
    In an additional series of 57 cases of spinal cord involvement by malignant
lymphomas, there were no instances of a primary tumor; all patients had either
primary lymphomas of the brain with secondary spread to the spinal subarachnoid space, or had spinal cord compression as a result of tumor in the vertebrae, the spinal epidural space, or the spinal dura. Hence the spinal cord
involvement was a secondary manifestation of a lymphoma elsewhere.
    Peripheral nerve involvement by lymphomas resulted in destruction of the
myelin sheaths and axons by tumor cell infiltration and the neuropathy was
always part of a generalized lymphomatosis.

Key words: Hodgkin's disease - lymphosarcoma - reticulosarcoma - plasmacytoma

INTRODUCTION

There is undoubtedly an increasing incidence in recent years of malignant
lymphomas in the body as a whole and also in the nervous system that at least
in part is associated with the generalized use of immuno-suppressive therapy
and with x-radiation. These lymphomas affect the central (1) and peripheral (2)
nervous systems and number among them Hodgkin's granulomas and sarcomas,
lymphosarcomas, reticulum cell sarcomas (reticulosarcomas) and plasmacytomas
(multiple myelomas).

MATERIALS

Over a period of more than 40 years this writer has collected some 7,000 cases
of neoplasms affecting the brain and spinal cord from various sources, including several hospitals and a large number of cases referred by private

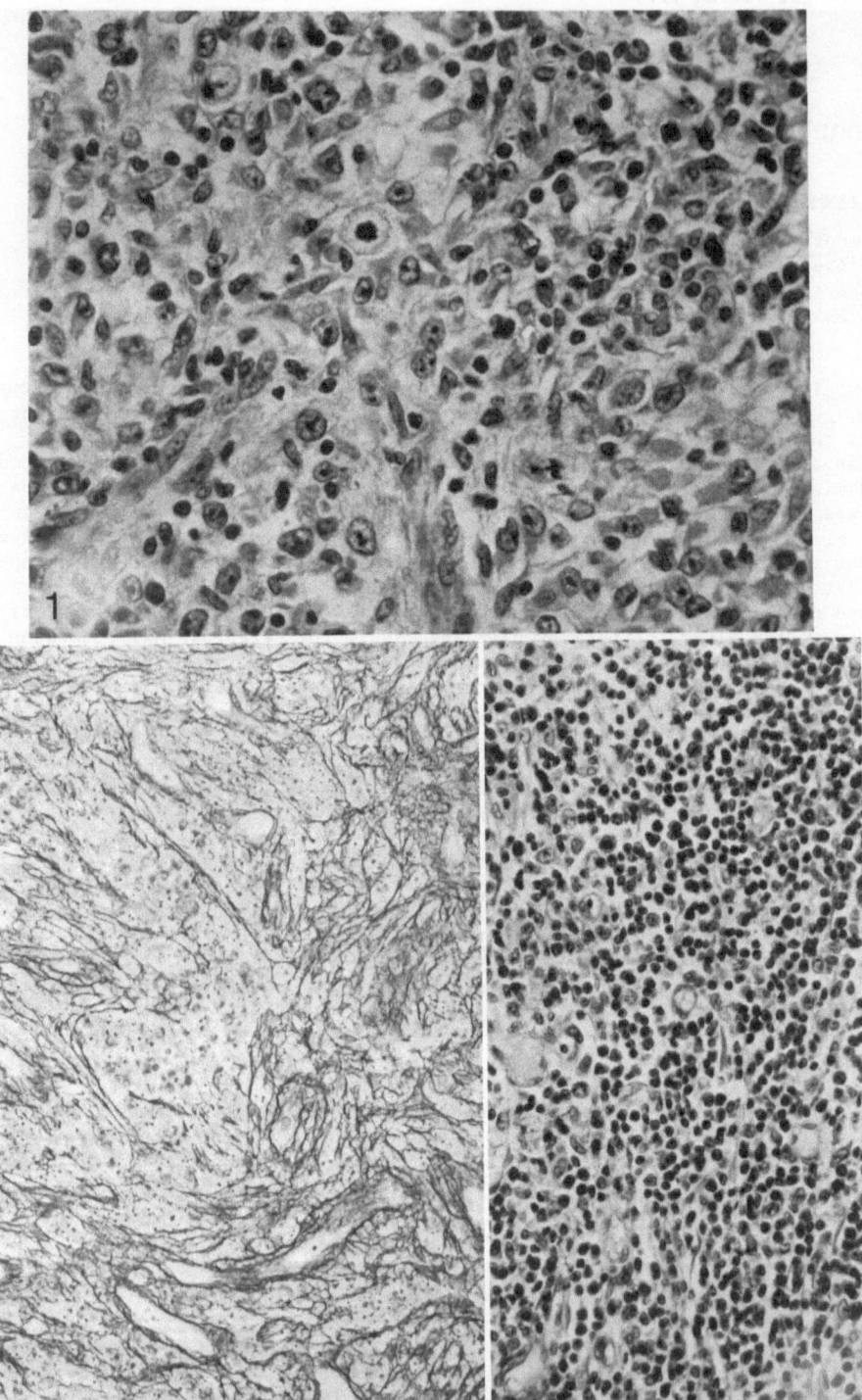

physicians for consultation. Among these tumors there were 208 malignant
lymphomas involving the brain and 57 affecting the spinal cord. In addition,
10 cases were studied in which there was significant peripheral neuropathy
occasioned by lymphomatous infiltration.

RESULTS

Hodgkin's disease

Fourteen patients had Hodgkin's disease, granuloma or sarcoma, confined to
the brain as verified by complete necropsies. Most of these tumors were circumscribed but not encapsulated. Some, however, invaded the brains diffusely
in the manner of an encephalitis. The circumscribed tumor masses were often
hemorrhagic and necrotic like certain glioblastomas. They were found in each
of the cerebral lobes, as well as in the basal ganglia, hypothalamus, tuber
cinereum, optic chiasm, brain stem and cerebellum. Of special interest was
the involvement of the septum pellucidum, but the other lymphomas - the lymphosarcomas and reticulosarcomas - had a similar predilection for this structure.

The tumor cells occurred with great frequency around blood vessels and
within their walls. They were quite pleomorphic, had numerous mitoses, and
numbered von Sternberg cells among them (Fig. 1). Eosinophilic mononuclear
and polymorphonuclear cells were often present, as were lymphocytes, fibroblasts, and newly formed capillaries. All of these tumors had a fibrillary
stroma of reticulin fibers of variable extent (Fig. 2). In different parts
of the tumor the microscopic appearance frequently varied to the extent of
resembling lymphosarcoma and reticulosarcoma (Fig. 3).

Lymphosarcoma

All the tumors of the malignant lymphoma variety in the brain, including the
lymphosarcomas, occurred either as discrete and circumscribed masses, or were
diffusely infiltrative. In any given case, of course, both types of involvement could sometimes be seen. The vessel walls in the brain and the Virchow-
Robin spaces were almost invariable sites of predilection for tumor cells.
The latter in some cases were of the small adult type, but some tumors were
composed predominantly of blast forms. A not inconsiderable number of the
lymphosarcomatous lesions contained reticulum cell sarcomatous portions, so
that classification became somewhat arbitrary. In spite of this, the most
frequent lymphoma in the brain was of the lymphosarcoma variety, and more
than one-third of the cases were confined exclusively to the intracranial
contents.

Reticulosarcoma

Representative of all the space-occupying, expanding and circumscribed lymphomas in the brain was the case ot a primary reticulum cell sarcoma in the

---

Fig. 1. Pleomorphic cellular composition of a primary Hodgkin's sarcoma in the
brain of a 33 year old man. Some tumor cells are in mitotic division. Hematoxylin-eosin; x 425

Fig. 2. Primary Hodgkin's sarcoma. Extensive meshwork of reticulin fibers in
tumor. Wilder's silver carbonate; x 180

Fig. 3. Same patient with primary Hodgkin's sarcoma whose tumor was shown in
figures 1 and 2. The small dark round cells suggest lymphosarcoma. Note newly
formed blood vessels as in granulation tissue. Hematoxylin-eosin; x 275

right frontal lobe illustrated in figure 4. This tumor in the centrum semi-ovale had the macroscopic appearance of a glioma, but was composed micro-scopically of large so-called reticulum cells as well as small, dark, round cells of lymphocytic appearance (Fig. 5). The former infiltrated the neural parenchyma mainly, and the latter surrounded the vessels and infiltrated their walls. As with all the lymphomas, a delicate reticulin stroma was found throughout the neoplasm.

In another patient the tumor mass replaced the entire septum pellucidum (Fig. 6). Both this and the previous case were instances of reticulosarcomas limited exclusively to the brain.
Diffusely infiltrating tumors of this variety were seen even more frequently than the solitary neoplasms (Fig. 7). In a number of cases they spread beneath the ventricular ependyma and even coated the ependymal lining. They found access to the cerebral and spinal subarachnoid space by way of the perivascu-lar spaces. Through this route some of the cranial nerves became involved (Fig. 8). The cytologic appearance of this neoplasm was the same in both its primary and metastatic forms, but it too had portions that resembled Hodgkin's disease and lymphosarcoma.

Plasmacytoma

This was the least commonly encountered of the intracranial lymphomas. The brain was directly involved by extension of the tumor from the calvarium, or the dura over the convex surfaces of the brain, or the falx cerebri except in two cases. In these, there seemed to be neither an osseous nor a dural involvement by tumor – the neural parenchyma alone was involved. And these two cases had no extracranial myelomatous (plasmacytomatous) neoplasms.

Malignant lymphomas of the spinal cord

Each of the 57 cases in this series had spinal cord involvement that was secondary to generalized lymphomatosis or to metastasis from a brain tumor. In the cases of Hodgkin's disease there was tumor in the vertebral bodies, the epidural space, or the spinal dura. The cord was merely compressed by the surrounding neoplasm. The cord itself was only rarely infiltrated by tumor cells and then only if these cells found a pathway through the subarachnoid space. The same facts pertained to the cord involvement in cases of multiple myeloma, lymphosarcoma and reticulosarcoma.

Malignant lymphomas in peripheral nerves

Peripheral nerve involvement by lymphomas was always in conjunction with generalized systemic disease. Examples of each type of tumor were found among the 10 cases of peripheral neuropathy. The tumor cells involved the nerves either by extension along the blood vessels as shown in figure 8 of the optic nerve or, more frequently, by invasion between the myelinated sheaths from an adjacent lymphoma mass. In either event the nerve sheaths and axons were disrupted and showed histologic evidence of breakdown.

DISCUSSION

The malignant lymphomas that involve the nervous system as primary newgrowths are in no wise different from those that occur extracranially and reach the brain by metastasis. This was made clear in the excellent article by SPARLING *et al.* in 1947 (3). The origin of the cell or cells of these tumors in the brain, however, is as yet obscure. Nor habe the techniques of light microscopy availed to resolve this important question. The invariable relationship of

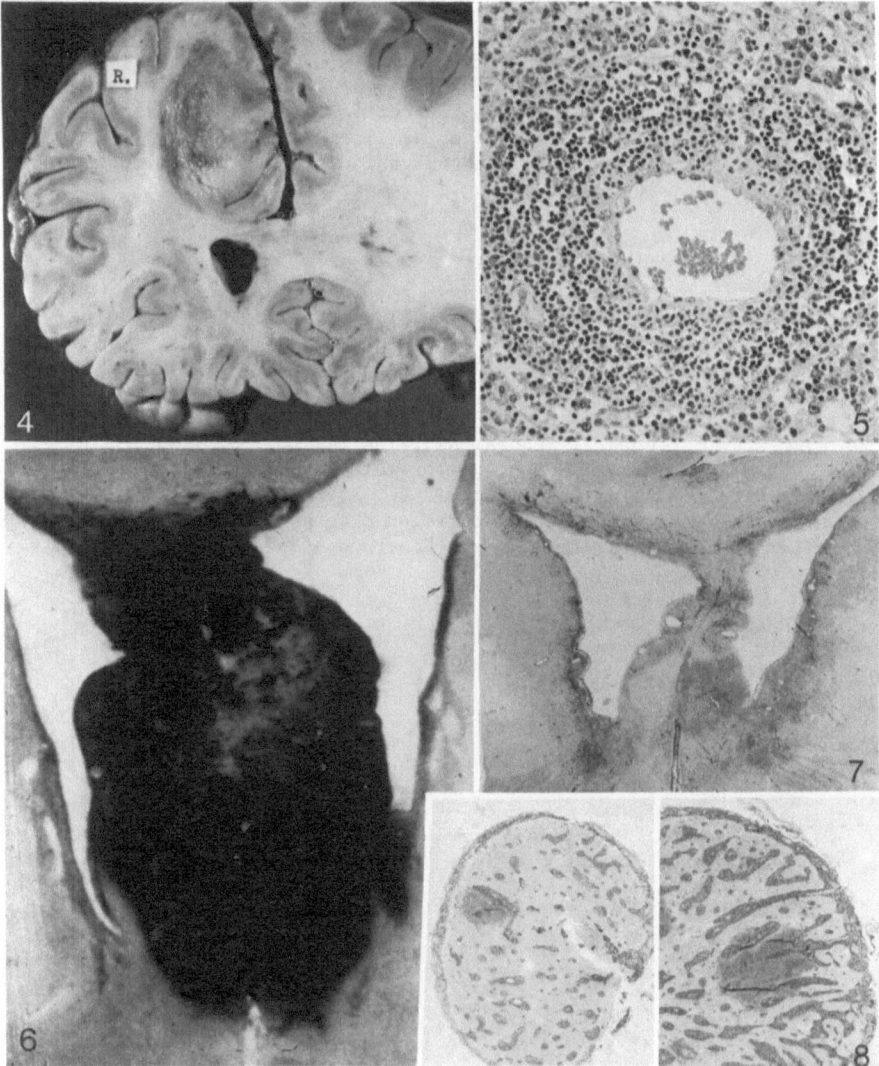

Fig. 4. Circumscribed primary reticulum cell sarcoma in subcortex of right frontal lobe

Fig. 5. Photomicrograph of tumor shown in figure 4. Note small dark tumor cells in vessel wall and the larger mononuclear tumor cells replacing neural parenchyma. Hematoxylin-eosin; x 200

Fig. 6. Primary reticulosarcoma in septum pellucidum. Nissl stain; x 2

Fig. 7. Primary reticulosarcoma beneath ependyma lining the lateral ventricles. Tumor cells infiltrate the corpus callosum and the periventricular gray matter in a manner resembling encephalitis. Nissl stain; x 2

Fig. 8. Metastatic malignant lymphoma infiltrating the leptomeninges and extending along the sheaths of blood vessels in the optic nerve. Hematoxylin-eosin; x 11

these tumors to the vascular and perivascular structures in the cases in this series perhaps suggests their origin in the reticular cells, but other methods will be necessary to resolve the problem.

Many of the lymphomas contained mixed cellular populations that made rigid classification arbitrary. Attention to this fact in cases of systemic lymphomatosis was called by HERBUT *et al.* (4) and by CUSTER and BERNHARD (5). These observations strongly suggest that the various lymphomas are not separate entities but rather stages of a single disease process.

REFERENCES

1. ZIMMERMAN, H.M.: Malignant lymphomas. *In:* MINCKLER, J. (ed.): Pathology of the Nervous System, p. 2165-2178. New York: McGraw-Hill (1971)
2. BARRON, K.D., ROWLAND, L.P., ZIMMERMAN, H.M.: Neuropathy with malignant tumor metastases. J. Nerv. Ment. Dis. *131*, 10-31 (1960)
3. SPARLING, Jr., H.J., ADAMS, R.D., PARKER, Jr., F.: Involvement of the nervous system by malignant lymphoma. Medicine *26*, 285-332 (1947)
4. HERBUT, P.A., MILLER, F.R., ERF, L.A.: The relation of Hodgkin's disease, lymphosarcoma and reticulum cell sarcoma. Am. J. Path. *21*, 233-253 (1945)
5. CUSTER, R.P., BERNHARD, W.G.: The interrelationship of Hodgkin's disease and other lymphatic tumors. Am. J. Med. Sci. *216*, 625-642 (1948)

Dr. H.M. ZIMMERMAN
Montefiore Hospital and Medical Center
111 East 210th Street
Bronx, New York 10467

Acta Neuropath. (Berlin), Suppl. VI, 75 - 79 (1975)

Lymphoreticular Proliferative Disorders of the CNS and Other Organs: Analogies and Differences

JOHN J. KEPES and MAGDA KEPES

Department of Pathology and Oncology
University of Kansas Medical Center
Kansas City, Kansas 66103, USA

Summary: Authors review *differences* between CNS and extraneural reticuloses, and consider the immediate threat to life by CNS lymphomas contrasting to other organ lymphomas, which usually become fatal only after generalization. Other special features of CNS reticuloses include the role of microglial cells, reactive astrocytosis, variations in meningeal vs. parenchymatous involvement and easier morphologic confusion with inflammatory processes.

Analogies exist between CNS and extranodal "organ" lymphomas in terms of relatively late or no generalization. The entire spectrum of lymphomatous and histiocytic proliferations may occur in the CNS, the latter including atypical fibrous xanthomas and xanthosarcomas.

A further analogy is seen in the presence of lymphocyte and plasma cells in cerebral and organ lymphomas that may well represent host defense reaction. When present in large numbers they may be responsible for the "inflammatory" appearance of some reticulum cell sarcomas of the brain.

Key words: CNS reticuloses - xanthomas - host reaction

For general pathologists who learned Neuropathology as a subspecialty, the analogies and differences between these two branches of our discipline have always been fascinating. Hence, we felt that perhaps it may be worthwhile to examine lymphoreticular proliferative disorders from this angle, i.e. discussing differences from and analogies with extraneural forms of reticuloses. Table 1 summarizes the differences we consider most important both from a biological standpoint and from the standpoint of certain morphological features which may create diagnostic problems in one group but not the other.

The analogies we considered important between CNS and extraneural lymphoreticular disorders are outlined in Table 2.

We have been particularly interested in histiocytic reticuloses and felt that Cline and Golde's (1) classification of these disorders as they occur at extraneural sites, would be useful. These authors classified the reticuloses by correlating a given disease process with the degree of differentiation of the proliferating cells. They list monocytic leukemia as representing proliferation of the least differentiated form of histiocytes. Such leukemia of course often involves the meninges and the brain. An example for proliferative disorder of better differentiated phagocytic histiocytes is familial erythrophagocytic lymphohistiocytosis. PRICE *et al.* (2) reported a similar familial condition affecting almost exclusively the CNS.

Proliferation of still better differentiated histiocytes is reflected in the three forms of histiocytosis X. Of these, Letterer-Siwe's disease has been seen to involve the brain and meninges as part of a generalized process (3) whereas Hand-Schüller-Christian disease and eosinophilic granuloma have both been re-

Table 1. *CNS and extraneural lymphoreticular proliferative disorders.*
Differences

1. cerebral lymphomas constitute a primary threat to life, other isolated "organ lymphomas" usually only after, and because of, generalization of the process.

2. Only the central nervous system has microglial cells, whose role in the genesis of CNS lymphomas needs further clarification.

3. Astroglial reaction to the tumor adds a specific histological dimension to CNS lymphoreticular disorders. (There appears to be more intense astrocytic reaction to proliferation of better differentiated histiocytes, e.g. histiocytosis X.)

4. Relative predominance of meningeal versus parenchymatous involvement creates morphological and clinical variations absent from extraneural lymphomas.

5. In the brain the perivascular genesis and spread of lymphomas is more likely to imitate inflammation than is the case in extraneural processes.

Table 2. *CNS and extraneural lymphoproliferative disorders*
Analogies

1. Malignant lymphomas may originate in lymph nodes or in solitary organs (e.g. stomach, uterine cervix, bone, etc.). The latter group usually shows late, or no generalization of the process. Most cerebral lymphomas appear to belong to this group of lymphomas.

2. All variants of malignant lymphomas (lymphosarcoma, reticulum cell sarcoma, Hodgkin's disease etc.) have been described to occur as primary lesions of the CNS, as have some forms of histiocytosis X. The occurrence of the tumors derived from more differentiated histiocytes: fibrous xanthomas and xanthosarcomas of the brain and meninges have also been observed.

3. In extraneural lymphomas (most notably in Hodgkin's disease) it has been postulated that some of the proliferating elements represent host reaction rather than tumor cells. We suggest that an analogous situation also exists in cerebral lymphomas.

ported as originating in the brain proper, with of without secondary involvement of other organs, the so-called Gagel's granuloma of the hypothalamus being a case in point (4, 5).

Cline and Golde's classification finally includes localized histiocytoma (or fibrous xanthoma) as representing a growth of the most differentiated form of histiocytes, (actually the type of cell, which is easily transformed into an even more mature cell type: the fibroblast; vide dermatofibroma, alias histiocytoma cutis). This last member of their list however is a tumor usually discussed as an entity involving the skin and/or soft tissues rather than the brain. In our experience such tumors of mature histiocytes with fibroblastic differentiation do sometimes involve the nervous system. One *fibrous xanthoma* that we have seen in the brain developed in the sphenoidal ridge area (unattached to the dura) in an 11 year old boy. It had the storiform pattern, large foamy cells, and Touton type giant cells characteristic of atypical fibrous xanthoma. This tumor recurred a few months after the first removal, the patient

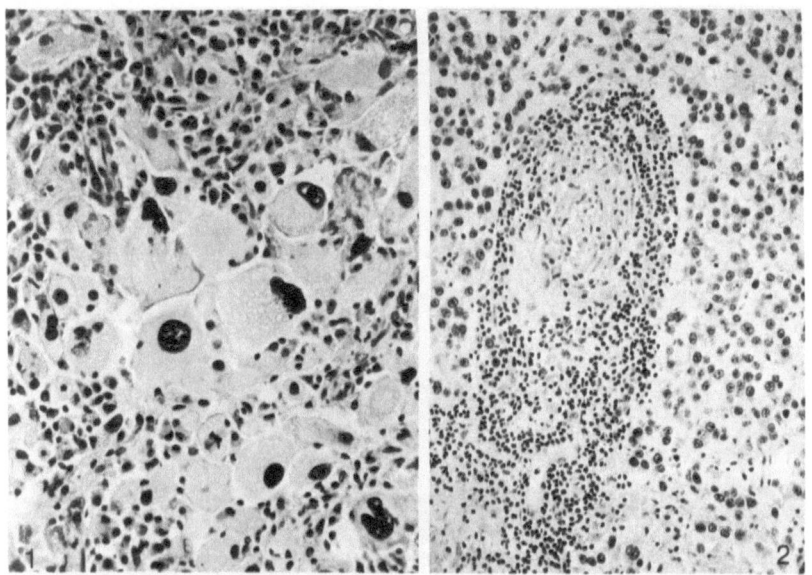

Fig. 1. Cerebral xanthosarcoma, 26 year old woman. Large neoplastic foamy histiocytes are intermingled with stromal lymphocytes and plasma cells. Hematoxylin-eosin, X 300

Fig. 2. Pineal germinoma, 12 year old boy. Perivascular lymphocytes and small histiocytic granuloma are in center, neoplastic germinal cells form the periphery. Hematoxylin-eosin, X 120

received radiation after the second resection and has been symptom-free now for more than 3 years (6).

It is well known that in reticulum cell sarcomas of the brain a certain contingent of foamy macrophages is often found. Are there brain tumors composed *entirely* of the neoplastic equivalents of foamy macrophages? We believe such entity does exist, although undoubtedly rare. We have seen a limited number of cases in consultation material from other hospitals and have in the past reported one of our own cases of *cerebral xanthosarcoma* (6). This was highly malignant right frontal lobe tumor in a 26 year old woman. The tumor was resected but a similar metastasis or perhaps second primary tumor in her cerebellum killed her one year later (Fig. 1).

As to the last point of the table of analogies, we feel that as is reportedly the case in extraneural lymphomas (7, 8), in cerebral *lymphomas* also, some of the more mature appearing proliferating elements may well represent cells of host reaction rather than tumor cells. Conglomerates of lymphocytes and/or plasma cells have long been regarded as a defensive cell line in such tumors as medullary carcinomas of the breast, in malignant melanomas of the skin and in germinomas of the testis and ovary. In general, particularly in the case of germinomas a better prognosis is anticipated if the tumor is rich in lymphocytes (some even have tubercle-like histiocytic granulomas). Similarly medullary carcinomas of the breast, which are rich in lymphocytic infiltrates, are regarded as tumors with statistically better prognosis than ordinary ductal carcinomas. It is easy of course to discern the difference between a group of carcinoma cells and the lymphocytes surrounding them, whereas in lymphomas "friend" and "foe" may look very much unlike. Nevertheless it has been sug-

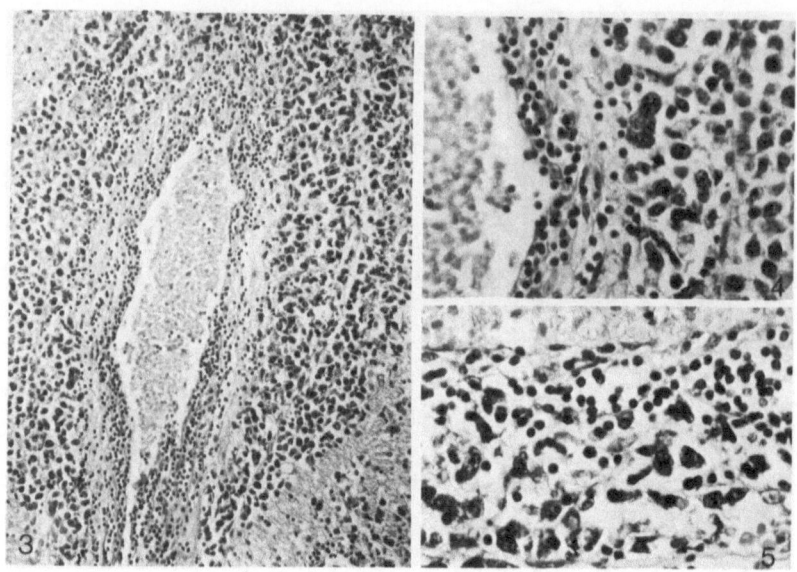

Fig. 3. Primary reticulum cell sarcoma, right parietal lobe, 65 year old man. Blood vessel in center is surrounded by inner collar of mature lymphocytes, these in turn are surrounded by sarcoma cells. Hematoxylin-eosin, X 100

Fig. 4. Same case as 3. Higher power illustrates differences between two cell types. In this case no transitons were seen between the two. Hematoxylin-eosin, X 400

Fig. 5. Another area of same tumor includes mature plasma cells in non-neoplastic perivascular infiltrate. Hematoxylin-eosin, X 400

gested and experimentally documented that such "lymphocytic civil war" exists in reality (7, 8). Fig. 2 is from a pineal germinoma of a 12 year old boy with lymphocytes forming a perivascular cuff, separating the blood vessel from the more peripheral larger and more pleomorphic tumor cells. Figs. 3 and 4 show a similar arrangement in a reticulum cell sarcoma of the parietal lobe. This perivascular collar of more mature lymphocytes has been described by RUBINSTEIN also (9). We believe these cells have an analogous role in germinomas, carcinomas and in lymphomas as well. The use of surface markers, distinguishing T from B lymphocytes will eventually make this distinction possible in cerebral lymphomas too. Some forms of cerebral reticuloses show such large numbers of non-neoplastic appearing lymphocytes and plasma cells that the true neoplastic nature of these lesions has been questioned and they have been regarded as transitional states between inflammatory proliferation and neoplasia ("granulomatous encephalitis" 10, 11, 12). We feel that one should consider the possibility that in those cases the truly atypical histiocytes, which may be few and for between, represent the neoplasm and the other inflammatory cells are indicative of an exaggerated host reaction.

REFERENCES

1. CLINE, M.J., GOLDE, D.W.: A review and re-evaluation of the histiocytic disorders. Amer. J. Med. 55, 49-60 (1973)
2. PRICE, D.L., WOOLSEY, J.E., ROSMAN, N.P., RICHARDSON, E.P.: Familial lympho-histiocytotsis of the nervous system. Arch. Neurol. (Chic.) 24, 270-283 (1971)

3. SCHOECK, V.W., PETERSON, R.D.A., GOOD, R.A.: Familial occurrence of Letterer-Siwe disease. Pediatrics *32*, 1055-1063 (1963)
4. KEPES, J.J., KEPES, M.: Predominantly cerebral forms of histiocytosis X. A reappraisal of "Gagel's hypothalamic granuloma", "Granuloma infiltrans of the hypothalamus" and "Ayala's disease" with a report of four cases. Acta Neuropath. (Berl.) *14*, 77-98 (1969)
5. ROSSENBECK, H.G.: Chronische disseminierte Histiocytosis X mit eosinophilen Granulomen in der Schädelkalotte, im Zwischenhirn - mit Diabetes insipidus - und in den Lungen. Frankfurt. Z. Path. *77*, 67-82 (1967)
6. KEPES, J.J., KEPES, M., SLOWIK, F.: Fibrous xanthomas and xanthosarcomas of the meninges and the brain. Acta Neuropath. (Berl.) *23*, 187-199 (1973)
7. VITA, V.T., de, Jr.: Lymphocyte reactivity in Hodgkin's disease: A lymphocyte civil war. (Editorial) New Eng. J. Med. *289*, 801 (1973)
8. SINKOVICS, J.G., SHIRATO, E., CABINESS, J.R., SHULLENBERGER, C.C.: Cytotoxic lymphocytes in Hodgkin's disease? Brit. Med. J. *268/1*, 172-173 (1970)
9. RUBINSTEIN, L.J.: Tumors of the central nervous system. p. 220. Armed Forces Institute of Pathology. Washington, D.C. 1972
10. VUIA, O., MEHRAEIN, P.: Primary reticulosis of the central nervous system. J. Neurol. Sci. *14*, 469-482 (1971)
11. STAMMLER, A., CERVOS-NAVARRO, J.: Die reticulohistiozytäre granulomatöse Enzephalitis. Fortschr. Neurol. Psychiat. *33*, 1-24 (1965)
12. WILKE, G.: Granulomatous encephalitis with reference to known and unknown aetiologies. Excerpta Med. (Amst.) Sect. VIII. *8*, 824-825 (1955)

John J. KEPES, M.D.
Department of Pathology and Oncology
University of Kansas Medical Center
Kansas City, Kansas 66103, USA

Acta Neuropath. (Berlin), Suppl. VI, 81 - 84 (1975)

Neoplastic Involvement of the CNS in Generalized Lymphomas

W. JÄNISCH, H. GERLACH, I. REMUS

Department of Pathology
Martin-Luther-University, Halle (GDR)

Summary: In 49 autopsies on patients with generalized malignant lymphomas a thorough histological examination of the CNS was performed. Isolated neoplastic foci were found in the CNS in 10 cases. It is believed that most of the tumour infiltrations in the CNS as a result of neoplastic transformation of local mesenchymal cells and are not blood-borne metastases.

Key words: CNS in malignant lymphomas - Hodgkin's disease - Mycosis fungoides - Reticulo-histiocytic granulomatous encephalitis

INTRODUCTION

In patients with malignant lymphomas, the central nervous system (CNS) can be damaged by the following processes:

1. Progressive multifocal leuko-encephalopathy,
2. Extradural tumour deposits, compressing or progressive infiltrating into the brain and spinal cord,
3. Neoplastic infiltration within the CNS unconnected with extraneural tumour (i.e. *separate* involvement).

It is often impossible to distinguish these three processes clinically, the precise diagnosis depending on a complete post-mortem examination. So far the frequency of separate CNS-involvement in generalized lymphomas has not been established. FANKHAUSER *et al.* (1) stress that in many accounts of generalized reticuloses, the brain is hardly mentioned and believe, therefore, that it would be premature to reach any conclusions about the frequency of CNS-involvement in generalized reticuloses. A retrospective study of 124 autopsies on patients with malignant reticuloses demonstrated separate intracerebral deposits in 16 (2). These findings, however, were mainly based on the gross appearance since microscopic examination of the CNS was not systematically performed. These results therefore provide on a rough estimate. To fill this gap in our knowledge, a thorough examination of the CNS was undertaken on patients dying with malignant lymphomas.

MATERIAL AND METHODS

In the last two years we have performed 49 autopsies on patients with malignant lymphomas. In every case the brain and spinal cord, including nerve roots and spinal ganglia, were fixed in formol for 2 - 3 weeks. The cerebrum, and the brain stem and cerebellum were sliced in the coronal plane and the spinal cord in the horizontal plane a 1 cm intervals. Bilateral frontal, parieto-temporal and occipital slices and slices of cerebellum and brainstem were embedded in paraffin wax. The spinal cord, nerve roots and adjacent spinal ganglia were histologically investigated at 10 levels. Longitudinal sections through the

Table 1. *Frequency of separate neoplastic CNS-involvement in generalized malignant lymphomas*

Types of lymphomas	number of autopsies	with CNS-involvment
Malignant reticulosis and reticulum cell sarcoma	26	5
Abt-Letterer-Siwe's disease	1	-
Hodgkin's disease	12	3
Mycosis fungoides	1	1
Lymphosarcomatosis	1	1
Plasmocytoma	8	-
Total	49	10

pituitary gland and at least two different pieces of the cranial dura mater were examined. In addition all areas of the CNS which were macroscopically abnormal and representative blocks from numerous extraneural organs were examined. The routine stain was hematoxylin-eosin. Where neccesary, the methods of NISSL, VAN GIESON and GOMORI were used. Involvement of the CNS was recorded only when separate deposite of neoplastic tissue were found. Infiltration via nerve roots or invasion of the CNS from foci in the bones and extracranial soft tissue were *not* counted.

RESULTS

The types of case examined and the results are summarized in Table 1.

Obvious macroscopic lesions were found in the CNS in only two cases. They appeared as poorly demarcated greyish-white soft areas (Fig. 1, 3). Histologically the neoplastic infiltrations were much more widespread than the naked-eye appearance suggested. In all the other cases with CNS-involvement no macroscopic abnormalities were found apart from non-specific brain swelling of slight thickening of the leptomeninges. There was no correlation between the extent of extraneural tumour and the presence of separate CNS-involvement. The microscopic distribution of the foci within the CNS often followed a definite pattern, infiltration of the leptomeninges (Fig. 2), involvement of the subependymal periventricular zones and perivascular cuffing being particularly common. In the case of lymphosarcomatosis the CNS-foci were situated exclusively in the dura mater. The perivascular lesions were sometimes confined to the adventitia but tumor cells often extended into the surrounding brain tissue, subsequently forming closely packed confluent masses (Fig. 4). The foci were composed of atypical reticular cells, histiocytes and lymphocytes and their histological appearance were usually very similar to those of the extraneural foci. In Hodgkin's disease, typical Reed-Sternberg giant cells were rare or completely absent in the CNS foci, even when giant cells were common in the extraneural deposits. Some lesions exhibited granu-

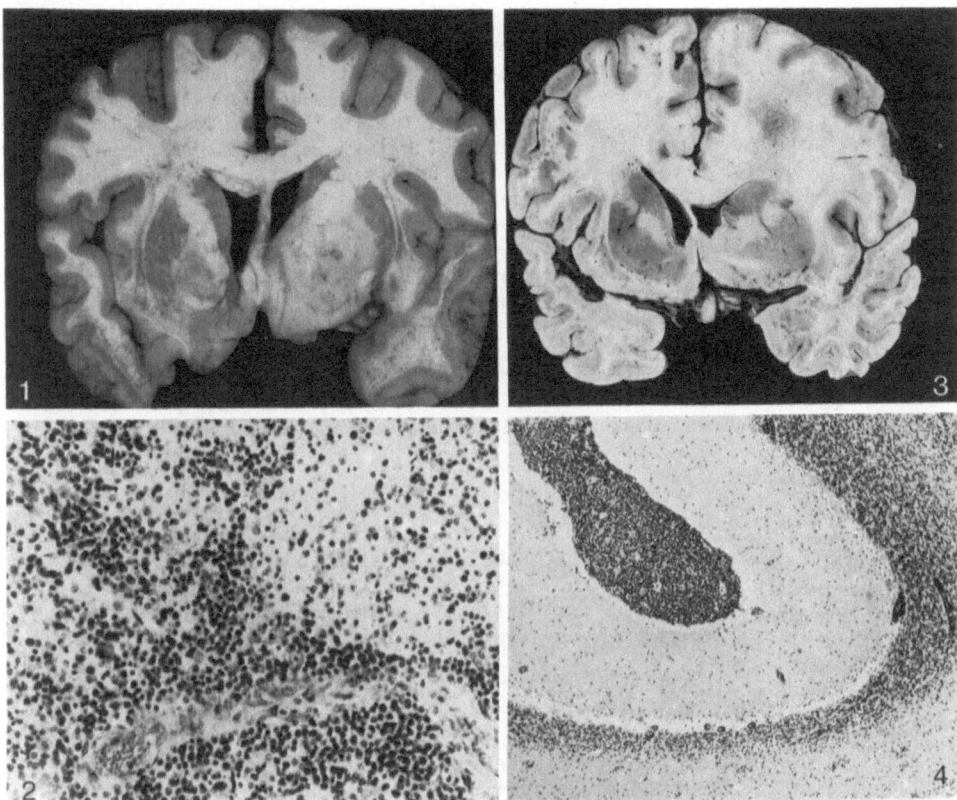

Fig. 1. Generalized reticulum cell sarcoma. Whitish tumour infiltrate in the
right pallidum and internal capsule. Autopsy nr. 832/74, female, 56 years

Fig. 2. Same case as Fig. 1. Microscopical appearances of the cerebral tumour
with aggregation of neoplastic cells around blood vessels. Hematoxylin-eosin,
200 x

Fig. 3. Mycosis fungoides. Greyish neoplastic infiltration in the white matter
of the right parietal lobe. Autopsy nr. 926/74, male, 56 years

Fig. 4. Generalized reticulum cell sarcoma. Leptomeningeal neoplastic infiltration and perivascular cuffing of tumour cells in the cerebellar cortex.
Autopsy nr. 1870/73, female, 10 years. Hematoxylin-eosin, 65 x

lomatous features, including plasma cells and a few polymorphonuclear leucocytes. In malignant reticulosis the tumour tissue in the CNS may contain a
dense network of reticulin fibres, but this is not related to the intensity of
fibre formation in extraneural deposits in the same case.

DISCUSSION

Separate tumour involvement of the CNS in generalized malignant lymphomas has
been occasionally described (3, 4, 5, 6, 7, 8). From these and other reports
based on individual cases the frequency of this occurrence is difficult to
assess. In the present investigation there was separate neoplastic tumour in
the CNS in about 20% of the autopsies on patients with malignant lymphomas.

The number of cases, however, is not yet large enough to draw any firm conclusions about the frequency of CNS-involvement in specified lymphoma types.
   Another controversial question is the pathogenesis of the CNS foci. They
might be blood-borne metastases or due to synchronous neoplastic transformation of lymphoreticular cells inside and outside the nervous system. The close
similar between the distribution patterns of primary malignant lymphomas of
the CNS and those observed in cases with generalized intra- and extra-neural
tumour suggests local rather than metastatic development. The similarity between both processes covers not only the distribution of tumour but also many
histo- and cytological details. In some cases, in addition to fully developed
neoplastic lesions, granulomatous alterations were found. They closely resembled reticulo-histiocytic granulomatous encephalitis (9). Similar granulomatous proliferations may also be found outside the CNS in malignant lymphomas
(10). This raises the question of the relationship between reticulohistiocytic granulomatous encephalitis and malignant lymphomas. Many morphological
details suggest that they might be different stages of the same process. A
final decision, however, cannot be made until more is known about the causative agents.

REFERENCES

1. FANKHAUSER, R., FATZER, R., LUGINBÜHL, H.: Reticulosis of the central
   nervous system in dogs. Advanc. vet. Sci. *16*, 35-71 (1972)
2. SCHOLTZE, P., JÄNISCH, W.: Zur Häufigkeit und Einordnung neoplastischer
   Retikulosen des Zentralnervensystems. Zbl. allg. Path. path. Anat. *114*,
   159-167 (1971)
3. LJUNGDAHL, I., STRANG, R.R., TOVI, D.: Intracerebral Hodgkin's granuloma.
   Report of a case and review of the literature. Neurochirurgia (Stuttg.)
   113-118 (1965)
4. ADAMS, J.H., JACKSON, J.M.: Intracerebral tumours of reticular tissue:
   the problem of microgliomatosis and reticuloendothelial sarcomas of the
   brain. J. Path. Bact. *91*, 369-381 (1966)
5. BARNARD, R.O.: Studies on cerebral tumours of lympho-reticular origin.
   In: VI. Internationaler Kongreß für Neuropathologie. S. 967. Paris:
   Masson et Cie 1970
6. BEBIN, J., HAQ, J.U.: Undifferentiated malignant reticuloendotheliosis
   ("Histiocytosis") with diffuse brain involvement. In: VI. Internationaler
   Kongreß für Neuropathologie. S. 968-969. Paris: Masson et Cie 1970
7. LHERMITTE, F., MARTEAU, R., DEROUESNE, C., POIRIER, J.: Un cas du mycosis
   fongoide avec atteinte du systeme nerveux central. In: VI. Internationaler
   Kongreß für Neuropathologie, S. 970-971. Paris: Masson et Cie 1970
8. PLAFKER, J., MARTINEZ, A.J., ROSENBLUM, W.I.: A neoplasm of the reticuloendothelial system involving brain (microglioma) and viscera (reticulum
   cell sarcoma). Sth. med. J. (Bgham, Ala.) *65*, 385-389 (1972)
9. CERVOS-NAVARRO, J., HÜBNER, G., PUCHSTEIN, G., STAMMLER, A.: Die Patho-
   morphologie der reticulo-histiocytären granulomatösen Encephalitis.
   Frankfurt. Z. Path. *70*, 458-477 (1960)
10. JÄNISCH, W., SCHREIBER, D., SCHOLTZE, P., GERLACH, H.: Über Beziehungen
    zwischen retikulo-histiozytärer Enzephalitis und neoplastischen Retiku-
    losen. Schweiz. Arch. Neurol. Neurochir. Psychiat. *112*, 263-270 (1973)

Prof. Dr. sc. med. W. JÄNISCH
Pathologisches Institut der
Martin-Luther-Universität Halle-Wittenberg
DDR 402 Halle/S., Leninallee 14

Acta Neuropath. (Berlin), Suppl. VI, 85 - 89 (1975)
© by Springer-Verlag 1975

Primary Lymphoreticuloses of the Nervous System in Animals

A. KOESTNER

Department of Veterinary Pathobiology
The Ohio State University
Columbus, Ohio 43210, U.S.A.

Summary: Lymphoreticular proliferative disorders occur in most species of animals including submammalian vertebrates but only occasionally affect the nervous system. Primary neoplastic lymphoreticular disorders of the nervous system have been recognized in chickens as a herpesvirus-induced avian neurolymphomatosis and in mammals, particularly in the dog, as reticulum cell sarcomas originating from perivascular mesenchymal precursor cells. Criteria have been discussed to distinguish neoplastic from inflammatory lymphoreticuloses but borderline cases exist where a clear distinction is not always possible.

Key words: Lymphoreticuloses - lymphomas of nervous system - peritheliomas - sarcomatosis-meningeal.

Lymphoreticuloses of the nervous system must be regarded as part of the general problem of lymphoreticular proliferative disorders although their isolated appearance in the nervous system has been recognized in animals and man. If one attempts to study lymphoreticuloses of the nervous system in various animal species one faces two inherent problems. One is to separate primary lymphoreticuloses of the nervous system from generalized lymphoreticular proliferative disorder affecting the nervous system and a second problem is to differentiate between inflammatory reticuloses and true neoplasms of lymphoreticular cells. It has been recognized by many who have studied this disease complex that no sharp line between inflammation and neoplasia can be drawn and that a continuous spectrum exists from unquestionable inflammatory reactions to unquestionable neoplasms (1. 2. 3). This report summarizes what is presently known about these disorders in vertebrates exclusive of man and subhuman primates.

INFLAMMATORY LYMPHORETICULOSES OF THE NERVOUS SYSTEM

These lesions consist of lymphoreticular cell accumulations reactive to known or unknown infectious agents such as certain viruses, *Mycobacterium tuberculosis*, some protozoa and fungi. Lower vertebrates such as fishes, amphibia and reptiles generally react with lymphoreticular proliferation to chronic infections regardless of the type of the agent. Fig. 1 depicts a nodule in the meninges of a turtle representing a proliferative nodule of lymphoreticular cells (granuloma) of unknown etiology. Infectious granulomas are well recognized in many species as responses to infections by *Mycobacterium tuberculosis* or fungi. Some viruses, particularly the virus of equine infectious anemia may stimulate proliferation of reticuloendothelial cells throughout the body including the central nervous system (CNS). In the course of equine

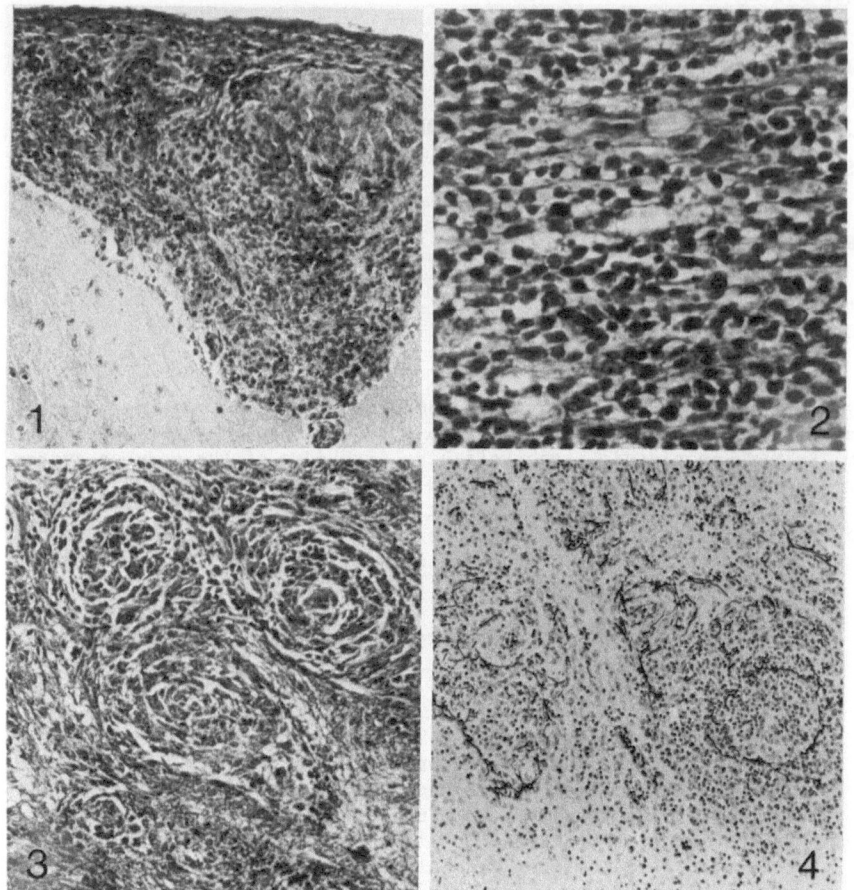

Fig. 1. Nodule in meninges of a turtle consisting of lymphocytes and reticular cells (Histiocytes). H ε E X 125

Fig. 2. Sciatic nerve of a chicken with Marek's disease. Diffuse lymphocytic infiltration of the nerve. H ε E X 500

Fig. 3. Space-occupying lesion in cerebrum of a dog classified as inflammatory reticulosis. Note perivascular arrangement of lymphoreticular cell infiltrates accentuated by intervascular necrosis H ε E X 125

Fig. 4. Same lesion as Fig. 3 illustrating the scarcity of reticular fibers. Wilder's reticulum X 125

infectious anemia tumorlike lymphoreticular proliferations may occur in the subependyma or around cerebral vessels either focally or diffusely (4). Inflammatory reticuloses of unknown origin have been observed in dogs, horses, cattle, and goats (3). Criteria in favor of inflammatory reticuloses over true neoplasms include: 1) the predominant perivascular arrangement of proliferating cells from simple cuffings by mature lymphocytes to perivascular granulomas (Fig. 2); 2) variety and maturity of cell elements, especially large numbers of plasma cells and lymphocytes; 3) scarcity of reticular fibers (Fig. 3); and 4) absence of pleomorphism, polyploidy, and mitoses.

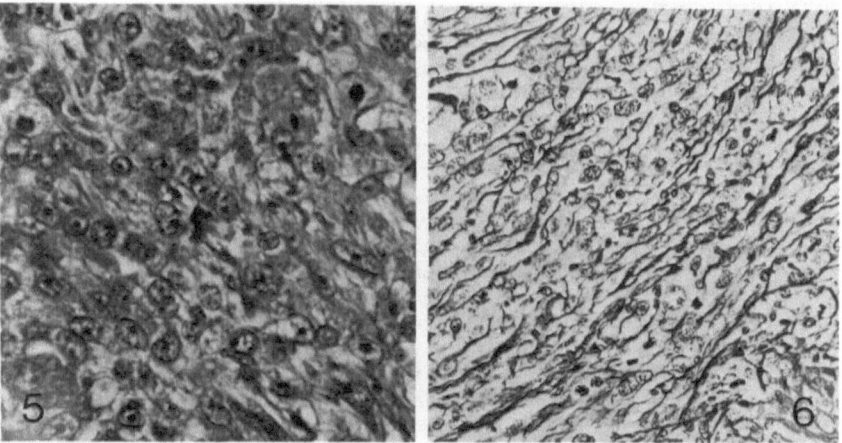

Fig. 5. Reticulum cell sarcoma in a canine brain. Notice pleomorphism of reticular cells and the large number of mitoses. H ε E X 500

Fig. 6. Same lesion as Fig. 5. Intensive staining of reticular fibers which
frame individual cells or groups of cells. Wilder's reticulum X 500

LYMPHORETICULAR PROLIFERATIVE DISORDERS WITH INVOLVEMENT OF THE CNS

Neoplastic lymphoreticular proliferative disorders have been recognized in
fishes (5), amphibia (6) and reptiles (7) but spread to the central nervous
system in these classes of animals has not been reported to our knowledge.
Neoplastic lymphomatosis has been well documented in birds and the viral
etiology has been well established. While neoplastic lymphomatosis in birds is
generally limited to non-neural organs, a form of lymphoproliferative disorder
affects the nervous system primarily or sometimes exclusively (Marek's disease)
and will be discussed separately as avian neurolymphomatosis.

Neoplasms of lymphoreticular cells have been described in most mammalian
species. As in chicken, RNA tumor viruses have been isolated as etiologic
agents of lymphomas in mice, rats, hamsters and cats. Infectious agents are
suspected as the cause of lymphoproliferative disorders in other species,
particularly in dogs and cattle. Occasional involvement of the nervous system
has been reported in most species in which generalized malignant lymphomatosis
occurs. In most cases only the meninges are infiltrated by neoplastic cells.
Whether the incidence of lymphoreticuloses in general and involvement of the
CNS in particular is increased in either inherited or acquired defective immunologic responsiveness, as it has been established in man (8), has to our
knowledge not been thoroughly investigated. There is substantial experimental
evidence that this be the case (8).

PRIMARY NEOPLASTIC LYMPHORETICULOSES OF THE NERVOUS SYSTEM

1. Avian Neurolymphomatosis (Marek's Disease)

First described by MAREK in 1907 as a polyneuritis in chicken the disease has
now been recognized throughout the world. The chicken seems to be the natural
host although lesions similar to those of Marek's disease in chicken have been
reported in turkeys, pheasants, and quails. Excellent reviews of this disease
have appeared in the literature during the past few years (9). A herpesvirus

was isolated in 1967 and later established as the etiological agent of Marek's disease. Herpesviruses have also been isolated from lymphomas of other species (guinea pigs, rabbits, man - Burkitt lymphoma)

There are factors influencing the course of Marek's disease in chickens either related to the viral strain (virulence) or to the host (age, sex, genetic resistance, and immune response). Generally, two forms of the disease have been recognized. The "acute" form is characterized by sudden onset, high mortality and tumors of visceral organs often exclusive of the nervous system. The "classical" form is characterized by low mortality and by clinical signs related to involvement of the nervous system. Although the nervous system is preferably affected in the so-called "classical" form tumors of the other organs, particularly of the ovaries but also of other viscera (liver, kidney, lung, heart), may occur. The lesions preferably affect the peripheral nervous system (brachial, sciatic, and celiac plexuses, the vagus and intercostal nerves) but also the CNS and occasionally the eye. The affected nerves are nodularly or diffusely enlarged due to massive infiltration of lymphocytes (Fig. 4). Lymphocytic infiltration may also be present around vessels of the brain and meninges. A vaccine derived from this herpesvirus or from an antigenically related herpesvirus of turkeys effectively protects chickens against this neoplastic disease.

2. *Primary Neoplastic Lymphoreticuloses of the CNS in Mammals*

They are space-occupying lesions occurring usually singly (occasionally multiply) in the brain but also in the spinal cord in the absence of lymphoreticular tumors of other organs. The species most frequently affected is the dog (2, 3). In our collection of 60 primary neoplasms of the CNS in dogs, 9 were reticulum cell sarcomas (perithelial sarcomas, adventitial sarcomas). These tumors seem to originate from undifferentiated adventitial cells (perithelial cells, polyblasts) of the vessels of the CNS. In distinguishing neoplastic from inflammatory reticuloses the presence of diffuse cellular infiltration, predominance of one cell type, large numbers of mitotic figures, pleomorphism and polyploidy were used as differential diagnostic criteria (Fig. 5). The arrangement of the reticulum (Fig. 6) framing individual cells or groups of cells is very similar to reticulum cell sarcomas in other organs. Occasionally a cell type with microglial characteristics appears to be the predominant cell type of this neoplasm. Such tumors have been classified as microgliomas or microgliomatosis (10). Both cell types (reticular cell and microglia cell) may derive from the same precursor cell and participate in various proportions in the same tumor (3).

A reticular cell population is recognized in some meningeal tumors classified as diffuse meningeal sarcomatosis (2). In this neoplastic disease reticular cells diffusely spread in preformed meningeal spaces with occasional peripheral cerebral infiltration along the course of the vessels. Histogenetically the neoplastic cells may also originate from perivascular precursor cells which are present in abundance in the meninges.

REFERENCES

1. WILKE, G.: Über primäre Reticuloendotheliosen des Gehirns. Dtsch. Zschr. Nervenh. *164*, 332-380 (1950)
2. KOESTNER, A., ZEMAN, W.: Primary reticuloses of the central nervous system in dogs. Am. J. Vet. Res. *23*, 381-393 (1962)
3. LUGINBÜHL, H., FANKHAUSER, R., McGRATH, J.T.: Spontaneous neoplasms of the nervous system in animals. *In:* KRAYENBÜHL, H., MASPES, P.E., SWEET, W.H. (eds.): Progress in Neurological Surgery *2*, 85-164 (1968)
4. FRAUCHIGER, E., FANKHAUSER, R.: Vergleichende Neuropathologie des Menschen und der Tiere. Berlin-Heidelberg-New York: Springer 1957

5. MAWDESLEY-THOMAS, L.E.: Some tumours of fish. In: MAWDESLEY-THOMAS, L.E.
   (ed.): Diseases of Fish. Academic Press 1972
6. RUBEN, L.N., STEVENS, J.M.: Lymphoreticular neoplasia and immunity in amphibia. Am. Zoologist. *11*, 229-237 (1971)
7. FRYE, F.L., CARNEY, J.D.: Acute lymphatic leukemia in a boa constrictor.
   J.A.V.M.A. *163*, 653-654 (1973)
8. KRÜGER, G.R.F.: Lymphoreticular neoplasia in immunosuppression: facts and
   fancies. Beitr. Path. *151*, 221-233 (1974)
9. BIGGS, P.M.: Marek's disease. *In:* KAPLAN, A.S. (ed.): The Herpesviruses,
   p. 557-594. Academic Press 1973
10. RUSSELL, D.S., MARSHALL, A.H.E., SMITH, F.B.: Microgliomatosis: a form of
    reticulosis affecting the brain. Brain *71*, 1-15 (1948)

Prof. A. KOESTNER
The Dept. of Veterinary Pathobiology
Ohio State University
1925 Coffey Road, Columbus, Ohio 43210

Acta Neuropath. (Berlin), Suppl. VI, 91 - 94 (1975)

Pathology of Primary Reticulum Cell Sarcoma of the Human Central Nervous System

M. REZNIK

Laboratoire d'Anatomie Pathologique
Université de Liège
(Belgium)

Summary: Among 6000 consecutive autopsies, 9 cases of primary reticulum cell
sarcoma of the central nervous system were discovered. There were 5 males
and 4 females from 17 to 68 years old, and the mean clinical duration was
5 months. Gross examination revealed a wide range of lesions in the cerebral hemispheres, cerebellum and spinal cord. Histologically, the same type
of malignant reticulum cell proliferation was encountered in every case.

Key words: Reticulum cell sarcoma - central nervous system

Regardless of terminology, the nosology of primary reticulo-sarcoma of the
central nervous system (CNS) has been controversial for many years. This
paper reports pathological observations that should contribute to the recognition of such an ambiguous disease.

MATERIAL AND METHODS

6000 consecutive autopsies performed in our department of general pathology
during the last 15 years were reviewed for neuropathological lesions resulting from reticulum cell sarcoma or Hodgkin's disease, cases with leukaemia
were excluded.
  Among 7 cases with Hodgkin's disease in lymph nodes who had been submitted
to neuropathological investigation, 2 had meningeal hemorrhage and 1 had microscopic infiltration of the meninges by tumour. Among 10 cases with visceral
reticulosarcoma, 1 had microscopic infiltration of the meninges by tumour, and
1 exhibited widespread deposits of tumor in the CNS appearing like foci of
softening. These cases will not be discussed in this paper.
  The diagnosis of *primary* reticulum cell sarcoma of the CNS, without visceral
involvement, was suggested in 9 cases which were reviewed for this presentation.

RESULTS

Case 1: M. 45 y. After one year of neurological symptomas, a parietal tumor was
removed and diagnosed as an undifferentiated metastasis. He died 3 days later
from pulmonary embolism. No other tumor was found. Re-examination of the cerebral tumor revealed a reticulum cell sarcoma (Fig. 1 and 2).

Case 2: M. 62 y.,admitted to a geriatric hospital because of rapidly progressive mental deterioration. He died one week later. An autopsy disclosed

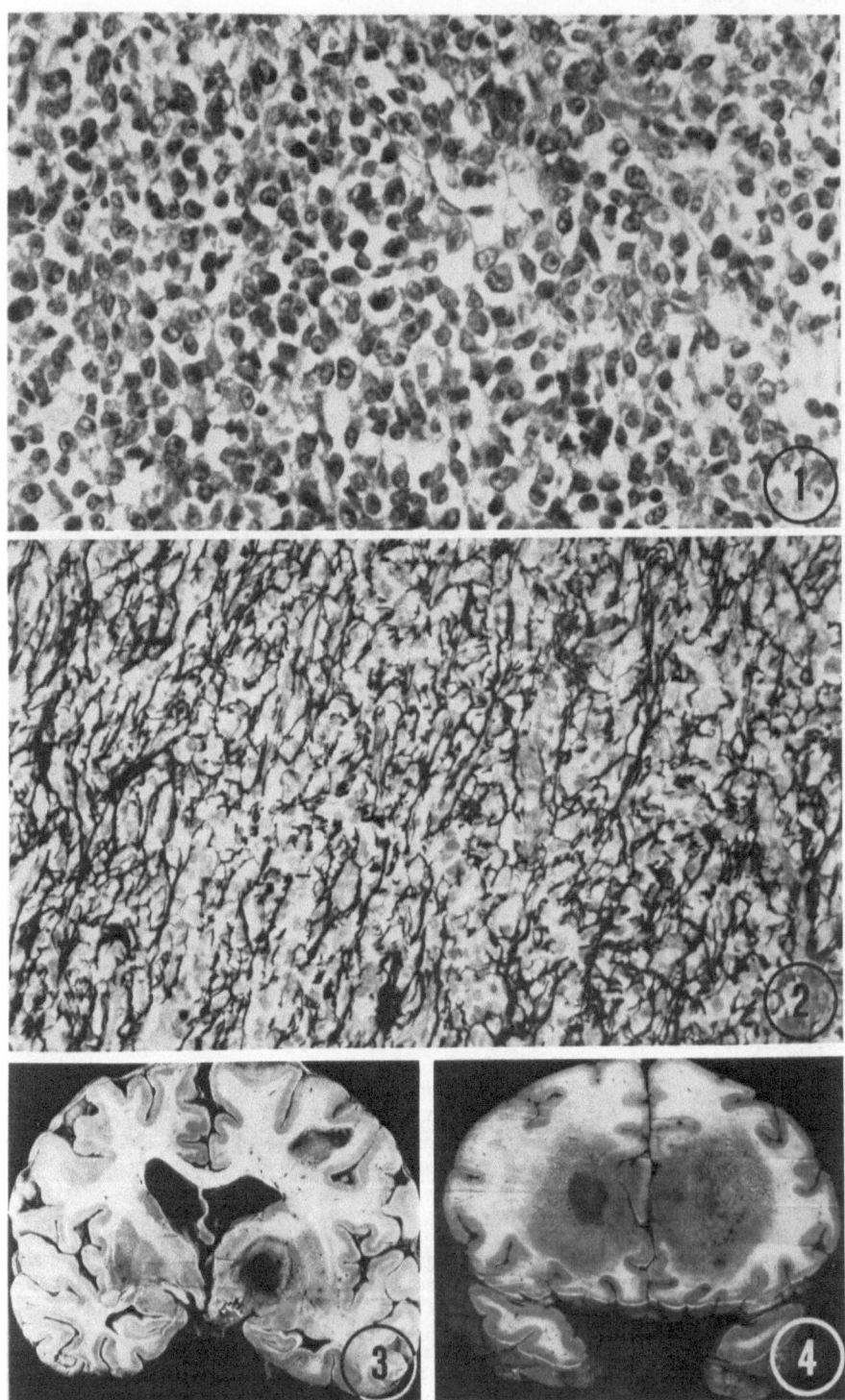

bilateral bronchopneumonia and atherosclerosis. No visceral tumor was seen.
In the cerebral hemispheres and in the cerebellum, several metastatic-like
tumors were found. It was a diffuse perivascular reticulosarcoma invading
the nervous parenchyma.

Case 3: F. 53 y.,with progressive paresis of the right leg. She was admitted
for treatment of a fracture. Because of neurological disturbance after ortho-
pedic surgery, investigations suggested left cerebral metastasis. An autopsy
6 months later did not reveal any visceral tumor. There were several deposits
of tumour in both cerebral hemispheres (Fig. 3) which were classified as
reticulosarcoma.

Case 4: F. 68 y., with syphilis since the age of 30. At the age of 61 y.,
after a transitory right hemiparesis attributed to hypertension, she developed
progressive dementia. At autopsy besides severe atherosclerosis, an old myo-
cardial infarct and a recent pontine hemorrhage, a butterfly-shaped cerebral
tumor was found (Fig. 4). This was a reticulum cell sarcoma similar to that
illustrated in Figs. 1 and 2.

Case 5: M. 43 y., admitted for psychiatric and neurological disorders. Bilateral
cerebral metastases were suspected clinically. At autopsy, the only macroscopic
abnormality was softening of both cerebral hemispheres which appeared to result
from a diffuse perivascular reticulum cell proliferation extending into the
cerebellum and the spinal cord. Reticulohistiocytic meningoencephalitis was
diagnosed.

Case 6: F. 60 y., who died 1 month after admission to a psychiatric hospital,
with a suspected diagnosis of a right cerebral tumor. At autopsy, a perforated
ulcer of the duodenum was found but no visceral tumor. Grossly, there was
extensive softening of the right cerebral hemisphere, but corpus callosum, part
of the left hemisphere and part of the cerebellum. microscopically, a diffuse
reticulosarcoma was found.

Case 7: M. 17 y., with recent neurological disturbances. Neuroradiological
examination suggested an infiltrating tumor of the brain stem. At autopsy,
restricted to the CNS, a necrotic lesion was found around the ventricles. While
a spongioblastoma was suspected at first, the tumor was a reticulosarcoma.

Case 8: F. 40 y., who died after a month illness thought to be a meningo-encephalitis caused by Listeria. Besides terminal lesions, the autopsy demonstrated
necrotic areas around the ventricles and in the brain stem and the cerebellum.
there was "malignant" reticulum cell proliferation in the meninges invading
the nervous parenchyma. Bacteriological investigation remained negative.

Case 9: M. 33 y., who underwent surgery for an intradural spinal tumor. This
tumor was considered to be an undifferentiated sarcoma. An autopsy 1 month

---

Fig. 1. Typical reticulum cell sarcoma invading the nervous parenchyma in the
brain. (H. E.; x 480)

Fig. 2. Reticulin fibres are abundant in all parts of the invading tumor.
(Foot; x 480)

Fig. 3. Several tumors are seen in both cerebral hemispheres

Fig. 4. A butterfly-shaped tumor that was a reticulum cell sarcoma

later demonstrated only a small pulmonary infarct with acute edema. Hemorrhagic softening of the cervical and dorsal spinal cord was found; microscopically, there was an invasion of the spinal cord by a reticulum cell sarcoma.

DISCUSSION

Among the last 6000 autopsies performed in our department of pathology, 9 cases were classified as primary reticulum cell sarcoma of the CNS. There were 5 males and 4 females, ranging in age from 17 to 68 years. The mean duration of clinical symptoms was 5 months (1 week to 1 year). These findings are similar to those of other series (1).

The clinical diagnosis was erratic in all cases.

As already described by others (1, 2, 3), gross examination revealed more extensive involvement of the CNS than had been expected clinically or radiologically. A wide range of pathological process was found: 1 solitary brain tumor that was removed surgically, 2 multiple tumors, 1 butterfly-shaped tumor, 2 bilateral softenings of the brain, 2 necrotic lesions around the ventricles or arising from the meninges and 1 intraspinal tumor. There seems therefore to be no predilection for a site of involvement.

Despite the wide range of gross appearances microscopic examination demonstrated very similar cytological morphology in almost every case. There was a predominant perivascular "malignant" proliferation of reticulum-like cells followed by invasion of the nervous parenchyma without tissue destruction. It is only in larger lesions that foci of necrosis are seen either in the tumor itself or in the nervous tissue.

Reticulin fibres were abundant in all cases, although intraparenchymal infiltrations have less reticulin than perivascular lesions. Astroglial reaction was often absent in the parenchyma. Although phagocytic cells could be found in necrotic areas, microglial impregnation was not conspicous in any case.

Whether all of these cases are true neoplasms (focal or diffuse) or some should be considered as reticulohistiocytic meningo-encephalitis remains uncertain.

REFERENCES

1. SCHAUMBURG, H.H., PLANK, C.R., ADAMS, R.D.: The reticulum cell sarcoma –
   microglioma group of brain tumors. Brain, 95, 199-212 (1972)
2. CONSTANTINIDIS, J., ESCOUROLLE, R.: Réticulose pallido-pédonculaire bilatérale et nécrosante. Arch. Suisses Neurol. Neuroch. Psych. 106, 223 –
   240 (1970)
3. EBELS, E.J.: Reticulosarcomas of the brain presenting as butterfly tumors.
   Europ. Neurol. 8, 333-338 (1972)

Dr. Michel REZNIK
Institut de Pathologie, Université de Liége
Rue des Bonnes Villes, I
4000 LIEGE - Belgium

Acta Neuropath. (Berlin), Suppl. VI, 95 - 102 (1975)

Primary Malignant Lymphomas of the Central Nervous System in Man

K. JELLINGER, TH. RADASKIEWICZ, F. SLOWIK

Neurological Institute and Department of Pathology,
University of Vienna, and Division of Neuropathology,
State Institute of Neurosurgery, Budapest

Summary: Sixty-eight primary malignant lymphomas of the CNS exclusively confined to the brain and its leptomeninges from a series of about 8000 intracranial neoplasms (incidence 0.85%) were examined and classified according
to current histopathologic criteria. Average age at onset of symptoms was
55 years, mean duration of illness to time of diagnosis was 3 months. Survival
averaged 1,8 months with supportive care, but 17,2 months with surgery, radiation and/or chemotherapy. CSF cytology was a useful and reliable tool for clinical diagnosis. The cerebral hemispheres were affected in about 50%, the
basal ganglia in 18%, posterior fossa in 10%, while multifocal lesions amounted to 22%. All CNS tumors were of the diffuse type of non-Hodgkin's lymphomas;
no follicular (germinal center) lymphomas were observed. Three histological
patterns comparable to extraneural lymphomas were distinguished: Immunoblastoma (reticulosarcoma) occurred most frequently (58.8%), lympho-plasmacytoid
immunocytoma constituted 28 percent, while lymphoblastic lymphoma occurred
least frequently (13.2%). There were no significant differences with regard
to onset, location, growth pattern or clinical course except for a much poorer
prognosis of lymphoblastic lymphoma. Although there are no definite cytological
differences between malignant lymphomas arising in extraneural sites or as primary lesions in the CNS, the latter showed a much greater proportion of phagocyting histiocytes (and microglia) and a frequent occurrence of plasmacytes
and their precursors which apparently exceeded pure host reaction. The prognostic value of modern classification schemes for CNS lymphomas needs further
critical evaluation.

Key words: Malignant Lymphoma - Primary CNS Tumor - Classification - Immunoblastoma - Immunocytoma - Lymphoblastoma

Primary (intrinsic) malignant lymphomas (ML) of the CNS confined exclusively
to the brain and its coverings are ranging in incidence from 0.3 to about
1.5 percent of all intracranial neoplasms (cf. 8). Although this group of
tumors often referred to as microgliomas/reticulosarcomas (cf. 6) shows an
appreciable degree of cytological variations, consistent histological patterns
comparable to ML arising in extraneural sites exist and, hence, can be classified according to current taxonomic concepts of non-Hodgkin's lymphomas (4, 5).
This paper presents clinico-pathological data and a preliminary classification
of 68 primary malignant CNS lymphomas found in a total of about 8000 intracranial neoplasms (incidence 0.85%)

MATERIAL AND METHODS

Among the intracranial tumors listed during the past 20 years in the files of
the Neurological Institute, Vienna, and the State Institute of Neurosurgery,

Budapest, all primary ML confined exclusively to the CNS and its leptomeninges were reviewed. Extradural growths and metastases from recognized extraneural ML were rejected. 33 cases had complete autopsies, 29 both biopsy and autopsy; biopsies alone were available in 9 patients without clinical evidence of systemic lymphoproliferative disease.

Routine stains (H.& E., K.V., Gomori, van Gieson's elastic method, Masson-Goldner, Giemsa, methyl-green-pyronine (pH 3.4 and 4.4), PAS, Sudanblack B, Oilred O, Hortega-Penfield), and in some cases cytochemical methods for peroxidase, acid and alkaline phosphatase, non-specific esterase, chloroacetate esterase, β-glucuronidase (see 2, 7) were performed. Vascular endothelial cells were identified by detection of blood group isoantigens by specific red cell adherence (SRCA) test (1). Frozen sections from 2 cases were examined by thin layer chromatography (3).

The Vienna series (36 cases of primary ML among 3800 intracranial tumors = 0.95%) was separately evaluated and classified (Table 2).

RESULTS

There were 40 males and 28 females ranging in age from 16 days to 76 years, but more than half of the patients were over 60. The mean age at onset of clinical symptoms was 55.4 ± 7.4 years. Non had received organ transplantation or immunosuppressive therapy. Non-specific clinical signs of space occupying intracranial lesion included mental symptoms, hemiparesis and aphasia or cerebellar and brainstem symptoms. The mean duration of symptoms from onset to the time of diagnosis was 3.3 ± 0.2 months. Survival from onset of symptoms to death averaged 1.85 ± 0.8 months with supportive care, 0.9 ± 0.3 months with surgery, and 17.2 ± 9.5 months with surgery, radiation and chemotherapy, or radiation and chemotherapy alone (Table 1). Six such patients are still alive and well after 12 months up to 12 years.

CSF examination performed in 40 cases showed increased protein in 85%, pleocytosis in 58% and neoplastic cells in 27.5%. CSF cytology showed either uniformely appearing medium-sized cells with large nuclei and sparse basophilic cytoplasm in lymphoblastic lymphoma (Fig. 11) or pleomorphic cells in immunoblastoma/reticulosarcome. Neither neoplastic cells nor paraproteinaemia were found in the peripheral blood.

Although all cases of malignant lymphoma originating in extraneural sites were excluded, two of the 62 autopsies with signs indicating primary CNS disease showed lymphoid microfoci in the skull and gall bladder, respectively. Three cases had secondary tumors of different type: mammary carcinoma, hypernephroma, and pituitary adenoma.

Grossly, the brain was involved in two ways, as localized tumors, resembling certain gliomas, either solitary or multiple, or as diffusely,infiltrating lesions. The cerebral hemispheres were affected in about 50%, with some predilection of the frontal and temporal regions. Butterfly-shaped tumors of the corpus callosum were seen in 8.6%. The basal ganglia were involved in 18%, the posterior fossa in 10% - including two connatal tumors. Multifocal lesions amounted to 22% (Table 1). The spinal cord was never affected.

Three histological patterns comparable to malignant lymphomas originating fron extraneural sites were distinguished and were classified according to the "Kiel classification 1974" of ML (5). All CNS lesions were of the *diffuse* type, with an apparent perivascular arrangement and diffuse invasion of the parenchyma. Neither nodular lymphomas nor primary Hodgkin's lymphomas were observed.

1. The most frequent cytological pattern 40 cases (58.8% ot the total series, only 41.7% of the Vienna series) was that of *immunoblastoma* (reticulosarcoma) showing a pleomorphic picture with different stages of differentiation. Pleo-

Table 1. *Primary Malignant Lymphomas of the Central Nervous System in Man*

	Immunoblastic Lymphoma ("Reticulosarcoma")	Lympho-plasmacyt. Immunocytoma (I. cytoma + blastoma)	Lymphoblastic Lymphoma (Lymphosarcoma)	T o t a l
Number Cases	40 = 58.8%	19 = 28%	9 = 13.2%	68
Males	24	11	5	40
Females	16	8	4	28
Age (Onset), mean	52.7 years	60.5 years	62.2 years	55.4 ± 7.4 yrs
Duration, mean (Onset-diagnosis)	3.5 months	2.6 months	3.0 months	3.3 ± 0.2 mo
Survival, mean (Onset-death)	1.7 months	1.6 months	1.7 months	1.85 ± 0.8 mo
Survival, mean (surgery)	0.9 months	0.75 months	0.5 months	0.9 ± 0.3 mo
Survival, mean (surgery/irrad)	25 months	14 months	6.0 months	17.2 ± 9.5 mo
Location				
Cer. hemispheres	16 = 40%	7 = 37%	5 = 56%	28 = 41.2%
Butterfly tumor	3 = 8%	2 = 11%	1 = 11%	6 = 8.6%
Bas. ganglia/ Brain stem	6 = 15%	5 = 36%	1 = 11%	12 = 17.7%
Multifocal	9 = 22%	4 = 21%	2 = 22%	15 = 22.0%
Posterior fossa	6 = 15%	1 = 5%	0	7 = 10.5%

morphic cells with large, oval nuclei, conspicuous nucleoli, and finely granular basophilic, PAS-, peroxidase-, alkaline and phosphatase- and esterase-
negative cytoplasm were admixed with various numbers of lymphocytes, plasmacytes or their precursors, and binucleated epitheloid or multinucleated giant

Table 2. *Primary Malignant Lymphomas of the Central Nervous System (Vienna Material)*

	Immunoblast. Lymphoma "Reticulosarcoma"	Immunocytoma Lympho-Plasmacyt. (cytoma-blastoma)	Lymphoblastic Lymphoma (Lymphosarcoma)	T o t a l
Number Cases	15 = 41.7%	16 = 44.4%	5 = 13.9%	36
Males	7	9	3	20
Females	8	7	2	16
Age (onset), mean	51.1 years	59.5 years	55.0 years	56.9 years
Duration, mean (onset-death)	3.4 months	3.4 months	3.3 months	3.5 months
Survival, mean (no therapy)	2.0 months	1.7 months	2.0 months	1.9 months
Survival, mean (Surgery)	0.9 months	1.0 month	0.5 month	1.0 month
Survival, mean (Surg., irrad.)	10.0 months	13.0 months	4.5 months	13.0 months
Location				
Cerebral hemispheres	5	5	3	12 = 33.3%
Butterfly tumor	–	2	1	3 = 8.3%
Basal ganglia/ Brain stem	4	4	–	9 = 25.0%
Multifocal	4	4	1	9 = 25.0%
Posterior Fossa	2	1	–	3 = 8.3%

cells resembling Reed-Sternberg cells (Fig. 1). Perivascular cuffing by neoplastic cells was accompanied by increase of reticulin and collagen fibers
(Fig. 2). SCRA-test was negative except for the endothelial cells lining the
stromal vessels. Histiocytes showing foamy cytoplasm with acid phosphatase and

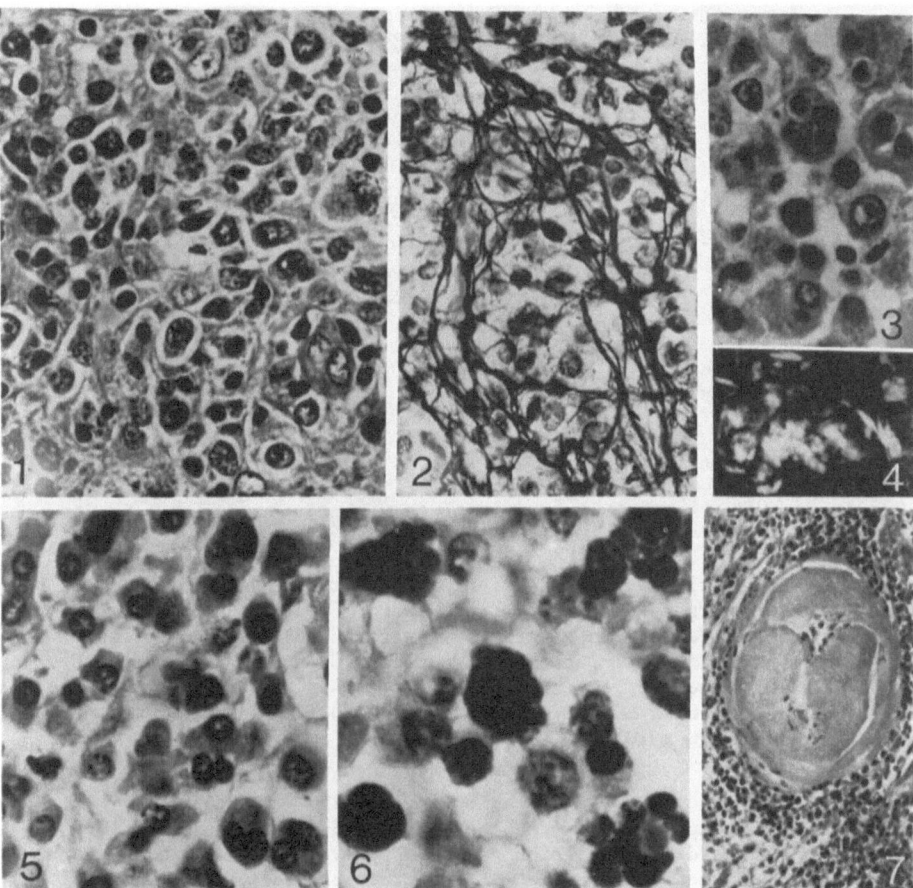

Figs. 1-4. Immunoblastoma in left temporal lobe of male aged 13 yrs; alive
12 years after surgery and radiotherapy. Pleomorphic picture with binucleated
epitheloid cells, a considerable amount of delicate stromal fibers, and
interspersed foamy histiocytes with lymphocytophagia and storage of birefringent lipids.
1) H.& E.x 400; 2) Gomori x 400; 3) H.& E. x 500; 4) Sudan-black B (Frozen
Section), Polarization x 500

Figs. 5-7. Immunocytoma in basal ganglia of male aged 52 years. Dense arrangement in the basal ganglia of plasmacytes, in places mimicking plasmacytoma (5),
many Russel bodies and PAS-positive globular cytoplasmic inclusions (6), and
congo-negative deposits in interstitial tissue (7).
5) H.& E. x 700; 6) PAS x 1100; 7) Congored x 100

strong non-specific esterase activity, frequent lympho- and plasmacytophagia,
and storage of sudanophilic, partly birefringent lipids were frequently interspersed (Fig. 3, 4). In places, lipid storage was excessive. Histochromatography
showed large amounts of cholesterol and cholesterol esters, and smaller amounts
of triglycerides and phospholipids. Activated metalophilic microglia and peripheral astroglial reaction were abundant.

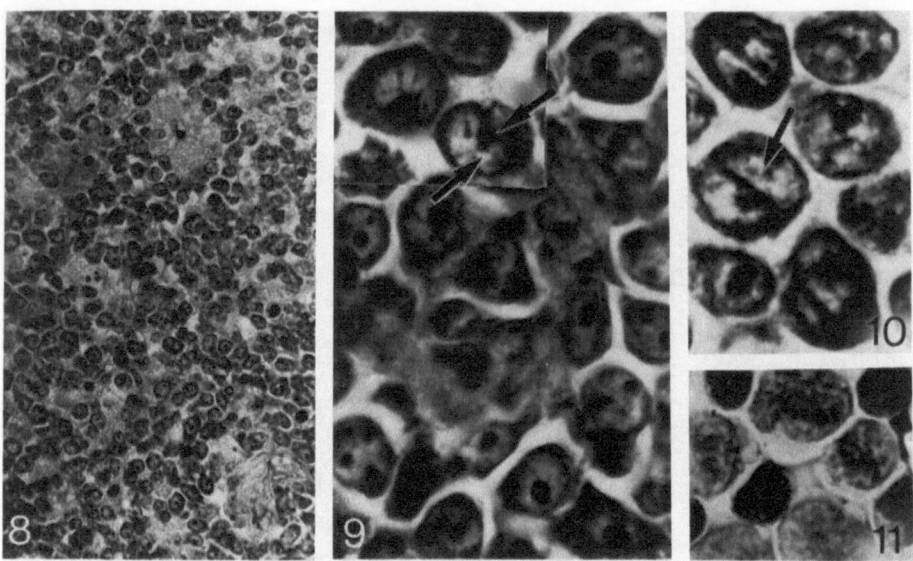

Figs. 8-11. Lymphoblastic lymphoma in right frontal region of male aged 63;
died 2 months after surgery and irradiation. Uniform picture of densely
arranged medium-sized cells with "starry sky pattern" (8), uniform cells
with large round nuclei with 1-2 prominent nucleoli, sparse cytoplasm, and
occasional cleaved nuclei (9, 10, arrows).
8- Giemsa x 420; 9 - Giemsa x 1400; 10 - Giemsa x 1500; 11- Lymphocytes and
lymphoblasts in CSF; MGG x 1050

2. Another pattern, comparable to lympho-plasmacytoid *immunocytoma* with various
degrees of cytological differentiation was seen in 19 cases (28% of the total
series, and 44.4% of the Vienna series). 12 of them showed predominance of
neoplastic lymphocytes, plasma cells and their pyroninophilic precursors, and
a variety of reticular cells and interspersed phagocyting histiocytes; multinucleated cell are usually absent (Fig. 5). Striking features were frequent
Russel bodies and plasmacytes or their precursors with strongly PAS-positive
globular cytoplasmic inclusions (Fig. 6) showing negative glycogen and lipid
reactions (glycoproteins, probably immunoglobulins produced by the tumor cells).
Occasional deposition in the interstitial tissue of PAS-positive, congo-negative, (par)amyloid-like material was seen (Fig. 7). Increased CSF IgG and IgG
immunofluorescence in CSF cells was seen in one case. Some foci of multicentric
tumors were transformed into connective tissue scars with perivascular cuffs
of neoplastic cells.

Seven cases of this group showed a similar, but more pleomorphic picture,
with increased numbers of mitoses, large reticular and occasional multinucleated giant cells. Due to the pronounced admixture of plasmacytes and their
precursors with PAS-positive cytoplasmic inclusions which in places may almost
mimic a plasmacytoma (Fig. 5), this type was considered to be a transitional
form between immunoblastic immunocytoma and plasmoblastic immunoblastoma.

3. An undifferentiated pattern, comparable to *lymphoblastic lymphoma* was seen
in 9 cases (13.2% and 13.9% of the Vienna series). No further subdivision of
this type of high-grade ML was made. It was featured by densely arranged, uniformly appearing, medium-sized cells with round nuclei showing occasional
cleavage planes, one or two prominent nucleoli, and poor basophilic, occasional-

ly PAS-positive, peroxidase-, esterase- and acid phosphatase-negative cytoplasm, numerous mitoses, and common absence of multinucleated giant cells, plasmacytes and mature microglia (Fig. 8 - 10). This type showed perivascular cuffing by neoplastic cells, often separated from the vessel itself by an inner ring of lymphocytes, or a densely diffuse arrangement of cells with varying amounts of phagocyting histiocytes with occasional "starry sky appearance". Reticulin stain showed no or very little perivascular stromal fibers.

There were no significant differences between these cytological types of primary CNS lymphomas with regard to age and sex distribution, site and growth pattern or clinical course, except for a much poorer prognosis of lymphoblastic lymphoma (Table 1 and 2).

DISCUSSION

The present light microscopic study of primary ML of the CNS, constituting 0.85 percent of a large consecutive series of brain tumors clearly demonstrates that this group of neoplasms can well be classified according to a modern histopatho-logical standard scheme of non-Hodgkin's lymphomas accepted by many general pathologists. Although there are no definite cytological differences between ML arising in extraneural sites of as primary lesions in the CNS, some cha-racteristic features of the latter should be emphasized:
1. No germinal center tumors, neither germinoblastomas (follicular lymphomas) nor germinocytomas (cleaved FCC tumors), were observed, as germinal centers are obviously absent in the CNS. In the present series, there were no instan-ces of primary Hodgkin's disease confined to the intracranial contents.
2. All types of primary malignant CNS lymphomas contain a much greater pro-portion of phagocyting histiocytes -and microglia - than those in extraneural sites. Although most of them may be considered as reactive phenomena, their role and origin need further clarification.
3. The frequent occurrence in many CNS lymphomas of plasmacytes and their pre-cursors, such as of mature lymphocytes, may well present a host reaction similar to that seen in other neoplasms. However, part of them may be neoplastic in nature and in places may even mimic the picture of plasmacytoma.
4. Perivascular spread of tumor, occasionally imitating an inflammatory process, predominance of meningeal and ependymal involvement, and peripheral astroglial reaction add further variations which, together with the above cytological reactions create particular histological dimensions to CNS lymphomas that may become sources of differential diagnostic confusion.
5. The prognostic value of classification of CNS lymphomas according to current concepts of low and high grade malignant lymphomas should be considered in the light of their intracranial location. Due to limited experience this problem needs further critical evaluation.

REFERENCES

1. DAVIDSON, I.: Early immunologic diagnosis and prognosis of carcinoma. Amer. J. clin. Path. 57, 715-730 (1972)
2. HENNEKEUSER, H.H.: Untersuchungen zur Klassifizierung akuter Leukämien. Erg. inn. Med. 33, 69-112 (1972)
3. HOLCZABEK, W.: Dünnschichtchromatographische Untersuchung von Gewebsschnit-ten. Dtsch. Z. gerichl. Med. 57, 211-214 (1966)
4. LENNERT, K.: Pathologisch-histologische Klassifizierung der malignen Lymphome, In: A. STACHER (edit.) Leukämien und maligne Lymphome pp. 181-194. München-Berlin-Wien: Urban & Schwarzenberg 1973

5. LENNERT, K.: Morphology and classification of malignant lymphomas and so-called reticuloses. Acta neuropath. (Berl.) Suppl. VI, 1 - 16 (1975)
6. RUBINSTEIN, L.J.: Tumors of the central nervous system. In: Atlas of tumor pathology. 2nd ser., Fasc. 6. Washington, D.C. Armed Forces Institute of Pathology 1972
7. SCHÄFER, H.E., KÄUFER, C., FISCHER, R.: Vergleichende ferment-cytochemische Untersuchungen an Blut- und Knochenmarkzellen bei Laboratoriumstieren. Virchows Arch. Abt. B Zellpath. *4*, 310-334 (1970)
8. ZIMMERMAN, H.M.: Brain tumors: their incidence and classification in man and their experimental production, Ann. New York Acad. Sci. *159*, 337-359 (1969)

K. JELLINGER, M.D.
Div. Spec. Neuropath.
Neurological Institute
University of Vienna
Schwarzspanierstraße 17
A-1090 Vienna / Austria

Acta Neuropath. (Berlin), Suppl. VI., 103 - 106 (1975)

Primary Lymphomas of the Central Nervous System; *in vitro* Culture Observations

L. GAZSO and F. SLOWIK

Institute of Neurosurgery
Budapest, Hungary

Summary: Out of 960 human brain neoplasms seven primary lymphomas were cultured and grown up to twenty-eight days. The monolayers had common cytological characteristics; /i/ immediately after explantation a high density of uniform cells was observed; /ii/ many cells were lost during subsequent medium changes; /iii/ the monolayers contained lymphocyte-like cells in different numbers. According to their individual characteristics the cultures could be classified into three categories: 1./ In the cultures of three tumours lymphocyte-like cells predominated. These tumours had low proliferative capacity *in vitro*. 2./ Cultures of three other tumours consisting mainly of tissue macrophages had a high proliferative capacity *in vitro*. 3./ Cultures of a single tumour showed the combined features of the former two categories: both lymphocyte-like cells, and tissue macrophages were present. These cultures showed the highest proliferative activity.

On the basis of these findings it is quite possible that besides other methods, tissue culture technique may be useful in the classification of brain lymphomas.

Key words: Brain tumour - Lymphoma - Tissue culture

INTRODUCTION

Since neoplastic cells maintain their morphological features at least during early culture periods, and since the dynamics of growth can be easily followed under *in vitro* conditions, cultivation of brain tumours offers great theoretical and practical advantages. Although the *in vitro* behaviour of most types of brain tumours is already known from monographs by KERSTING /1/ and LUMSDEN /2/, some varieties of brain neoplasms are not yet described in the literature. Primary lymphomas belong to this kind of tumour.

At the Neurosurgical Institute of Budapest tissue cultures are regularly prepared from the operative material. During the last seven years out of 960 brain neoplasms of different types, seven tumours histologically proved to be primary lymphomas. Studies were performed in order to identify the types of cells these tumours consisted of, and at the same time to observe their proliferative capacity.

MATERIAL AND METHODS

Immediately after surgical removal the tumour tissue was divided into two parts. One part was put to explantation, the second part to routine histology.

Tissue Culture Technique. After removing blood and necrotic parts, the solid tumours were cut into 1-2 mm fragments under sterile conditions and washed several times with Tyrode-solution. These pieces were transferred to cover-

slips which were coated with a mixture of chicken plasma and chick embryo
extract. Coverslips were inserted into Leighton-tubes containing two milli-
liters of nutritive medium (80 per cent TC-M-199 /DIFCO/ and 20 per cent
foetal calf serum) and incubated at 37°C. The medium was changed every other
day. After having checked the growth in its native state every day, cultures
were fixed at different time intervals and stained according to May-Grünwald-
Giemsa. Cultivation time has been extended up to twenty-eight days at the
longest.

Histological Technique. After formalin fixation the tumour tissue was embedded
in paraffin. Three micron thick sections were stained with hematoxylin-eosin.
Parallel sections were subjected to silver impregnation.

RESULTS

All cultures exhibited common cytological characteristics: all explants showed
a high density of tumour cells without any stroma; during the early culture
period a large proportion of the cells was damaged and lost during medium
changes; in all culture lymphocyte-like cells occurred in different numbers.
   In spite of the low number of cases investigated the cultures could be distinguished form each other according to their individual characteristics and classified into three categories.
   In cultures of three tumours small and round lymphocyte-like cells predominated /Fig. 1a/. They were mostly found individually around the original explants without forming monolayers. Real monolayers did not develop even by
the end of the culture period. Some solitary cells had "hand mirror"-shape,
characteristic for moving lymphocytes. The cytoplasm of some larger cells with
eccentric nuclei possessed vacuoles containing dead lymphocyte-like cells.
Some round cells - probably in a passive way - formed cell groups. Mitoses were
not visible. In tissue sections of these tumours immature lymphoblast-like
cells predominated, among them small mature lymphocytes were also visible
/Fig. 1b/. In tissue sections treated with silver impregnation a few reticulin
fibers could be seen.
   Three other tumours formed monolayers consisting of two types of cell. One
type was small and spindle-shaped with elongated nuclei. These cells had a
strong similarity to microglial-macrophages described by KERSTING /1/ in cultures of certain brain tumours. In high-power magnification elongated nuclei
and cell bodies with fine processes could be observed. Mitoses could not be
seen, but cell grouping and multinucleated cells did occur, suggesting the probability of cell fusion. The second type of cells was larger and abundant in
cytoplasm and contained a big and round nucleus. In younger cultures these
larger cells were arranged in rows; in older ones they formed monolayers with
closely packed cells having polymorphous nuclei /Fig. 2a/. Round- and comma-
shaped nuclei were equally visible. Mitotic figures could be frequently observed. Proliferative activity was higher than in cultures consisting mainly
of lymphocyte-like cells. Tissue sections of these tumours showed pleomorphous
cell pictures of reticulum cells, lymphoblast-like cells and lymphocytes.
Transitional forms of these cells were also present /Fig. 2b/. Tumour cells
were arranged in nests separated from each other by very few reticulin fibers.
   The cultures of a single tumour were characterized by the highest proliferative activity. These cultures showed the combined character of the former two
categories. Large cells having nuclei of different sizes and shapes formed
continuous monolayers; on their surface groups of lymphocyte-like cells could
be seen /Fig. 3a/. Not only the nuclei but also the cytoplasms of the cells
had unusual outlines. Cytoplasmic fragments indicated heavy clasmatocytotic
activity. In tissue sections large reticulum cells with round nuclei, and
small mature lymphocytes were visible /Fig. 3b/.

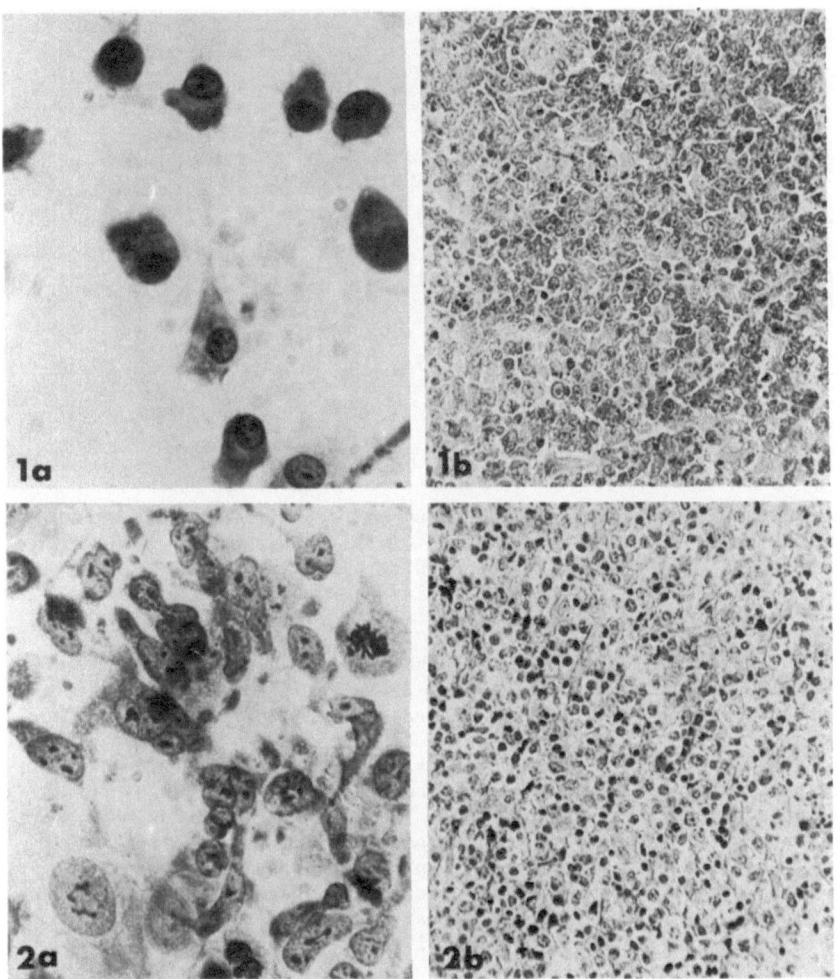

Fig. 1 a and b. 13-day-old culture a) originating from a tumour b) abundant
in lymphocyte-like cells. a) Isolated cells of lymphocytic type with "hand
mirror" outlines (arrow). May-Grünwald-Giemsa staining, x 630. b) Tumour
tissue consisting mainly of lymphoid cells. H.E.-staining, x 250

Fig. 2 a and b. 21-day-old monolayer a) of a tumour b) of macrophage type.
a) Closely packed cells. Note cell bodies and nuclei of bizarre shapes.
May-Grünwald-Giemsa staining, x 630. b) Tumour tissue with predominance of
reticulum cells. H.E. - staining, x 250

DISCUSSION

Identification of cells present in our cultures is quite difficult. Illustra-
tions of other authors cannot help us in this respect, because primary brain
lymphomas have not been cultured hitherto - at least not to our present knowledge. Although MURRAY and STOUT /3/ described the *in vitro* characteristics
of various lymphomas these, however, did not originate from the central nervous system. We think the recognition of cells is all the more difficult, be-

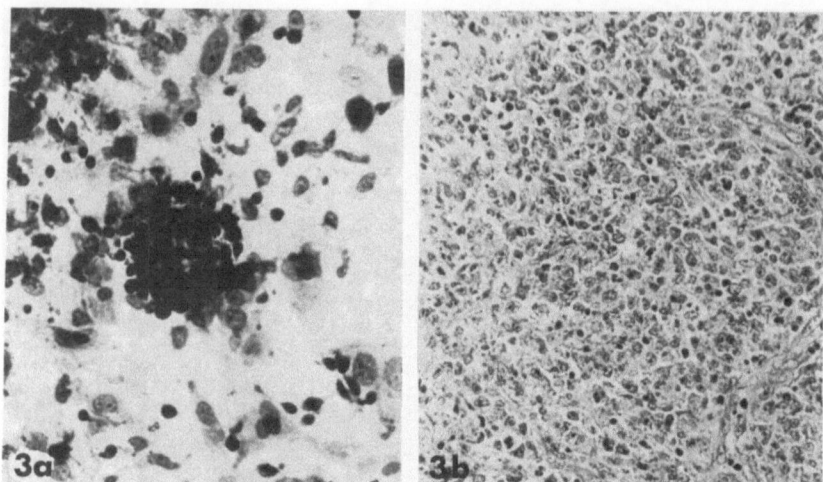

Fig. 3 a and b. 21-day-old culture *a)* of a tumour *b)* having a mixed character. *a)* Group of lymphocyte-like cells on surface of the monolayer. May-Grünwald-Giemsa staining, x 250. *b)* Tumour tissue showing pleomorphous cell picture of lymphoid and reticulum cells. H. E. - staining, x 250

cause the cells these tumours consist of, exhibit perhaps the highest trans-mutability of all the cells of the organism. It is quite possible that, be-sides mature and immature cells, series of transitional cell forms have also to be taken into consideration. In our seven cases the brain lymphomas showed a different behaviour under *in vitro* circumstances. It seems to be quite plau-sible, that there were differences not only among the types of cells, but among the degrees of their maturity as well. The tumours consisting mainly of lymphocyte-like cells possessed low proliferative capacity *in vitro*. Their small, round, mature cells were not able to proliferate, only to survive. Cultures of tumours consisting mainly of tissue macrophages grew actively. Cultures of a single tumour were of mixed character, as far as their cellular composition is concerned, however, their proliferative activity made them rather similar to cultures of the macrophage type.

Up to now our observations were made on fixed and stained cultures of lymphomas. Our findings left many uncertainties. Phase-contrast examinations of living cells with immune response experiments may offer further information about types and origins of the cells in question.

REFERENCES

1. KERSTING, G.: Die Gewebszüchtung menschlicher Hirngeschwülste. Berlin-Göttingen-Heidelberg: Springer 1961
2. LUMSDEN, C.E.: The study by tissue culture of tumours of the nervous system. In: RUSSEL, D.S. and RUBINSTEIN, L.J.: Pathology of tumours of the nervous system, p. 334-420. London: Arnold, E., Ltd. 1971
3. MURRAY, M.R., STOUT, A.P.: The classification and diagnosis of human tumors by tissue culture methods. Texas Rep. Biol. Med. *12*, 898-915 (1954)

Lenke GAZSO
Institute of Neurosurgery
Amerikai ut 57
H-1145 Budapest/Hungary

Acta Neuropath. (Berlin), Suppl. VI, 107 - 113 (1975)

Primary and Borderline Brain Lymphosarcoma:
A Neuropathological Review of Nine Cases

Jean-François FONCIN and Jean-Noël FAUCHER

Laboratoire de Physiologie et Psychologie Neurochirurgicales,
Ecole Pratique des Hautes Etudes
La Salpêtrière, and Unité 106, I.N.S.E.R.M., Paris

Summary: Brain lymphosarcoma may be devided into the circumscribed forms, surrounded by marked oedema with fibrin, and the diffuse or infiltrating forms.
Cytology of the former is more uniformly lymphocytic, its clinical course is
more rapidly fatal. Anatomically primary diffuse lymphosarcoma of the brain
may be secondary to 'cured' systemic lymphoma.

Key words: Brain lymphosarcoma - microglioma - neuropathology - classification

INTRODUCTION

The present paper details a series of brain lymphosarcomas from a neuropathological, as distinct from a cytological or cytogenetical, point of view. This
approach has been chosen because the primary consideration of topography and
brain reaction was expected to correlate better with the clinical data and
prognosis, and with the biological properties of tumour cells, than would the
method of morphological cytology.

MATERIAL AND METHODS

Nine cases were collected during the period 1963-1973 at the Clinique de Chirur-
gie Neurologique, La Salpêtrière. The total number of autopsies during the same
period was 827. The cases were selected according to the following criteria:
1. Histological diagnosis of lymphosarcoma or lymphoreticulosarcoma of the
   brain.
2. Complete autopsy failed to show any evidence of systemic involvement. In 6
   cases out of 9 the gross findings were supplemented by the histological
   examination of multiple visceral specimens.
Table 1 presents the main clinical data. Age range was 34-66, mean 54 years:
distribution was equal between both sexes. Focal or pseudo-focal neurological
signs were a constant finding, although mental disturbances were the main
presenting symptom. Brains were sectioned after formalin fixation. Histological
examination was carried out on multiple large paraffin sections (H.E., Masson's
trichrome) and celloidin sections (NISSL, LOYEZ, VAN GIESON, Mallory's P.T.A.H.).
Metallic impregnation was attempted at an early stage of the study, but failed
to yield consistent results. In cases 5 and 9, biopsy tissue was processed for
electron microscopy (glutaraldehyde, osmium, araldite, uranyl acetate-lead
citrate). Tumour was observed in case 9 only.

Table 1.

Case	Sex	Reference	Age	Preoperative course	Postoperative course	Presenting symptom
1	F	13/66	66	3 weeks	3 weeks	Drowsiness
2	M	259/63	62	3 weeks	1 day	Dysarthria
3	F	345/72	52	1 week ?	no operation	"Tiredness"
4	F	99/74	50	2 weeks	1 month	Disorientation
5	M	8/66	56	2 1/2 months	1 1/2 month	Emotional disturbances
6	M	123/67	53	5 months	1 1/2 month	Hemiplegia
7	F	7/71	34	1 month	4 months	Cephalalgia
8	M	13/64	59	6 months	1 month	Disorientation
9	F	4/72	50	1 month	3 days	Cephalalgia

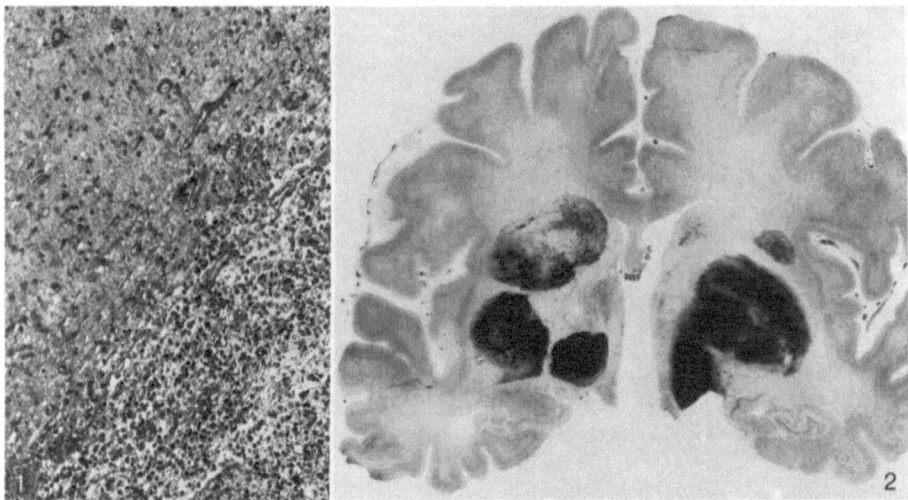

Fig. 1. Case 3 (x 140) Masson's trichrome. Clear-cut border of tumor surrounded by oedema

Fig. 2. Case 4 Nissl. Multicentric infiltration of grey nuclei

RESULTS

Two main groups may be distinguished.

The first group is remarkably homogeneous, and may be described as one entity, comprising 3 cases (Nos. 1, 2, 3). It is characterized macroscopically by well-defined tumours, solitary in cases 1 (right frontal) and 2 (left central), double in case 3 (left putaminal and left parietal). Oedema is marked in the whole hemisphere with corresponding midline shift and tentorial herniation. Histologically the tumour cells are rather uniform, lymphocyte-like, but often with uncompletely split of bizarre, although not enlarged, nuclei. Collagenous fibres are prominent between the tumour cells. The histological boundary of the tumour is sharp, with occasional lymphocytic cuffing around vessels at some distance (Fig. 1). Oedema with fibrin (blue stained with Masson's trichrome) is very marked even at a considerable distance from the tumour, with a conspicuous astroglial reaction.

The second group is less homogeneous. The common feature of cases 4 to 9 is the diffusion of neoplastic infiltration to the point where no true tumour can be distinguished either with the naked eye or histologically. The cytology is more varied in these cases. Various types of 'reticular' cells coexist with large macrophages exhibiting phagocytic activity. Lymphocytic proliferation may appear cytologically malignant in part of a specimen, and reactive, interspersed with plasmocytes, in another. Necrosis or demyelination may occur without apparent direct connection with the neoplasm, but no concomitant multifocal leucoencephalopathy was found. Oedema is minimal, and the brain is not markedly deformed.

This group may be further sub-divided according to the topography of the tumorous infiltration. In cases 5, the process affects primarily the corpus callosum, with extension along the white tracts into the centrum semiovale: "Leucophilic" form. In cases 4 and 8, the process mainly affects the grey nuclei bilaterally and appears multifocal at low magnification (Fig. 2). Widespread infiltration of the central grey matter is revealed at closer scrutiny: "Poliophilic" form.

In cases 6 and 7 the process is widespread above and below the tentorium. Neoplastic proliferation tends to be more perivascular in the white matter and

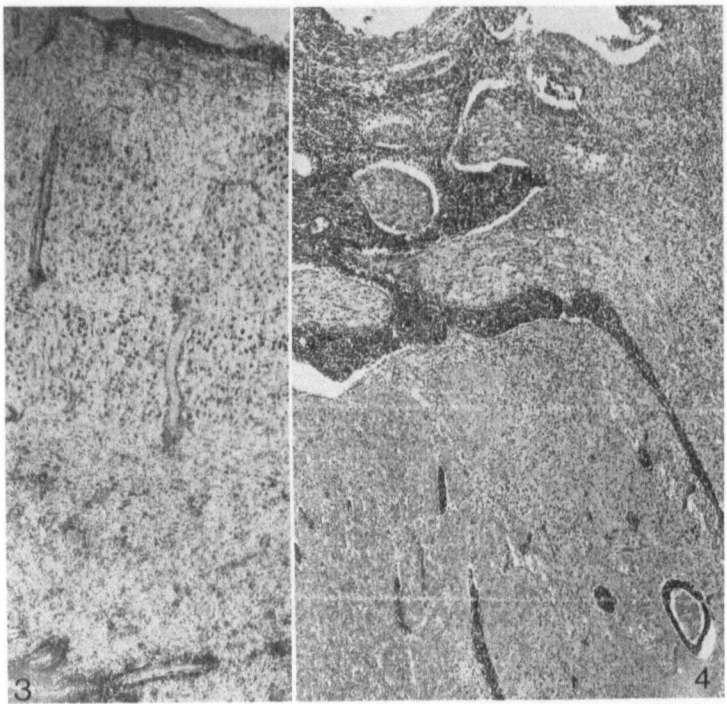

Fig. 3. Case 7 (x 35) Nissl, Uncus. Diffuse infiltration with bipolar accumulation (subpial and white matter)

Fig. 4. Case 9 (x 38) Masson's trichrome. Dense interfascicular infiltration of the emerging third nerve. Loose marginal infiltration with perivascular cuffing

diffuse in the grey matter, but careful examination reveals its ubiquity. Meningeal infiltration is more marked than in the two preceding subgroups (Fig.3). The cerebellar cortex is the least affected part of the encephalon. Case 9 represents a special problem. It apparently fulfils the usual criteria for primitive brain lymphosarcoma. The absence of systemic involvement was confirmed by histological examination of multiple visceral specimens. Yet it was later learned that the patient had been submitted in another hospital to chemotherapy for "histiosarcoma" diagnosed by bone marrow aspiration (complete records or reports could not be obtained). Topographically, tumour cell proliferation is diffuse, but with a pattern distinct from that observed in cases 4 to 8. Meningeal infiltration is prominent (Fig. 4); the peripheral part of the nerve roots is selectively infiltrated, with a well-defined boundary at the glio-schwannian junction. Infiltration is diffuse all over the subpial and subependymal regions. The supraoptic nuclei are picked out by the infiltration. The rest of the central nervous system shows perivascular cuffing by tumour cells; the central grey nuclei are relatively spared. Cytologically, the cells are rather uniform, small, with dense nuclei and scanty cytoplasm. At the ultrastructural level, neuronal and glial changes are moderate and non-specific. The tumour cells have irregular, sometimes partly split nuclei with a large nucleolus. The cytoplasm is scanty, dense, homogeneous, with numerous dispersed ribosomes, and occasional small clumps of glycogen-like granules. A few ergasto-

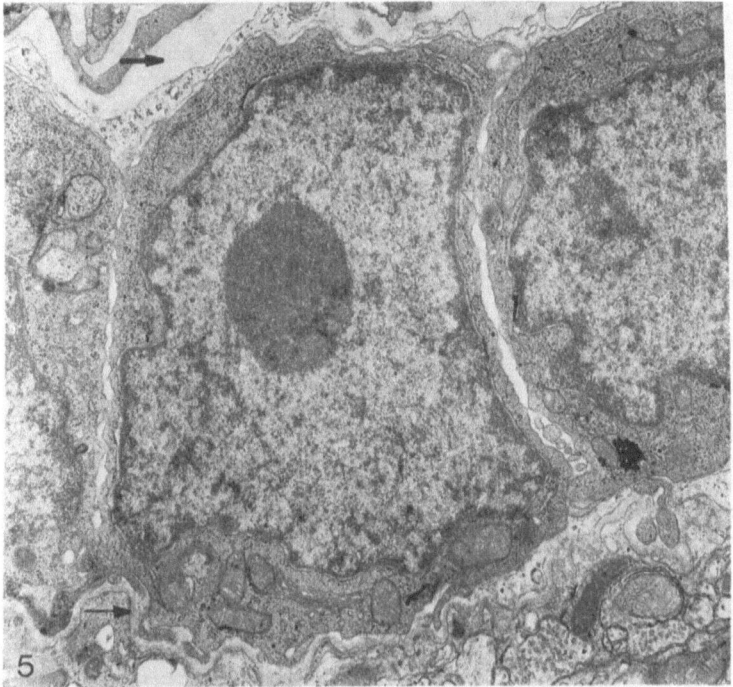

Fig. 5. Case 9 (x 24.000) Thick arrow: vascular basal lamina. Thin arrow: peripheral lamina

plasmic cisterns, normal Golgi apparatus and mitochondria are found. The cell outlines are usually rounded but there are occasional villi. The tumour cells are exclusively perivascular. Around venules they are free-lying in the Virchow-Robin spaces and interspersed with collagen fibres. Around capillaries they are tightly packed around a normal endothelial basal lamina; they are separated from the parenchyma by another basal lamina, thinner, very irregular, which appears to be newly-formed (Fig. 5). Occasional pericytes with secondary lysosomes may be seen in the same space, and they are quite distinct from the tumour cells.

DISCUSSION

1. Clinico-pathologic correlation

The age and sex distribution are similar among the various types of lymphosarcoma, and comparable with data in the literature (1). Symptoms were completely non-specific; in particular, localized tumours exhibited no more focal symptoms than diffuse proliferations. The course of the illness was more rapid in the localized forms, measured in a few weeks, instead of months in the diffuse forms. This can be correlated with the massive brain oedema which is a feature of the localized forms, whereas in the diffuse forms infiltration takes place without much gross displacement. Our autopsy material does not warrant any therapeutic discussion. Surgery does not appear to be useful, even in the presence of a localized tumour. Radiation therapy was used in case 7 only, which happens to have the longest post-operative survival (4 months).

2. Correlation with data from the literature

Most of the literature on the subject of brain lymphosarcoma, "lymphoreticu-loma" or "microgliomatosis" is oriented towards a discussion of the nature of the tumour cell, especially since the introduction of the latter concept (2). Accordingly, localized forms did not attract as much attention; they are nevertheless represented in some large series: case 6 in the series of ABBOTT & KERNOHAN (3) is quite comparable with our cases 1, 2, 3 and represents an instance of this type.

Analogies for the various subtypes we have distinguished among the diffuse form are readily found. Case 4 is comparable with the cerebral sarcoma with multifocal localisation described by VAN GEHUCHTEN & BRUCHER (4); case 8 corresponds to those of LOSLI (5), and WILLIAMS & PETERS (6), case 6 to the one of MAGE & SCHERER (7), case 7 to case 6 of RUSSELL *et al.* (2), and to the case of KÖRNYEY (8). Obviously, most of the cases previously reported could be reclassified according to the criteria used in the present paper, bringing together cases reported under various denominations. This semantic confusion seems inevitable as long as classification and denomination are based on hypotheses concerning the origin of tumour cells, hypotheses which cannot be proved by purely morphological methods.

Cases were selected for the present paper so as to exclude the problem of the borderline between "brain reticulosis" and "granulomatous encephalitis" for which the reader is referred to a previous publication (9).

3. Discussion of case 9: Borderline case

Full interpretation of this case is made difficult by the fragmentary nature of information regarding the history of systemic involvement by the malignant process. Nevertheless, the extraneous nature of the tumour may correlate with its topography, for it is the only example in our series in which the meningeal spaces appear to be the origin of the tumorous proliferation, and the neuraxial involvement secondary. This topography is however not a specific feature of secondary tumours, and is found, for instance, in the "peritheliosarcoma" (10).

Electron microscopic examination confirms the impression gained with the light microscope: a thin, newly-formed basal lamina separates as "strangers" tumour cells from the parenchyma. Their ultrastructure further confirms that the tumour cells are lymphoid, and distinct from pericytes: lymphosarcoma is a valid denomination for the whole group and synonyms like "histiosarcoma" or "peritheliosarcoma" are unnecessary (11). A further point worthy of notice is the complete absence of detectable systemic relapse at the time of death. The meningeal space is now well known as main reservoir to tumour cells and the main obstacle to the eradication of malignant leucocytes. But interest in this phenomenon has been mainly as a cause of later systemic relapse. The sequence of facts observed in our case, on the contrary, suggests a tentative hypothesis about the origin of "primary" brain lymphosarcomas, the origin of which has always been mysterious in an organ normally devoid of lymphoid tissue: apparently primary brain lymphosarcoma could be in effect a localisation of minimal systemic lymphoid neoplasia, either spontaneously healed by immunological processes, or, more prosaically, too small to be found even by the most painstaking autopsy.

REFERENCES

1. HANBERY, J.W., DUGGER, G.S.: Perithelial sarcoma of the brain: a clinico-pathological study of 13 cases. Arch. Neurol. Psych. *71*, 732-761 (1954)
2. RUSSELL, D.S., MARSHALL, A.H.E., SMITH, F.B.: Microgliomatosis: a form of reticulosis affecting the brain. Brain, *71*, 1 - 14 (1948)

 3. ABBOTT, K.H., KERNOHAN, J.W.: Primary sarcomas of the brain. Review of the literature and report of 12 cases. Arch. Neurol. Psych. *50*, 43-66 (1943)
 4. VAN GEHUCHTEN, P., BRUCHER, J.M.: Sarcome cérébral à localisation multiple et à extension périvasculaire diffuse, pouvant donner l'aspect d'une encéphalite. Revue neurol. *102*, 671-680 (1960)
 5. LOSLI, E.J.: Primary intracerebral pleomorphic reticulum cell sarcoma; report of a case. Arch. Path. *1*, 322-328 (1956)
 6. WILLIAMS, J.L, PETERS, H.S.: Malignant reticulosis limited to the central nervous system. J. Neurosurg. *26*, 532-535 (1967)
 7. MAGE, J., SCHERER, H.J.: Tumeur cérébrale parvicellulaire se propageant dans l'espace de Virchow-Robin (la question des sarcomes adventitiels, périvasculaires ou périthéliaux). J. Belge Neurol. Psych. 731-746 (1937)
 8. KÖRNYEY, ST.: Eine sich entlag den Gefäßwandungen ausbreitende Hirngeschwulst (Adventitielles Sarkom). Z. ges. Neurol. Psychiat. *149*, 50-67 (1933)
 9. LE BEAU, J., FONCIN, J.-F., DAUM, S.: Encéphalite granulomateuse aiguë primitive (à propos de deux cas anatomocliniques). Rev. Neurol. *103*, 381-395 (1960)
10. COSTE, F., BRION, S. Etude anatomoclinique d'un cas de péritheliosarcome du système nerveux central. Sem. Hôpitaux, Paris *28*, 3305-3312 (1952)
11. HORVAT, B., PENA, C., FISHER, E.R.: Primary reticulum cell sarcoma (microglioma) of the brain: an electron microscopic study. Arch. Path. *87*, 609-616 (1969)

Additional references may be found in the doctoral dissertation of the junior author: FAUCHER, J.N.: Contribution à l'etude des lymphoreticulosarcomes primitifs du système nerveux central, à propos de neuf cas. Thèse, Université de Paris VI, Fac. Med. Pitié-Salpêtrière, 63 pp., 96 ref. (1974)

J.-F. FONCIN
Laboratoire de Physiologie
et de Psychologie Neurochirurgicales
Ecole Pratique des Hautes Etudes
Hôpital de la Salpêtrière
Paris 13 E
47, Blvd de l'Hôpitel
France

Acta Neuropath. (Berlin), Suppl. VI, 115 - 118 (1975)
© by Springer-Verlag 1975

Microglioma and/or Reticulosarcoma of the Nervous System

M. POLAK

Registro Latinoamerican de Tumores del
Sistema Nervioso, Buenos Aires, Argentina

Summary: 49.microgliomas of nervous parenchyma were studied, all of them with
aniline techniques in part of the material embedded in paraffin, and the rest
with Del Rio Hortega- Polak's technique in frozen sections. It is considered
that the microglia is the representative of the R.E.S. in the nervous tissue,
and is characterised by its cytoplasmic argentophilia. The existence of a non-
argentophilic primitive reticular cell is denied, and it is maintained that
microglioma and reticulosarcoma are synonymous thus refuting the concept of
the existence of a reticulosarcoma consisting of non-argentophilic cells and
a microglioma consisting of argentophilic cells, as different neoplasms.

Key words: Microglioma - Reticulosarcoma - Argentophilia - Microglia

In a number of papers (1, 2, 4) published on different occasions, dealing with
the study of the normal and pathological R.E.S. and its representative in the
nervous system (microglia), we maintained that this system was a true morphological entity. We affirmed that the main and specific characteristic of its
constituent cells, whichever their localization, is the argentophilia they
show when frozen sections are impregnated with a variant of the silver technique
of Del Rio Hortega, modified by us (3).
However, some authors (specifically those who follow Maximow's (5) ideas)
point out that - in particular on the level of the hemopoietic organs - the cells
with nuclei of the type accepted as of reticuloendothelial lineage in sections
stained with routine aniline techniques, surpass in number the argentophilic
ones, and that those non-argentophilic cells in normal as well as in pathologic
material, correspond to those cells called primitive reticular elements by the
previous authors (undifferentiated reticular syncytial cells).
The scientists who follow this author accept the existence of those cells,
interpret them as germinal corpuscles of the reticular tissue and as multipotential elements, that is to say capable of originating connective, hemopoietic and metalophil cells. The latter are not considered by MARSHALL (6)
as being able to differentiate into other cells, except fibroblasts in healing
processes, tuberculosis and in Hodgkin's disease. However in our experience
such situations are not exceptional but occur frequently in many physiological
conditions and pathological processes.
We think also that in numerous situations, only the existence of reticuloendothelial cells can explain the presence of normal and pathological leucocytic nests in non-hemopoietic organs.
We have studied the cells described by MAXIMOW with many techniques simple
and combined, as well as with the silver technique already mentioned and
arrived to the conclusion that those cells correspond to hemocytoblasts and
young lymphoid and myeloid cells, and that the syncytial groups are artefacts
generally produced by paraffin embedding.
FEIGIN (7), employing a modification to Del Rio Hortega's technique for microglia, applicable to material embedded in paraffin, does not confirm the investigations of DEL RIO HORTEGA (8) with regard to the presence of microglial cells

in human brains, since he textually says "we found very few and at time, no
such cells in normal human tissues". FEIGIN considers that the description of
microglial cells in nervous organs of animals is due, besides other things, to
the existence in them of infectious processes. He maintained therefore that the
very small quantity of microglial cells, which exist-according to his investi-
gations- in the nomal nervous tissue, its rapid apparition in great quantities
and its uniform distribution when mobilizing,is related to the existence of a
precursory cell of which the microglial cells, with their characteristic morphology and argentophilia would came from. FEIGIN therefore supports BLOOM and
FAWCET's (9) concept, which is that of MAXIMOW's about the existence of fixed
cells with unlimited mesenchymal potentialities in connective tissue, that would
also be present in the nervous system.

In this manner he agrees with MARSHALL when he defends the existence of the
"primitive reticular cell", and accepts its presence in the central nervous
tissue. The cytoplasm of this cell, according to FEIGIN is not impregnated by
the silver solution, but can be recognized by the small nucleus, moderately
or intensely stained, and stretched or irregular like that of the microglia
in its first stages.

These cells under the influence of different noxae react by proliferating
or acquiring argentophilia (7). They would thus adopt a microglial morphology,
whatever its original shape may have been, to transform themselved later into
macrophages. It seems unwise, says FEIGIN, to use the same word, microglia,
for these precursor cells and also for the stage described by DEL RIO HORTEGA,
since those cells differ in their staining reactions and, what is even more
important, in their cytological characteristics. We prefer, he says, the word
"primitive reticular cell", relating these cells to similar mesenchymal multipotential cells of other organs.

This concept about the existence of two different types of cells of mesenchymal origin in the central nervous tissue is also shared by others (10, 11,
12, 13, 14) who therefore consider that two types of blastomas may originate
from them: the *reticulosarcoma* formed by non-argentophilic cells and the
microglioma formed by cells which are impregnated by the DEL RIO HORTEGA's
silver solution. KERNOHAN and UIHLEIN (12) refering to the sarcomas of R.E.S.,
describe 40 cases which they divide into three sub-groups: 25 reticulosarcomas,
8 Hodgkin sarcomas and 7 microgliomas. The blastomas of the two first sub-groups
consisted of cells of little or no affinity for the silver solution. In their
final comments about the sarcomas of the R.E.S. the authors recognize that in
the majority of the cases they could not carry out the specific silver technique.

RUSSELL and RUBINSTEIN (14) arrive at similar conclusions and although they
point out the difficulties they find in differentiating the reticulosarcomas
from the microgliomas, they conclude by affirming that "the requisite criteria
for the acceptance of reticulum cell sarcomas must be based on the recognised
cytological characters of the reticulum cell, its lack of affinity for silver
and the architecture of its neoplasms". When refering to the microglioma they
say that "their cytoplasm is satisfactorily visualised only with appropiate
silver methods".

We don't share these opinions and we believe that only through the use of
a deficient technique the non-existence of microglia in the human normal nervous
system can be upheld. It is important to bear in mind that at present there is
no technical variant to Del Rio Hortega's method applicable to sections from
material embedded in paraffin and comparable with results obtained on frozen sections be it for the study of the R.E.S. in general or the microglia in particular.

On the other hand it is a well known fact that to obtain good results, Del
Rio Hortega's technique must be applied on each animal species with slight
modifications in time, concentration and type of the mordant. It is not the
same to investigate the microglia in the rat, the mouse, guinea-pig or the
rabbit. The impregnation is easy in the rabbit, it is harder in the others. In
humans it is easier in the newborn and in the child than in the adult. We do not
think that the theory of FEIGIN and others about the action of different noxae

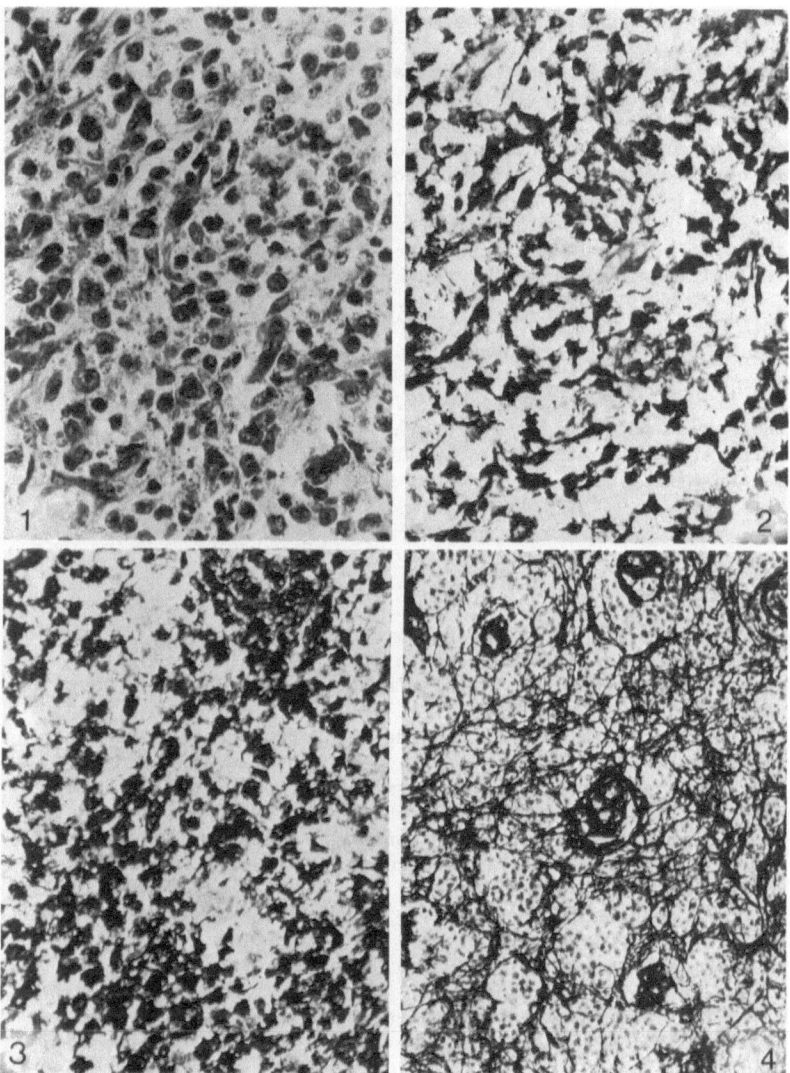

Fig. 1. Cell morphology of a microglioma of the frontal lobe stained with hematoxylin-eosin

Fig. 2. Blastomatous microglia with its characteristic argentophilia (frontal lobe). Del Rio Hortega-Polak's technique

Fig. 3. Argentophilia of blastomatous microglia in a microglioma localized in the brain stem. Del Rio Hortega-Polak's technique

Fig. 4. Distribution of the reticulin fibers in a microglioma of occipital lobe. Del Rio Hortega's technique

transforming the supposed non-argentophilic primitive reticular cells into argentophilic ones is valid according to those observations.

Our studies on normal material make us deny the existence of the non-argentophilic primitive reticular cells of MARSHALL, this view being based on the microscopic analysis of a huge pathologic and normal R.E.S. material observed during more than 30 years.

For similar reasons we don't accept the existence of brain reticulosarcomas (non-argentophilic) and microgliomas (argentophilic), as different blastomatous entities.

All our 49 cases are formed by proliferation of argentophilic cells, which is similar to that observed in the reticulosarcomas originating in different sites of the body (Fig. 1-4). Cases sent to us for consultation with the diagnosis of brain reticulosarcoma behaved in the same way. Others referred with this diagnosis proved to belong in some cases to the neuronal blastomas, and sometimes to neuroglial tumors as demonstrated by appropriate silver techniques.

From what we have said we may draw some conclusions which we find of interest:

1. A non-argentophilic primitive reticular cell does not exist in the central nervous system.
2. The microglia is the representative of the R.E.S. in the nervous system.
3. The reticuloendothelial cells and therefore also the microglia have its fundamental characteristic in the argentophilia of its cytoplasm.
4. Reticulosarcoma and microglioma are synonyms when referring to the blastomas originating from the microglial cells.

REFERENCES

1. POLAK, M.: Consideraciones sobre la histologia de la amigdala, en especial relacion con el s.r.e. Rev. Med. Cienc. afin. 5; 270, 1941
·2. POLAK, M.: Sobre la histopatologia de los microgliomas cerebrales. Arch. de Hist. norm. pat. 5; 41, 1953
3. POLAK, M.: Sobre una variante a la tecnica de Rio Hortega para la impregnacion de celulas. etc. Arch. de Hist. norm. y pat. 6; 220, 1956
4. POLAK, M.: El sistema reticuloendotelial normal. (Entidad morfologica o estado funcional del tejido conjuntivo?) Arch. Fund Roux Ocefa. 3;1, 1969
5. MAXIMOW, A.: Der Lymphocyte als gemeinsame Stammzelle der verschiedenen Blutelemente in der embryonalen Entwicklung und in postfetalen Leben der Säugetiere. Folia Haemat. 8; 125, 1909
6. MARSHALL, A.H.E.: An outline of the Cytology and Pathology of the Reticular Tissue. London: Oliver and Boyd, 1956
7. FEIGIN, I.: Mesenchymal Tissues of the Nervous System (Presidential Adress). J. Neuropath. Exp. Neurol. 28; 6, 1969
8. DEL RIO HORTEGA, P.: Histogenesis y evolucion normal; exodo y distribucion regional de la microglia. Mem. Real Soc. Esp. de Hist. Nat. 11; 213, 1921
9. BLOOM, W., FAWCETT, A.: A textbook of Histology. 8th. ed. W.B. SAUNDERS, Philadelphia, 1962
10. BURSTEIN, S.D., KERNOHAN, J.W., UIHLEIN, A.: Neoplasms of the Reticuloendothelial System of the Brain. Cancer 16; 289, 1963
11. PEIRSON, B., VORIS, D.: Primary Sarcoma of the R.E.S. of the Brain. J. Neurosurg. 23; 630, 1965
12. KERNOHAN, J.W., UIHLEIN, A.: Sarcomas of the Brain. Springfield: Charles C. Thomas, 1962
13. BRAND, M.M., MARINKOVICH, V.A.: Primary malignant Reticulosis of the Brain in Wiskott-Aldrich Syndrome. Arch. Dis. Child. 44; 536, 1969
14. RUSSELL, D., RUBINSTEIN, L.J.: Pathology of Tumours of the Nervous System. 3rd. ed. London: Edward Arnold, 1971

Prof. Dr. Moises POLAK
Registro Latino Americano de tumores del Systema Nervioso
Terrada 1164 BUENOS AIRES, Argentinia

Acta Neuropath. (Berlin), Suppl. VI, 119 - 123 (1975)

The Classification of Microgliomatosis with Particular Reference to Diffuse Microgliomatosis

J. HUME ADAMS

Institute of Neurological Sciences, Glasgow, Scotland

Summary: In 13 of 14 autopsied cases of microgliomatosis, there was macroscopic evidence of tumour in the brain. In 11 of these 13 cases, microscopical examination disclosed many other small foci of microgliomatosis. In the brain which appeared normal macroscopically, there was only diffuse microgliomatosis. This was histologically indistinguishable from that found in the cases with distinct masses of tumour.

Key words: Microgliomatosis - Tumoural Form - Diffuse Type - Reticulum Cell Sarcoma - Lymphoproliferative Disorders

INTRODUCTION

There is a distinctive group of intrinsic tumours in the nervous system that can be classified as being associated with the lymphoreticular system. There has been considerable argument about the nomenclature of this group of tumours (1, 2, 3) but the argument tends to have been one of semantics rather than of any difference in opinion as to the clinical behaviour or basic histological appearances of these tumours. The adoption of the term "reticulum cell sarcoma - microglioma" (RCS-M) by RUBINSTEIN (4) is probably a generally acceptable compromise. The term microgliomatosis has been retained here since in every tumour of the RCS-M group that we have observed, the cytoplasm of a proportion of the tumour cells has impregnated specifically with the NAUOMENKO and FEIGIN (5) technique for demonstrating microglia.

MATERIAL AND METHODS

This report is based on a series of 14 cases with microgliomatosis (Table 1). A full autopsy was undertaken on each case. In 12 of the cases the brain was fixed intact prior to dissection: in 2 only representative parts of the brain were submitted to the Institute for examination. Multiple representative blocks were embedded in paraffin wax and sections stained by a wide variety of techniques. In some cases representative large blocks of brain embedded in celloidin were also examined.

RESULTS

The macroscopic appearance of the brain varied widely (Table 1); in 5 there were solitary fairly well-defined masses (Fig. 1); in 7 there were multiple lesions, some of which showed a remarkable similarity to diffuse astrocytoma (Fig. 2); in 1 there was diffuse softening of both frontal lobes, the abnormal areas being in continuity across the genu of the corpus callosum; and in 1 the brain appeared normal.

Table 1. *Principal Findings in 14 Cases of Microgliomatosis*

Case No.	Sex	Age	Neurological Illness	Brain Macroscopic Appearances	Microscopic Findings Diffuse Changes	Meningeal Tumour	Systemic Lesions
1 (61028)	M	28	3W	Mass in right anterior striatum and pallidum extending into median eminence.	d	-	Lymphosarcoma of stomach 1 yr previously. Deposits in liver, kidneys, adrenal glands.
2 (63011)	M	52	6M	No tumour seen.	D	+	Nil
3 (22/64)	M	73	3W	Moderately well circumscribed mass in hypothalamus (Fig. 1).	d	+	Deposits of lymphoid neoplasm in gastro-intestinal tract and in lymph nodes.
4 (64045)	F	57	5M	Diffuse soft granular tissue in frontal lobes and genu of corpus callosum.	D	+	Nil
5 (201/66)	M	7	3M	Multiple soft granular masses.	D	+	"Subacute leukaemia".
6 (67015)	M	45	3M	Soft granular masses in occipital and parietal lobes and in mid-brain.	d	-	Nil
7 (114/67)	F	57	6W	Mass in cerebellum.	d	+	Nil
8 (103/68)	F	57	17M	Multiple lesions rather like diffuse astrocytoma — cerebrum, cerebellum and brain stem (Fig. 2).	D	+	Nil
9 (68017)	M	58	6M	Mass centred on left putamen	-	-	Nil
10 (68135)	F	66	2W	Deposits of tumour on either side of third ventricle.	-	-	Systematised lymphosarcoma for 20 years.
11 (67318)	F	71	21M	Mass of tumour in right frontal lobe.	D	-	Nil
12 (69170)	M	74	6M	Deposits of tumour in right occipital lobe and in basal ganglia.	d	-	Nil
13 (22/73)	M	68	3W	Deposits of tumour in frontal lobes and in median eminence.	D	+	Malignant lymphoid neoplasm in pharyngeal tonsil.
14 (209/73)	F	32	2M	Deposits of tumour in right temporal lobe and in median eminence.	D	+	Disseminated lymphosarcoma.

Key: W = week; M = month; D = obvious diffuse changes; d = slight diffuse changes.

There was a wide range of histological abnormalities, our experience being virtually identical to that of RUBINSTEIN (4). In the centres of the macroscopically abnormal areas there was densely cellular tumour, the most frequent type being fairly small, round or oval, and containing a slightly twisted or convoluted nucleus with a well-defined nuclear membrane and conspicuous chromatin stippling (Fig. 3). Other cells were larger and more like primitive reticulum cells, and in some cases binucleate or multinucleated types were seen (Fig. 4). Reticulum-like cells predominated in occasional tumours. There were also variable numbers of lymphocytes. Plasma cells were infrequent. In every case the cytoplasm of a proportion of the tumour cells impregnated with silver techniques designed specifically to demonstrate microglia (Fig. 5).

The edge of the tumour mass, or masses, had a particularly characteristic appearance viz. a gradual thinning out of tumour cells except around vessels

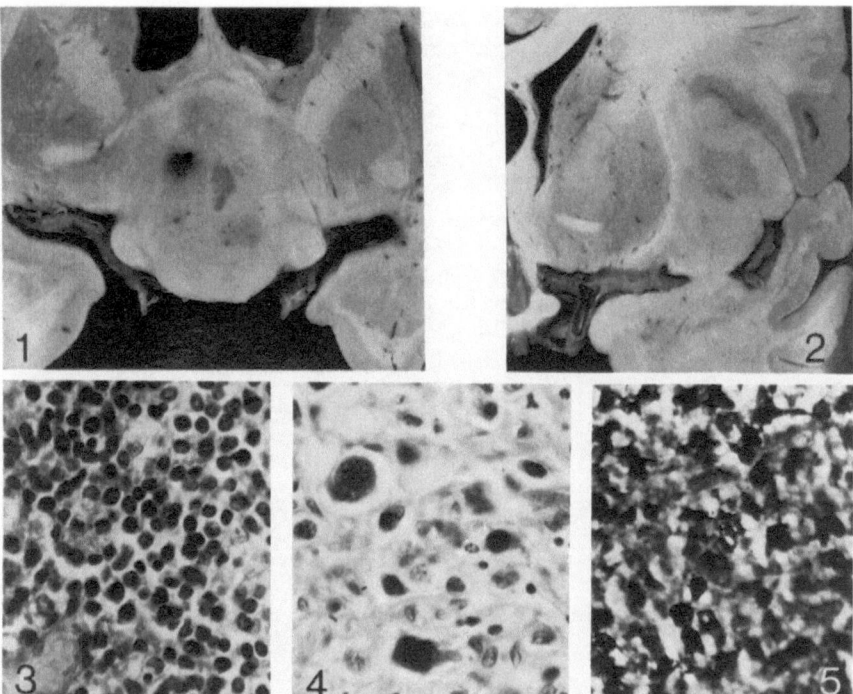

Fig. 1. (Case 3) There is moderately well circumscribed solitary mass of tumour in the hypothalamus

Fig. 2. (Case 8) The cortex of the insula and the adjacent temporal lobe is expanded by pale tumour. Note the loss of demarcation between cortex and white matter

Fig. 3. (Case 7) Centre of main tumour to show small cells with dark and rather convoluted nuclei. Haematoxylin and eosin, x 300

Fig. 4. (Case 12) Note the presence of large binucleate cells. H. and E., x 300

Fig. 5. (Case 3) The cytoplasm of many of the tumour cells has impregnated selectively by the Nauomenko and Feigin technique (5)

where there were accumulations of tumour cells which also infiltrated into the adjacent brain (Fig. 6). These cells showed the same degree of agyrophilia as those in the main tumour masses. There were varying numbers of lymphocytes usually close to the vessel wall, but plasma cells again tended to be infrequent. Large reactive astrocytes were usually prominent. The reticulin pattern was highly distinctive, concentric rings of reticulin enclosing small groups of tumour cells (Fig. 7).

Histological abnormalities identical to those seen around tumour masses were found diffusely throughout the brain in 11 of the 13 cases with obvious macroscopic abnormalities (Table 1) and were the only abnormality in the case in which the brain appeared normal (Fig. 8). In 8 cases there was also local or diffuse infiltration of the subarachnoid space, and in one there was widespread subpial tumour (Fig. 9).

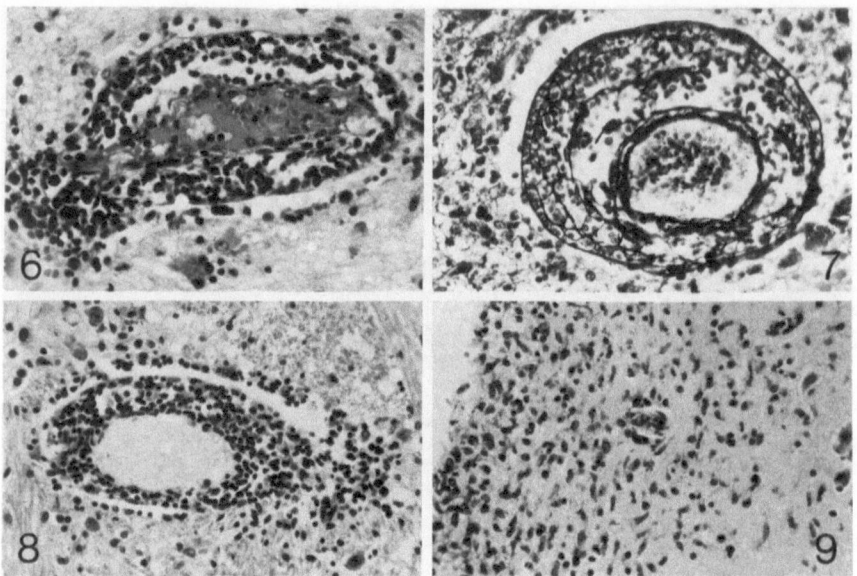

Fig. 6. (Case 1) This vessel adjacent to the main tumour mass is cuffed by lymphocytes and tumour cells. H. and E., x 200

Fig. 7. (Case 4) In this vessel adjacent to the main mass of tumour there is concentric reduplication of reticulin. Reticulin x 200

Fig. 8. (Case 2) Vessel in brain stem from case of diffuse microgliomatosis. Note the tumour cells infiltrating into the perivascular tissue. Compare with Fig. 6. H. and E., x 100

Fig. 9. (Case 14) In this case there was diffuse subpial tumour. H. and E., x 100

In 6 of the 14 cases there were *systemic* lympho-proliferative disorders (Table 1). The histological appearances of the systemic deposits of tumour were not always identical to those in the brain (6), and in only 4 were argyrophilic cells conspicuous in the systemic tumour.

DISCUSSION

One of the most characteristic features of the RCS-M group of tumours is the presence of diffuse changes throughout the brain. Though divorced from an obvious macroscopic lesion, the appearances of these diffuse changes are indistinguishable from the histological abnormalities invariably seen at the edge of a discrete mass of tumour. Even when lymphocytes are numerous around blood vessels, aberrant and primitive microglial cells stream out from the vessels into the adjacent brain. The characteristic reticulin pattern in small vessels is also common to both lesions.

There has been considerable discussion in the past about granulomatous reticulo-histiocytic encephalitis (2, 3, 6). It is not clear to me if this term has been used to describe histological abnormalities identical to those seen in diffuse microgliomatosis. At a purely morphological level, however, there is an entity properly termed diffuse microgliomatosis which cannot be confused with a purely inflammatory process because of the perivascular proliferation of primitive cells' which clearly infiltrate into the adjacent brain tissue. The appearances throughout the brain are identical to those seen around masses of RCS-M tumour, and identical to those seen throughout the brain in the majority of cases with solitary or multicentric masses of RCS-M tumour. Diffuse microgliomatosis should therefore be classified as a malignant process.

REFERENCES

1. KERNOHAN, J.W., UIHLEIN, A.: Sarcomas of the Brain,120-153. Springfield, Illinois: Thomas 1962
2. RUBINSTEIN, L.J.: Microgliomatosis. *In:* ZÜLCH, K.J., WOOLF, A.L. (eds.): Classification of Brain Tumours. Acta Neurochir. Suppl. X, 201-217, 1964
3. ADAMS, J.H., JACKSON, J.M.: Intracerebral tumours of reticular tissue; the problem of microgliomatosis and reticuloendothelial sarcomas of the brain. J. Path. Bact. *91*, 369 - 381, 1966
4. RUBINSTEIN, L.J.: Tumours of the Central Nervous System, 215 - 225. Washington, D.C.: Armed Forces Institute of Pathology, 1972
5. NAOUMENKO, J., FEIGIN, I.: A modification for paraffin sections of silver carbonate impregnation of microglia. Acta Neuropath. (Berl.) *2*, 402 - 406 (1963)
6. ADAMS, J.H.: The various forms of microgliomatosis. *In:* Proc. VIth Inter. Congr. Neuropath., 437 - 438. Paris: Masson et Cie 1970
7. BRUCHER, J.M.: The classification and diagnosis of intracranial sarcomas. *In:* ZÜLCH, K.J., WOOLF, A.L. (eds.): Classification of Brain Tumours. Acta Neurochir. Suppl. X, 190 - 200 (1964)

Prof. Hume ADAMS
Department of Neuropathology
Institute of Neurological Sciences
Southern General Hospital
GLASGOW G 51 4 TF, Scotland

Acta Neuropath. (Berlin), Suppl. VI, 125 - 130 (1975)

Patterns of Proliferation in Cerebral Lymphoreticular Tumours

R.O. BARNARD and T. SCOTT

Maida Vale Hospital for Nervous Diseases,
London W. 9, England

Summary: A study of eighteen cases of primary lymphoreticular tumours in the
brain is described. In four of these there were extraneural lesions and in one
macroglobulinaemia. The use of whole brain sections embedded in celloidin, and
of metallic impregnation methods, revealed certain constant patterns of proliferation. The tumours were diffuse and multicentric; the leptomeninges and
perivascular spaces especially in the subependymal regions were frequently involved. Mature microglia were active both in infiltrated and in apparently
tumour-free regions.

Key words: Lymphoreticular - Microglioma - Subependymal - Perivascular space

Of the 18 cases examined (Table 1) eleven subjects were male and seven female;
the age varied from 37 to 73; and, with one exception (case 12), the duration
of symptoms was less than one year. In four patients small foci of lymphoma
were found in extraneural sites such as lymph node and lung; in one patient
abnormal globulins were present in the serum and in one patient the cerebral
tumour appeared shortly after a renal transplant.

MATERIAL AND METHODS

The brains were sliced in the coronal plan after formalin fixation, and whole
brain slices embedded in celloidin were used as well as paraffin-wax blocks and
frozen sections for metallic impregnations. An extensive microscopical examination was carried out on all parts of the brain.

FINDINGS

In fifteen cases a tumour mass was recognized naked-eye, though only four of
these were of large size (Table 1). In some cases a swollen, congested appearance
with blurring of the normal anatomical structures suggested infiltration; in a
few softening and brown discoloration mimicked infarction. In every case microscopical examination revealed diffuse cerebral infiltration apart from any
localised tumour, though in four cases it was slight.

Despite individual differences certain patterns of proliferation were constant
throughout the series. In the majority of cases tumour cells coated the leptomeninges, but usually only in regions close to underlying infiltration. Widespread leptomeningeal involvement was rare. The most common type of appearance
was for a heavy concentration of cells to distend the perivascular spaces in
the white matter over a certain area, with cuffs of cells extending from the
infiltrated leptomeninges to the cortex via the sleeves of the penetrating
vessels (Fig. 1). The parenchyma away from the vessels was infiltrated diffusely,
and where many affected vessels were packed closely the intervening tissue was

TABLE 1.

Case	Sex	Cerebral symptoms	Diffuse infiltration	Obvious tumour mass	Extraneural lesions
1	58 F	few weeks	++	O	Lymph nodes; lung
2	51 M	few weeks	++	+	Liver; bone marrow
3	54 M	4 months	++	+	Lymph nodes
4	56 M	6 months	++	++	None
5	41 F	few months	+	+	None
6	61 F	2 months	++	+	None
7	39 F	6 weeks	++	++	None
8	56 M	8 weeks	++	++	None
9	73 M	4 weeks	++	O	None
10	57 M	4 months	++	O	None
11	50 M	12 months	++	+	None
12	53 M	6 weeks (5 yr)*	++	+	None
13	40 F	3 weeks	++	+	Lymph node; lung
14	58 M	4 weeks	+	++	None
15	58 M	3 months	++	+	None
16	49 F	3 weeks	+	+	None
17	37 F	6 weeks	+	+++	None (renal transplant case)
18	69 M	4 months	++	+	Macroglobulinaemia

* Spontaneous remission of symptoms 5 years.   Rapid recurrence.

necrotic. This perivascular distribution, characteristic of all cases in the series, was emphasized by the appearance displayed in reticulin impregnations. The affected perivascular spaces were greatly enlarged, and the reticulin fibrils stretched and fragmented by the proliferating cells with the formation of a concentric lamella pattern.

Subependymal localisation was frequent in lesions unrelated to cortex and leptomeninges; in a few the choroid plexus was involved. The corpus callosum and the fornices (Fig. 2), were frequently affected. The posterior parietal white matter around the occipital horn of the lateral ventricle was sometimes the site of a large tumour (Fig. 3) or, more often, contained small aggregates of cells close to the ependyma. Close to the temporal horn, the white matter was infiltrated in some cases. In Case 9 many perivascular spaces bore cuffs of tumour cells, but diffuse infiltration of neural tissue was relatively

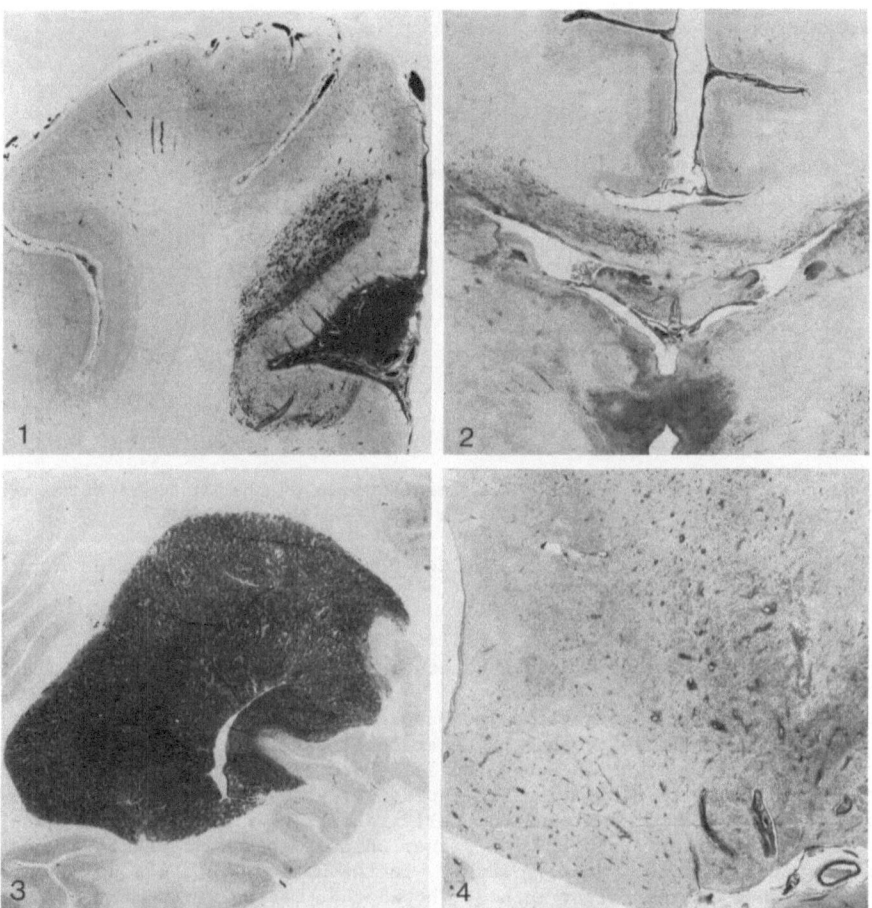

Fig. 1. (Case 2) Focal aggregation of cells in frontal leptomeninges, with cuffing of penetrating cortical vessels and perivascular infiltration of the underlying white matter. Cresyl violet x 3.8

Fig. 2. (Case 1) Infiltration of the corpus callosum, fornix, and subependymal regions of the lateral and third ventricles. The leptomeninges are involved. Cresyl violet x 2.7

Fig. 3. (Case 8) A well-circumscribed dense tumour mass surrounds the occipital horn of the lateral ventricle. The mottled appearance results from necrosis between the cuffs of tumour cells. Cresyl violet x 2.0

Fig. 4. (Case 9) Perivascular infiltration of the central grey matter. Each of the prominent blood vessels has a cuff of neoplastic cells. Cresyl violet x 4.7

sparse (Fig. 4). In the brain-stem the grey matter round the aqueduct and round the fourth ventricle were the commonest sites and Case 8 exemplifies the remarkable symmentry sometimes found (Fig. 5). This mode of distribution, un-like that of any other cerebral tumour, suggests similarity with the original

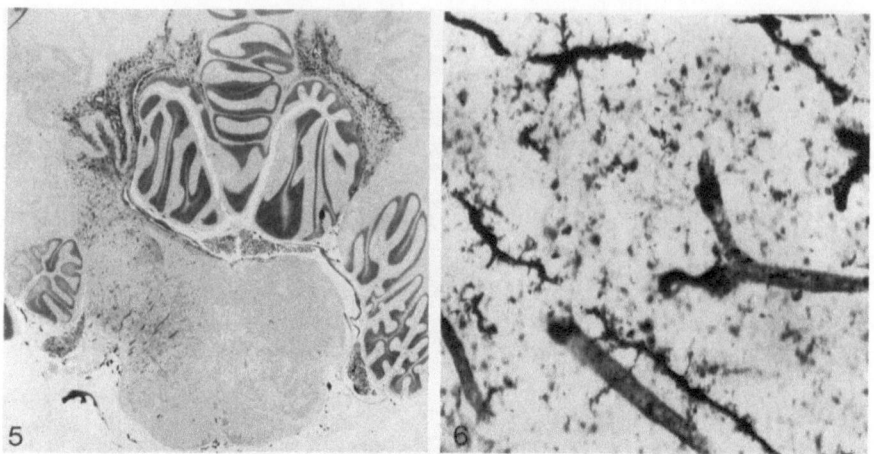

Fig. 5. (Case 8) Symmetrical perivascular infiltration of the white matter around the fourth ventricle. Cresyl violet x 1.9

Fig. 6. (Case 2) Hypertrophic microglia in the cortex remote from obvious neoplasm. Weil-Davenport x 1,200

points of entry of the microglia into the nervous system as described by DEL RIO-HORTEGA (4).

The results of metallic impregnation methods revealed another aspect of the neoplastic process. Primitive lympho-reticular cells usually congregated in the perivascular spaces, with large oval nuclei containing prominent nucleoli, sparse cytoplasm, and with a high mitotic incidence, showed varied degrees of metallophilia: some were not impregnated. Cells resembling microglia more and more closely, and staining strongly with silver salts, were found within the perivascular spaces and, to a greater extent, in the nearby brain tissue. But, remote from the tumour, the silver methods showed that microglia in many places were abnormally numerous and hypertrophic; they tended to elongate, lying parallel with capillary vessels and adopted the rod-cell form. Often, reactive and neoplastic microglial cells tended to merge and no clear distinction was possible. Other cells sometimes present in the infiltrate included lymphocytes, plasma cells and phagocytes laden with Schiff-positive material.

In the majority of cases large astrocytes were conspicuous in the infiltrated regions and often a dense feltwork of fibres surrounded tumour cells. This reaction was often most obvious near the margins of the infiltration where lymphocytic cuffing was also common. These changes, however, were less marked in Case 17, (the transplantation subject).

In addition one case of a cerebral deposit from systemic reticulum-cell sarcoma was examined. The tumour was well circumscribed; the cell type fairly uniform; and there was an overall network of fine reticulin fibrils. It could easily be distinguished from those of the 'primary' group for the perivascular concentration, meningeal involvement, and distant microglial activity were not found.

DISCUSSION

The variety of nomenclature, and the relative importance given by different authors to different pathological features, have confused the recognition of

TABLE 2. *Patterns of Proliferation and Distribution of Lesions*

Cases	Meninges	Perivasc. spaces	Sub-ependy.	Choroid plexus	Brain-stem	Remote microgl.	Astro. reaction	Lymphocytic cuffing
1	+	+	+	O	+	+	+	+
2	+	+	+	O	+	+	+	+
3	+	+	+	O	+	+	+	+
4	+	+	+	O	+	+	+	+
5	L	+	+	+	O	+	+	+
6	+	+	+	O	+	+	+	+
7	+	+	+	O	+	+	+	+
8	+	+	+	O	+	+	+	O
9	+	+	+	?	+	+	+	+
10	+	+	+	O	+	+	+	+
11	+	+	+	+	+	+	+	+
12	+	+	+	O	+	+	+	+
13	+	+	+	O	O	+	+	+
14	L	+	+	O	O	+	O	+
15	O	+	+	O	+	+	+	+
16	+	+	+	O	O	+	S	+
17	+	+	+	O	+	+	S	S
18	+	+	+	+	+	+	+	+

S - Slight   L - Lymphocytes only

cerebral lymphoreticular tumours as an overall group. Certain distinct patterns of proliferation, recognized one after another in published reports over the last five decades, are present in our series (Table 2).

A large tumour may be obvious, but often the naked-eye appearances are somewhat inconclusive and, microscopy may reveal unexpected dense perivascular infiltration (2). A multifocal and diffuse mode of growth, only appreciated in large brain sections, is characteristic (3). In our cases the perivascular spaces were always involved; the meninges frequently; and the subependymal regions, especially close to the genu and splenium of the corpus callosum, were sites of predilection.

Microglial activity with rod-cell formation (1) is conspicuous both at the margins of the neoplasm and in regions of the brain distant from identifiable tumour. Reactive and neoplastic microglia tend to merge, providing excellent examples of 'secondary structures' within the meaning of SCHERER (3) - one of the salient features of tumours derived from cells indigenous to the brain (5).Reactive astrocytic hypertrophy with fibre-formation is frequent and peri-vascular lymphocytic cuffing, common at the periphery of the infiltration, may also be found in the dense tumour masses, where the lymphocytes form an inner ring. In Case 17, (the transplantation subject), lymphocytic and astro-cytic changes were less notable.

The rarity of brain deposits in systemic reticulum cell sarcoma has been noted (6). In the one case that we examined the pathological features could easily be distinguished from those of the 'primary' tumours.

Acknowledgements

Fifteen of the cases described were under the care of the staff of the Maida Vale Hospital for Nervous Diseases to whom we are indebted. We would like to thank Dr. H.C. GRANT (Middlesex Hospital Medical School), Dr. P.D. LEWIS (Royal Postgraduate Medical School) and Professor H. SPENCER (St. Thomas's Hospital Medical School) who allowed us to study the brains of Cases 12, 17 and 18.

REFERENCES

1. AWZEN, A.P.: Du type spécial des tumeurs mésenchymes non muries du système nerveux central. (Un cas de mésoglioblastome). Acta med. Scand., *87*, 470 - 486 (1936)
2. CASSIRER, R., LEWY, F.H.: Zwei Fälle von flachen Hirntumoren. Zschr. Neurol. *61*, 119 - 144 (1920)
3. MAGE, J., SCHERER, H.J.: Tumeur cérébrale parvicellulaire se propageant dans l'espace Virchow-Robin. J. belge, Neurol. Psych., *37*, 731 - 746 (1937)
4. RIO-HORTEGA, P., del: In: Cytology and cellular pathology of the nervous system. Ed. by W. PENFIELD. New York, Paul B. Hoeber, Inc. pp. 483 - 536 (1932)
5. RUBINSTEIN, L.J.: Tumors of the Central Nervous system. Atlas of Tumor Pathology. 2nd series. Fasc. 6 Armed Forces Institute of Pathology (1972)
6. SCHAUMBURG, H.H., PLANK, C.R., ADAMS, R.D.: The reticulum cell sarcoma - microglioma group of brain tumours. A consideration of their clinical features and therapy. Brain, *95*, 199 - 212 (1972)

Dr. R.O. BARNARD
Maida Vale Hospital
London, W. 9 1TL
England

Acta Neuropath. (Berlin), Suppl. VI, 131 - 133 (1975)

„Malignant Lymphoma" of the Brain Following Renal Transplantation

G. KERSTING and J. NEUMANN

Institut für Neuropathologie der Universität Bonn, BRD

Summary: A patient is described who was thought to have developed a malignant lymphoma of the brain after renal transplantation. The correct diagnosis was toxoplasmosis.

Key words: Renal transplantation - Cerebral "Lymphoma" - Granuloma - Toxoplasmosis

Among the numerous reports of generalised or localised malignant lymphomas developing after renal transplantation (5, 6) there have been some cases with lymphomas restricted to the brain. A further case is reported.

CASE REPORT

A 44 year old man suffering from cystonephrosis underwent renal transplantation in February 1972. Immunosuppressive therapy was administered. Three weeks after the operation a transient right-sided hemiparesis accompanied by inflammatory changes in the CSF developed. The tentative diagnosis was virus encephalitis. The condition improved after treatment with gamma globulin and high doses of corticosteroids. The hemiparesis reappeared three month later and remained static until november 1972. The patient then detoriated progressively and developed complete hemiparesis, involvement of the cranial nerves and psychic alterations. The EEG showed a left temporal focus. The echoencephalogram showed a shift to the right. Bilateral arteriography was normal. There was an increase of cells and protein in the CSF. Serological and microbiological examinations were negativ. Other laboratory findings including tests of renal function were normal.

Despite intensive antibiotic and cardiovascular therapy and continuation of immunosuppression, the patient progressively deteriorated and died 10 month after the transplant from respiratory failure.

At autopsy the transplanted kidney showed some oedema and a mild interstitial sclerosing nephritis indicative of mild chronic rejection. Macroscopic examination of the brain showed extensive infarction of the cortex and white matter, within the territory of the left middle artery. In the inferior part of the left putamen there was a granular neoplastic mass of the size of a cherry. Histologic examination revealed a mass of proliferating tissue composed of pleomorphic lymphocytes, plasma cells, reticulohistiocytes and gigant cells, the appearances being identical to many of the previously described malignant lymphomas occurring after renal transplantation and immunosuppressive therapy (Fig. 1 - 4).

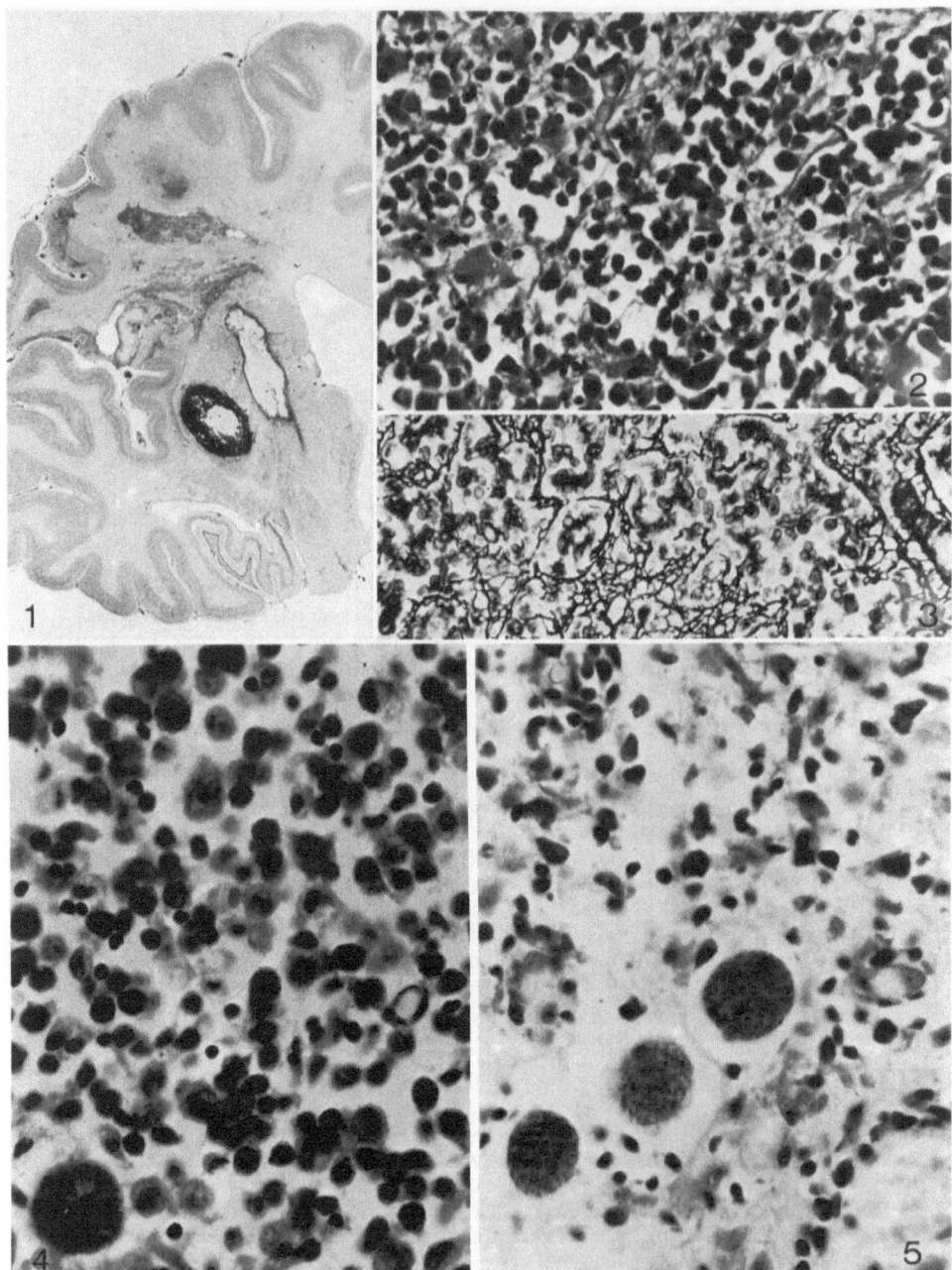

Fig. 1. Cerebral hemisphere with extensive cortical and subcortical infarction within the area of the left middle artery. There is a well circumscribed highly cellular mass with central necrosis in the lower part of the left putamen

Fig. 2. The characteristic histological picture of a so called malignant pleomorphic lymphoma. V. GIESON 200:1

DISCUSSION

The nature of malignant lymphomas after renal transplantation and immunosuppressive therapy remains obscure.

Four different theories are offered to try an interpretation:

1. The formation of the neoplasm might be due to the direct carcinogenic effect of some cytostatic agents used in immunosuppressive therapy.

2. Immunosuppressive therapy itself might result in the activation of oncogenic viruses.

3. Immunosuppressive therapy might result in a lack of surveillance, thus preventing the early elimination of malignant cells which are thought to occur during normal cell division.

None of the theories however, would account for the very high incidence of lymphoproliferative disorders compared with other neoplastic processes.

4. A further possibility is, that the antigenic stimulus of the graft, i.e. the transplanted kidney itself, forces the lymphoreticular tissue into neoplastic transformation.

We would like to suggest that at least some of the isolated malignant lymphomas of the brain which occur after renal transplantation and immunosuppressive therapy are not of neoplastic nature but -as in the present case- might realy be infectious granulomas produced by cerebral toxoplasmosis (Fig. 5).

One must always remember that during intense immunosuppressive therapy, the nervous system may be invaded by a variety of agents which cannot be detected clinically or serologically but which can produce granulomas morphologically very similar to malignant lymphomas. In such cases a thorough histological search for infectious agents is strongly indicated (1, 2, 3, 4).

REFERENCES

1. BARLOTTA, F.M. et al.: Toxoplasmosis, Lymphoma or both? Ann. Intern. Med. 70, 517 - 528 (1969)
2. BOBOWSKI, S.J., REED, W.G.: Toxoplasmosis in an Adult Presenting as a Space-Occupying Lesion. Arch. Path. 65, 460 - 464 (1958)
3. DIEZEL, P.B., SEITELBERGER, F.: Erwachsenen-Toxoplasmose mit produktiv-granulomatöser Enzephalitis vom Charakter einer reaktiven Retikulose. Verh. Ges. Pathol. 37, 270 - 278 (1954)
4. GHATAK, N.R., POON, T.P., ZIMMERMAN, H.M.: Toxoplasmosis of the Central Nervous System in the Adult. Arch. Path. 89, 337 - 348 (1970)
5. PENN, I., STARZEL, T.E.: Malignant Lymphomas in Transplantations. A Review of the World Experience. Int. J. clin. Pharmacol. 3, 49 - 54 (1970)
6. SCHNECK, ST.A., PENN, I.: De-novo Brain Tumors in Renal-Transplant Recipients. Lancet 1, 983 - 986 (1971)

Dr. J. NEUMANN
Institut für Neuropathologie d. Univ.
Annaberger Weg
5800 Bonn-Venusberg, BRD

Fig. 3. Fine network of reticulin fibers surrounding small groups of proliferating cells. GOMORI 200:1

Fig. 4. The different cell types in the proliferating tissue range from small lymphocytes to mono- or multinucleated giant cells. NISSL 360:1

Fig. 5. Masses of toxoplasms in huge pseudocysts from peripheral parts of the granuloma. NISSL 360:1

Acta Neuropath. (Berlin), Suppl. VI, 135 - 140 (1975)

Human and Experimental Reticulum Cell Sarcoma (Microglioma) of the Nervous System [1]

H. CRAVIOTO

Department of Pathology (Neuropathology),
New York University School of Medicine
New York, N.Y. 10016

Summary: The histology and ultrastructure of primary central nervous system
and metastatic (epidural) reticulum cell sarcoma is described. The tumors
showed varying numbers of argyrophilic microglial cells which in all cases
constituted a minority of all tumor cells. A primitive, undifferentiated cell,
common to all tumors, was a small cell with a large dense nucleus and a narrow
rim of poorly structured cytoplasm. These cells frequently showed small fatty
inclusions and were tentatively identified as primitive multipotential cells
from which all other tumor cells develop. It is concluded that reticulum cell
sarcoma of the nervous system (primary or metastatic) and microglioma or
microgliomatosis are one and the same tumor.

Key words: Reticulum Cell Sarcoma - Microglioma - Phagocytes - Central Nervous
System - Ultrastructure

INTRODUCTION

Pial and perivascular histiocytes and free microglial cells can be identified
on brain sections. However, when these cells react to noxious stimulation,
(injury, inflammation, neoplasia) they become histologically indistinguishable
from one another (1-4). It is also known (1, 2) that microglia originates from
pial cells during fetal development.These cells (histiocytes for some authors)
enter the neural parenchyma along pial and choroidal blood vessels and once in
the depths of the brain become microglia. For some investigators (5, 6) reticulum cell sarcoma of the nervous system and microglioma, are two separate
entities. For others (4) they are subgroups of a neoplastic process of reticuloendothelial cells. The dispute as to when a brain tumor is a microglioma
or a reticulum cell sarcoma revolves around the demonstration (or lack of it)
of "metalophilia". According to MARSHALL (7) only the microglia can be impregnated with Hortega's silver carbonate, (metalophilic cells) not the primitive
reticulum cells. Thus, for RUSSELL *et al.* (5) a microglioma is a tumor in which
the metalophilic microglial cells undergo neoplastic proliferation, and a reticulum cell sarcoma a tumor in which primitive cells (non-metalophilic) undergo
neoplastic proliferation.
  Electron microscopic study of these tumors can help to clarify this dispute.
If it can be shown, as apparently our observations do, that the metalophilic
microglial cells, are but a stage in the evolution of primitive cells (reticulum cells), it could be persuasively argued that these tumors are indeed

1 This work was supported in part by USPHS Research Grant CA-10887, and contract
  USPH 43-67-1174 from the U.S. National Cancer Institute and from The New York
  University Neurosurgical Research Fund.

reticulum cell tumors. Ultrastructural studies of these type of tumors have been reported by others (8, 9)

MATERIAL AND METHODS

Two human tumors and one rat tumor, diagnosed as reticulum cell sarcoma were studied.

Case 1. A woman aged 53 entered the hospital with a 3 month history of speech difficulties evolving into aphasia, right hemiparesis and "akinetic mutism". Neurological work-up disclosed a tumor in the left centrum semiovale and the corpus callosum. Part of it was surgically removed. Histologically it was a reticulum cell sarcoma (Figs. 1 - 2). The patient received x-ray therapy and was discharged from the hospital with no evidence of tumor outside the CNS. She was lost to follow-up.

Case 2. A 32 year old man entered the hospital with one month history of low back pain radiating to the thigh, and progressive numbness of the left toes and leg. A myelogram showed a complete block at T_{9-10}. An epidural tumor mass was removed. Histologically this was a reticulum cell sarcoma (Figs. 3 - 4). There was no evidence of tumor elsewhere. The patient received X-ray therapy, was discharged from the hospital and appeared well 6 months after surgery.

Rat experimental tumor (EA-227). A one day old male Long-Evans rat was given an intracerebral injection of ethylnitrosourea (0.15 mg). There were no ill effects following this, and the rat grew and developed well. He died on the 368th day of life. At autopsy a one cm. intracranial, extracerebral tumor mass was found between the tips of the frontal lobes. It was histologically diagnosed as reticulum cell sarcoma. The brain showed in addition an undifferentiated glioma.

HISTOLOGY

With minor variations the two human tumors showed a similar histological appearance (Figs. 1-4). There was a variety of cells intermixed with each other. The majority of the cells were of medium size, with a round, ovoid or irregular nucleus with moderate amount of evenly distributed chromatin, and a small amount of eosinophilic cytoplasm, and no distinct processes. Other cells had a dark round nucleus and were indistinguishable from lymphocytes. Other cells had an eccentric nucleus, and a round or ovoid finely granular or vacuolated cytoplasm; these had the general appearance of phagocytes. Other cells appeared spindle-shaped with relatively long cytoplasmic processes. Mitotic figures were seen here and there. With a silver stain both tumors showed areas where a slight to moderate number of cells appeared metalophilic (Figs. 2 and 4). These cells had a large elongated irregular nucleus, and a moderate amount of cytoplasm, forming short stubby processes, giving to the cell an ameboid appearance. These cells were seen only in some areas of the tumors. Even in the areas where they were found, they constituted a minority of all the cells in those areas. In some places the mediumsized cells, constituted the larger number of

Figs. 1 - 4. Reticulum cell sarcoma. Note preponderance of small and medium sized, round to ovoid cells in H & E stains (1 and 2). Note that the minority of cells are silver positive (metalophilic) cells (2 and 4). Pictures were taken from same areas in adjacent sections from paraffin block. 1 and 3 H & E stain; 2 and 4 silver carbonate stain (NOUMENKO-FEIGIN) Figs. 1 and 2 from Case One, Figs. 3 and 4 from Case two. All pictures x 300

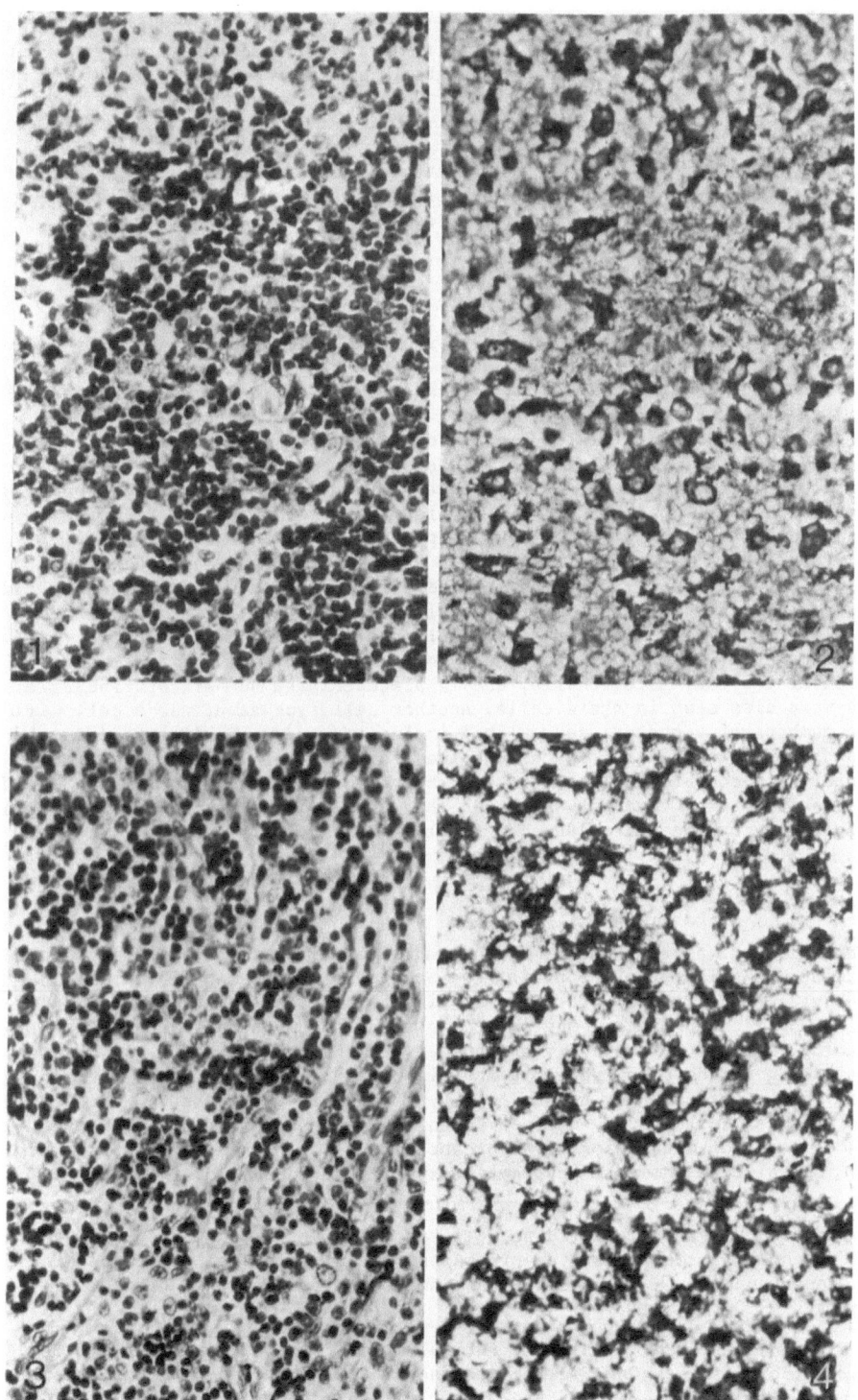

all cells encountered. It was predominantly among these cells where the metalophilic cells were seen. In some places, there was considerable amount of reticulin surrounding blood vessels. Although in some areas there were a few reticulin positive fibers in between tumor cells, for the most part there were none.
In case two there was considerable amount of dense connective tissue forming
septae.

The histology of the rat experimental tumor differed from the human tumors
just described, in that it had a considerable amount of reticulin fibers among
tumor cells, and the silver carbonate stain was negative.

ULTRASTRUCTURE

Fragments of the human tumors only were prepared for electron microscopy.
Several cell types were identified (Figs. 5 and 6). There were small cells
with a round, large, moderately dense nucleus, with some areas of marginated
chromatin; their cytoplasm consisted mostly of RNP-granules, an occasional
mitochondrion, and a profile or two of rough endoplasmic reticulum (RER).
Other cells had a larger, irregularly shaped nucleus, and more abundant cytoplasm; this formed frequently either multiple small processes, and/or one long
broad process. The contents of the cytoplasm were predominantly RNP-granules,
an occasional Golgi complex, a few more profiles of RER, and, regularly, a
few mitochondria. Inclusions, apparently the result of phagocytosed material
were seen frequently in these cells. Other, larger cells, were apparently the
same type of cells as those described, although the cell surface contained
many small processes which were apparently actively phagocytic; their cytoplasm
contained larger amounts of membrane bound inclusions and varying amounts of
well developed RER. Mitochondria, and in places, large numbers of fine filaments were also seen in these cells. Another cell type seen, was a cell with
large numbers of vacuoles, dense lipid inclusions and a highly infolded cell
periphery. The intercellar space contained cellular debris, fine granular
material, and conspicuously, wisps of a heavily osmiophilic fibrillary material
occasionally matted together. Although this material was mostly extracellular,
it apparently originated in some of the larger phagocytic cells.

DISCUSSION

The histological picture of the human tumors described was essentially the same.
One tumor was primary in the brain, the other was extracerebral (epidural). The
histological and ultrastructural similarity favors a common cell origin. The
presence of metalophilic microglial cells in both tumors favors the diagnosis
of microglioma (5, 6). However, the number of metalophilic cells constituted
the minority of the tumor cells in any microscopic field. It would not appear
proper to classify a tumor by the cell type which is the minority. Furthermore,
the microglial cells observed appeared to represent a better differentiated or
advanced stage of maturation of a more primitive cell (the small cells) which
early in evolution showed a phagocytic capacity, evidenced by the formation of

Fig. 5. Primary cerebral reticulum cell sarcoma (Case 1). Major cell types are
illustrated. Small cells with no processes, medium-large cells with several
processes, and cells with vacuoles and inclusions (phagocytes). Electron
micrograph x 3000

Fig. 6. Spinal epidural metastatic reticulum cell sarcoma (case 2). Similar
cells as those of case one Fig. 5, are shown. Note light and black inclusions
and short thin processes in same cells. Electron micrograph x 5000

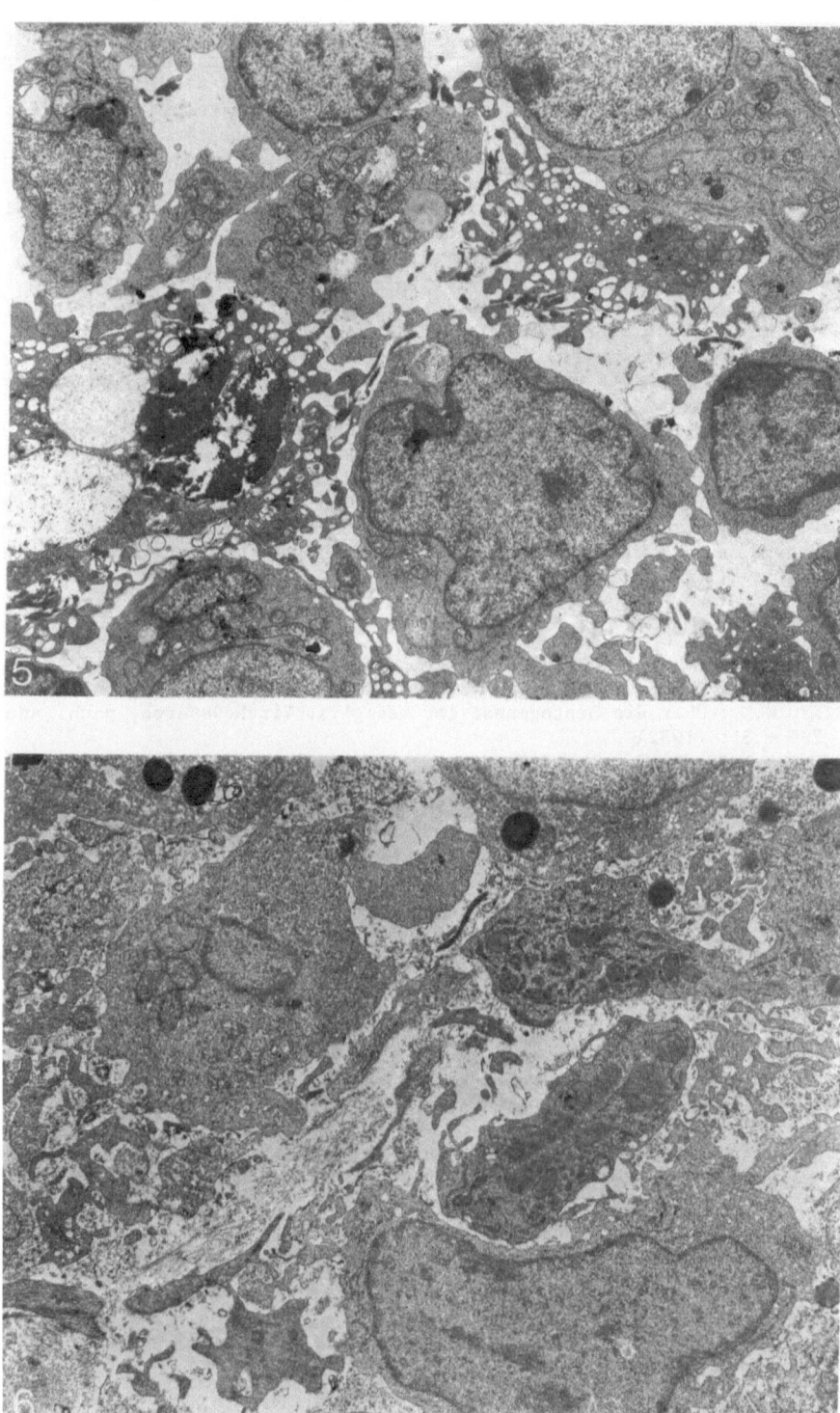

cell processes with engulfed extracellular material. It would be more proper to classify the tumors described by the small more primitive, and potentially more malignant cells observed.

It is reasonable to assume that of the cells found in the tumors the smallest undifferentiated cell is a primitive cell from which all other tumor cells developed. This evolution was characterized by increase in the amount of cytoplasm, development of cytoplasmic organelles, and fundamentally, of phagocytic properties. This satisfies the cytologic criteria for reticuloendothelial cells, especially histiocytes. The name reticulum cell, seems appropriate for these cells. It is unlikely that the highly developed metalophilic microglial cells gave rise to more of the same cells or to the smaller undifferentiated cells. It is more reasonable, that the neoplastic process starts in reticuloendothelial cells (4), some of which may become microglial cells, rather than in highly differentiated microglial cells.

The present study supports the thesis of DUNNING and FURTH (10) which states that microglial cells and histiocytes (Kupffer's cells, reticulum cells of spleen and lymph nodes) are morphologically and functionally identical and constitute a single cell type. It also corroborates the ultrastructural study (8) in which the conclusion is made that microgliomas are tumors derived from reticulum cells. Finally this work tends to substantiate at the ultrastructural level the thesis proposed by FEIGIN (11) of the existence in the brain of primitive mesenchymal multipotential cells from which mesenchymal elements found in pathological states of the nervous system can arise.

REFERENCES

1. DEL RIO HORTEGA, P.: In: PENFIELD, W. (ed.): Cytology and Cellular Pathology of the Nervous System. Vol. 2, p. 483-534. New York: Paul B. Hoeber Inc. 1932
2. BELEZKY, W.K.: Über die Histogenese der Mesoglia. Virchows Arch. path. Anat. 284, 295 - 311 (1932)
3. DOUGHERTY, T.F.: Studies on Cytogenesis of Microglia and their relation to cells of the reticuloendothelial system. Am. J. Anat. 74, 61 - 95 (1944)
4. BURSTEIN, S.D., KERNOHAN, J.W., UIHLEIN, A.: Neoplasms of the Reticuloendothelial system of the brain. Cancer 16, 289 - 305 (1963)
5. RUSSELL, D.S., MARSHALL, A.H.E., SMITH, F.B.: Microgliomatosis: form of reticulosis affecting brain. Brain 71, 1 - 15 (1948)
6. RUSSELL, D.S., RUBINSTEIN, L.J.: Pathology of tumors of the nervous system, p. 66 - 69. London: Edward Arnold 1963
7. MARSHALL, A.H.E.: An Outline of the Cytology and pathology of the reticular tissue. Edinburgh: Oliver and Boyd 1956
8. HORVAT, B., PENA, C., FISHER, E.R.: Primary Reticulum cell sarcoma (microglioma) of brain. An electron microscopic study. Arch. Path. 87, 609 - 616 (1969)
9. VUIA, O., HAGER, H.: Primary Cerebral Blastomatous Reticulosis. Clinical Pathohistological and Ultrastructural Study. J. Neurol. Sci. 19, 407 - 423 (1973)
10. DUNNING, H.S., FURTH, J.: Studies on the relation between microglia histiocytes and monocytes. Am. J. Path. 11, 895 - 913 (1935)
11. FEIGIN, I.: Mesenchymal tissues of the nervous system. The indigenous origin of brain macrophages in hypoxic states and in multiple sclerosis. J. Neuropath. Exp. Neurol. 28, 6 - 24 (1969)

Humberto CRAVIOTO, M.D.
Department of Pathology
(Neuropathology)
N.Y.U. Medical Center
550 First Avenue
New York, N.Y. 10016
USA

Acta Neuropath. (Berlin), Suppl. VI, 141 - 145 (1975)
© by Springer-Verlag 1975

A Comparison of the Fine Structure of Malignant Lymphoma and Other Neoplasms in the Brain

A. HIRANO

Montefiore Hospital and Medical Center
Bronx, New York, U.S.A.

Summary: The fine structure of a primary intracranial lymphoma was examined and compared with that of a group of central nervous system tumors comprised of medulloblastoma, oligodendroglioma, ependymoma and ependymoblastoma. The principal difference was the absence of any junctional devices on the principal tumor cells of the lymphoma and their presence in the other tumors. It is suggested that this difference reflects the difference in origin of these tumors.

Key words: Brain - Electron Microscope - Desmosome - Hemidesmosome - Lymphoma

INTRODUCTION

The fine structural features of intracranial lymphomas have already been studied in some detail (1, 2). Furthermore, the same can be said of various other central nervous system tumors which bear a superficial resemblance to malignant lymphomas, namely medulloblastoma (3, 4), oligodendroglioma (5), ependymoma (5) and ependymoblastoma (6).

The purpose of the present communication is to compare the fine structure of the malignant lymphomas to the latter group and to point out the similarities and differences we consider significant. Special attention will be paid to the junctional specializations, or the lack thereof, of the tumor cells.

MATERIAL AND METHODS

Specimens included a primary malignant lymphoma (2), medulloblastoma (3), oligodendroglioma (5), ependymoma (5) and ependymoblastoma (6). All the tumors examined were obtained by surgical excision. Portions of each were prepared for both optical and electron microscopy.

RESULTS

Optical microscopy revealed the expected histological features associated with the various tumors. The electron microscopic findings were similar to those previously reported (2, 3, 5, 6).

The cells comprising the bulk of the malignant lymphoma were rather closely-packed and displayed a high nucleocytoplasmic ratio. The generally narrow extracellular space usually contained an electron dense fluid. The rounded, scanty cytoplasm contained rather few organelles including scattered mitochondria and a few elongated elements of rough endoplasmic reticulum. Abundant, free ribosomes were present. Despite persistent search, no junctional device could be detected on the surfaces of these cells (Fig. 1). In addition to these primitive-appearing cells, a few phagocytes were found within the mass of the lymphoma. These extended irregular processes among the more common tumor cells and, in general, showed a more well developed organization. In addition, unlike the main tumor cells, hemidesmosomes, sometimes quite large, could often be found at the surfaces of the phagocytes which abutted large, collagen-containing extracellular spaces (Fig. 2).

The other tumors examined all showed a basic similarity to the malignant lymphoma in that they displayed the primitive characteristics of the main tumor cell of the malignant lymphoma. Nevertheless, each retained its own characteristic fine structure (3 - 6). More important, however, was the presence of surface specializations on the tumor cells. Whereas such structures were limited in the malignant lymphoma to the relatively few phagocytic cells, they were found to varying degrees on the predominant cell type in the medullo-blastoma, oligodendroglioma, ependymoma and ependymoblastoma.

The medulloblastoma showed scattered punctate adhesions holding adjacent cells together. The number and size were variable but usually several could be found in a single field (Figs. 3 and 4). Similar attachments, both in type and frequency, were found in the oligodendroglioma. The ependymoma showed significant variations from area to area in this regard. In some regions, few surface attachments could be detected while in other areas scattered punctate adhesions were present, similar to that seen in medulloblastoma and in the oligodendroglioma. Some parts of the ependymoma, however, showed interdigitation and prominent, well-developed junctional complexes, including desmosomes, identical to those seen between adjacent ependymal cells (3, 5). In the ependymoblastoma, intercellular junctions were the most common of all the tumors examined (Figs. 5 and 6). Desmosomes were frequent as well as punctate adhesions and a less well characterized junctional device similar to that found in the developing neural tube.

DISCUSSION

One of the most obvious features of the central nervous system is that most of the cells are fixed and show specific intercellular junctions. Even oligodendroglia display intercellular junctions (7). Thus, the presence of junctional devices on the surface of the tumor cells of medulloblastomas, oligodendrogliomas, ependymomas and ependymoblastomas is not surprising. Evidently, these features are retained after the neoplastic transformation although they may be reduced in quantity and some of their characteristics altered.

On the other hand, the absence of such specialization from the surface of most of the tumor cells of the malignant lymphoma confirm the hypothesis that these tumors derive from either the so-called microglia of an extraneuronal lymphoid cell, both of which are devoid of junctional specializations whether in a resting or reactive state. This inference is further strengthened by

---

Fig. 1. A section through the malignant lymphoma showing the sparse distribution of cytoplasmic organelles, the scanty cytoplasm with many free ribosomes and the dense material filling the extracellular space. Junctional devices are absent. x 13.000

Fig. 2. A phagocytic cell within the malignant lymphoma showing hemidesmosomes (arrow). x 15.000

Figs. 3 and 4. Tumor cells of a medulloblastoma showing large and small junctional devices (arrows). Fig. 3, x 20.000. Fig. 4, x 25.000

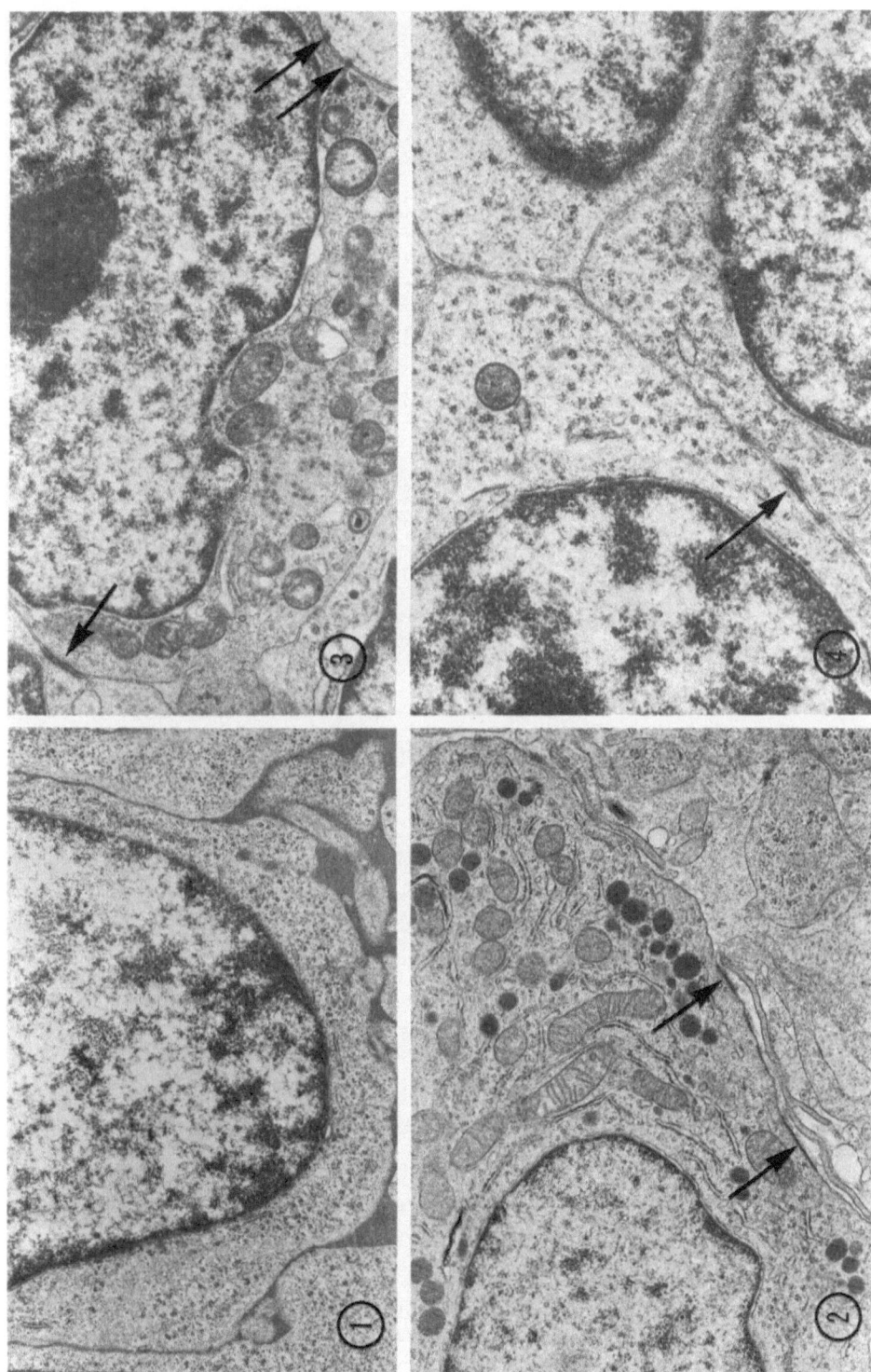

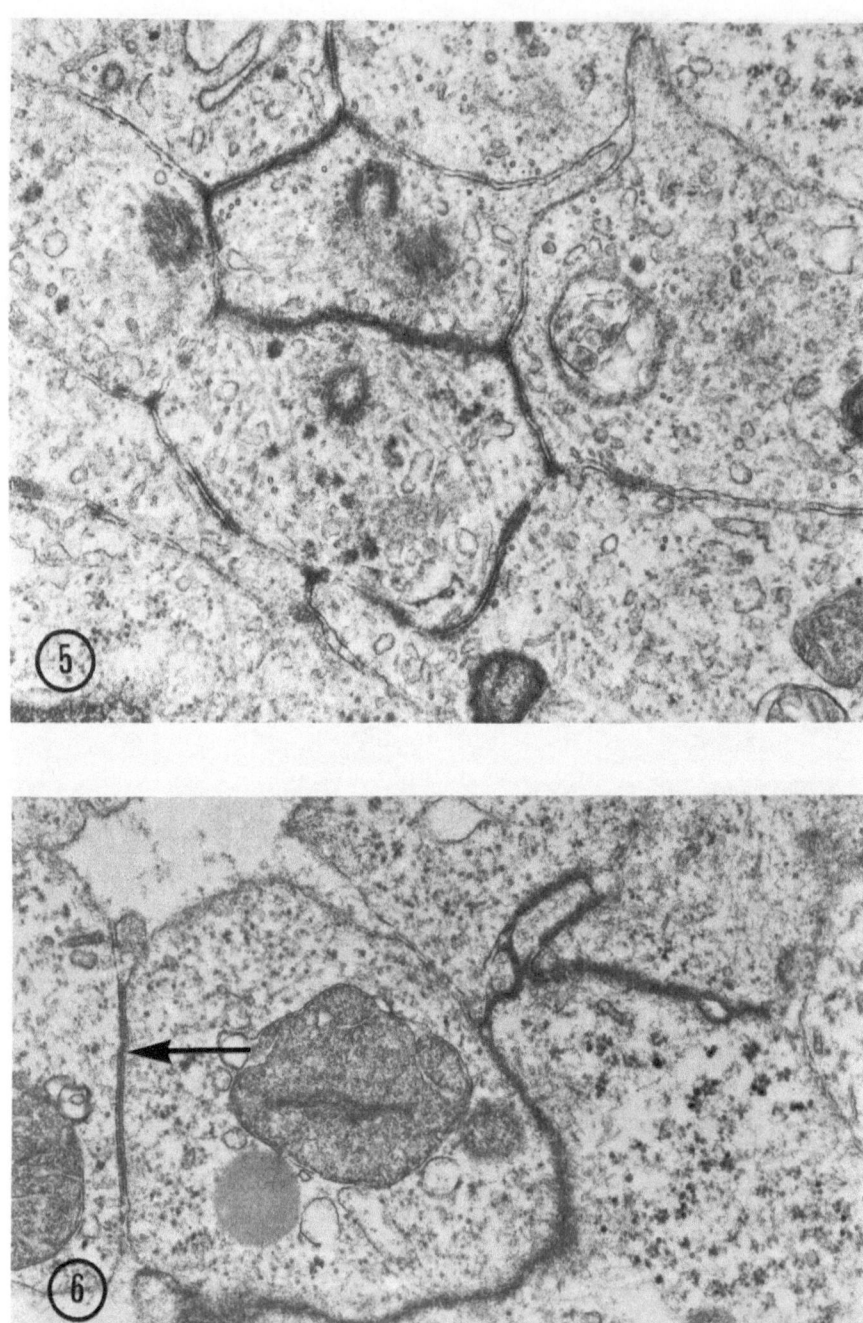

Figs. 5 and 6. Tumor cells of an ependymoblastoma showing a variety of junctional devices including one which is characterized by a dense line between the two apposing plasma membranes (arrows). x 25.000

the observation that even primary intracranial lymphomas are almost identical
to those seen outside the central nervous system (2).

We must now, however, overlook the phagocytic cells of the malignant lymphoma
which do, indeed, bear quite elaborate hemidesmosomes. These presumably are
the counterparts of the reticular cells of normal lymphoid tissue where they
seem to separate the lymphocytes into lobular and where they also show intercellular junctions (8). Such junctions are retained in the reticular elements
of follicular lymphomas in lymph nodes (2, 9).

REFERENCES

1. HORVAT, B., PENA, C., FISHER, E.R.: Primary reticulum cell sarcoma (microglioma) of brain. Arch. Path. *87*, 609 - 616 (1969)
2. HIRANO, A., GHATAK, N.R., BECKER, N.H., ZIMMERMAN, H.M.: A comparison of
   the fine structure of small blood vessels in intracranial and retroperi-
   toneal malignant lymphomas. Acta neuropath. (Berl.) *27*, 93 - 104 (1974)
3. MALAMUD, N., HIRANO, A.: Atlas of Neuropathology, 2nd Ed. Berkeley and
   Los Angeles, University of California Press 1974
4. SOEJIMA, T.: Fine structure of medulloblastoma. Gann *61*, 17 - 26 (1970)
5. POON, T.P., HIRANO, A., ZIMMERMAN, H.M.: Electron microscopic atlas of
   brain tumors. New York: Grune and Stratton 1971
6. HIRANO, A. GHATAK, N.R., ZIMMERMAN, H.M.: The fine structure of ependymoblastoma. J. Neuropath. exp. Neurol. *32*, 144 - 152 (1973)
7. SOTELO, C., ANGAU, P.: The fine structure of the cerebellar central nuclei
   in the cat. I. Neurons and neuroglial cells. Exp. Brain Res. *16*, 410 - 430
   (1973)
8. MOE, R.E.: Fine structure of the reticulum and sinuses of lymph nodes.
   Am. J. Anat. *112*, 311 - 335 (1963)
9. LENNERT, K., NIEDORF, H.R.: Nachweis von desmosomal verknüpften Reticulum-
   zellen im follikulärem Lymphom (Brill-Symmers). Virchows Arch. Abt. B.
   Zellpath. *4*, 148 - 150 (1969)

A. HIRANO, M.D.
Division of Neuropathology
Montefiore Hosp. and Medical Center
111 East 210th Street
BRONX, N.Y. 10467, U.S.A.

Acta Neuropath. (Berlin), Suppl. VI, 147 - 153 (1975)
©by Springer-Verlag 1975

Fine Structure of Primary Reticulum Cell Sarcoma of the Brain

Y. ISHIDA

Department of Pathology
Gunma University School of Medicine, Maebashi, Japan

Summary: An electron microscopic study was made on two cases of reticulum cell
sarcoma (microglioma) of the brain. In both, the tumour was composed of several
type of cells; cells with an undifferentiated appearance and cells with ultrastructural features of the reticulum cell and histiocyte. There seemed to be
no significant difference in the fine structure between the tumour cells in
reticulum cell sarcoma of the brain and extracerebral forms. The ultrastructure
of a lymphosarcoma of the spinal epidural space was also examined and resembles
that of such tumours occurring elsewhere in the body.

Key words: Reticulum cell sarcoma - Microglioma - Electron microscopy - Lymphosarcoma, spinal epidural

In reviewing case reports it seems that various forms of the lymphoreticular
tissue tumours, including reticulum cell sarcoma, lymphosarcoma and the
Hodgkin's disease, among which, however, reticulum cell sarcoma is most common,
may involve primarily the nervous system. Primary reticuloendothelial tissue
tumours of the brain have been described under a variety of names: Perivascular
or perithelial sarcoma, reticulum cell sarcoma and microglioma, because controversy exists as to the origin of this type of tumours. We studied the ultrastructure of two cases of reticulum cell sarcoma of the brain to determine
the kind of cells forming the tumour. Electron microscopic observations were
also made on a lymphosarcoma of the spinal epidural space. Its features were
compared with those of the reticulum cell sarcoma of the brain.

MATERIAL AND METHODS

Surgically excised fresh tumour tissue from two cases of reticulum cell sarcoma
of the brain and a case of lymphosarcoma of the spinal epidural space were
studied. For electron microscopy, specimens were fixed in 2% osmium tetroxide
solution buffered with sodium veronal and acetic acid at pH 7.4 for two hours,
after dehydration the tissues were embedded in epon resin. Sections were cut
on a LKB ultratome, stained with uranyl acetate and lead citrate, and observed
with a JEM 7A electron microscope. For light microscopy paraffine and frozen
sections were made from the formalin-fixed tumour. They were examined with
the following stains: hematoxilin-eosin, Luxol fast Blue, Nissl, Pap silver,
Penfield and Tsujiyama silver, and Oil red O. Epon embedded thick sections
were stained with 0.1% buffered toluidine blue. Cryosections were made from
Case 2 tumour tissue and studied histochemically with NADH and NADPH diapho-
rases, succinic dehydrogenase, and alkaline and acid phosphatase. The patients
clinical data are summarized in Table 1.

Table 1. *Clinicopathological Summary of Cases*

Case No.	Pt. Age and Sex	Location of tumor	Total duration of symptoms before surgery	Therapy	Postoperative course	Histological diagnosis
1	31 yrs. F	Right fronto-parietal lobe (No. 22445)	7 months	Radical surgery X ray	Death 4.5 months	Reticulum cell sarcoma
2	52 yrs. M	Right parietal lobe (No. 28139)	1 year	Radical surgery X ray	Death 9 months Hepatic metastasis at autopsy (No. S 3903)	Reticulum cell sarcoma
3	10 yrs. M	Spinal epidural space from Th 5 to Th 12	2 months	Non-radical surgery, X ray	Death, 2 months Metastasis to paravertebral tissue and cervical lymph nodes at autopsy (No. S 4107)	Lymphosarcoma

RESULTS

1. *Reticulum cell sarcoma of the brain*

Light microscopy: Light microscopic findings were similar in the two cases. The tumour was densely cellular. The dominant cell type was a medium-sized cell with a round to oval nucleus containing relatively pale nucleoplasm and frequent well-defined nucleoli. The reticulin fibers formed a network. In addition to this type of cell dark lymphocyte-like cells, large cells with abundant foamy cytoplasm and those containing phagocytic material were variously intermingled as tumour constituents. Mitotic figures were abundant. The tumour contained also areas with the histology of so-called perivascular sarcoma, where the cells formed thick sleeves around the vessels. On reticulin staining, the fibers formed characteristic perivascular rings. With Penfield and Tsujiyama silver carbonate method for demonstration of microglia, varying proportions of tumour cells showed a positive affinity for silver impregnation. A reactive proliferation of plump astrocytes was marked in areas where the neoplastic cells invaded diffusely the nervous parenchyma. Histochemically, acid phosphatase activity was marked in the neoplastic cells, whereas diaphorase and dehydrogenase activities were demonstrated chiefly in the reactive astrocytes.

Electron microscopy: Electron micrographs showed that the tumour was comprised of cells with varied ultrastructural features.

Some cells appeared undifferentiated (Type 1 cell). The nucleus had an irregular outline with occasional deep indentations. The nuclear-cytoplasmic ratio was high. One or two fairly large nucleoli were demonstrated. A large number of free ribosomes were disseminated throughout the cytoplasm. The cytoplasmic organelles were generally few in number. Only a few mitochondria were seen, unevenly distributed. The Golgi apparatus appeared inconspicuous. In some cells a finely vesicular endoplasmic reticulum was fairy well developed.

Occasional cells were found in contiguity to the intercellular fibrillated matrix (Type 2 cell). This matrix consisted of collagenous fibers and amorphous or filamentous materials. The cytoplasmic membrane of the cells was occasionally deeply indented and the fiber matrix appeared embraced by the cytoplasmic processes.

There were also cells characterized by an ample amount of cytoplasm with an eccentric nucleus (Type 3 cell). The cytoplasm contained a large number of vesicles, vacuoles, lysosomes, and inclusions of diverse internal structures varying from dense granules to myelin figures. Occasional cells were found to include whole cell figures. The Golgi apparatus was prominently displayed.

Electron micrographs taken from Case 1 showed that the tumour contained the additional fourth cell type whose cytoplasm was filled with a multitude of dilated membranous profiles of rough-surfaced variety. They contained dense fibrous material with banded structure. The cells with ultrastructural features of fibroblast, plasma cell and leucocyte were present within the tumour. They were, however, few in number and not of intrinsic value as tumour constituents. In areas where the light microscopy presented perivascular invasion of cells, electron microscopy showed the perivascular space to be packed with cells of similar ultrastructure. This space was, in electron micrographs, bordered internally by the vascular basement membrane and externally by the glial basement membrane. Intervascular neuronal tissue was also the site of neoplastic cell proliferation. They were characterized by a large nucleus with prominent nucleoli or by an abundant cytoplasm filled with a multitude of lysosomes and lysosome-like particles. Fine pseudopodial processes protruded from the cellular membrane of these cells. There were cells with the ultrastructure of an astrocyte. The cytoplasm of these cells was filled with fine glial fibrils. Occasional astrocytic nuclei were found to contain nuclear inclusions. They

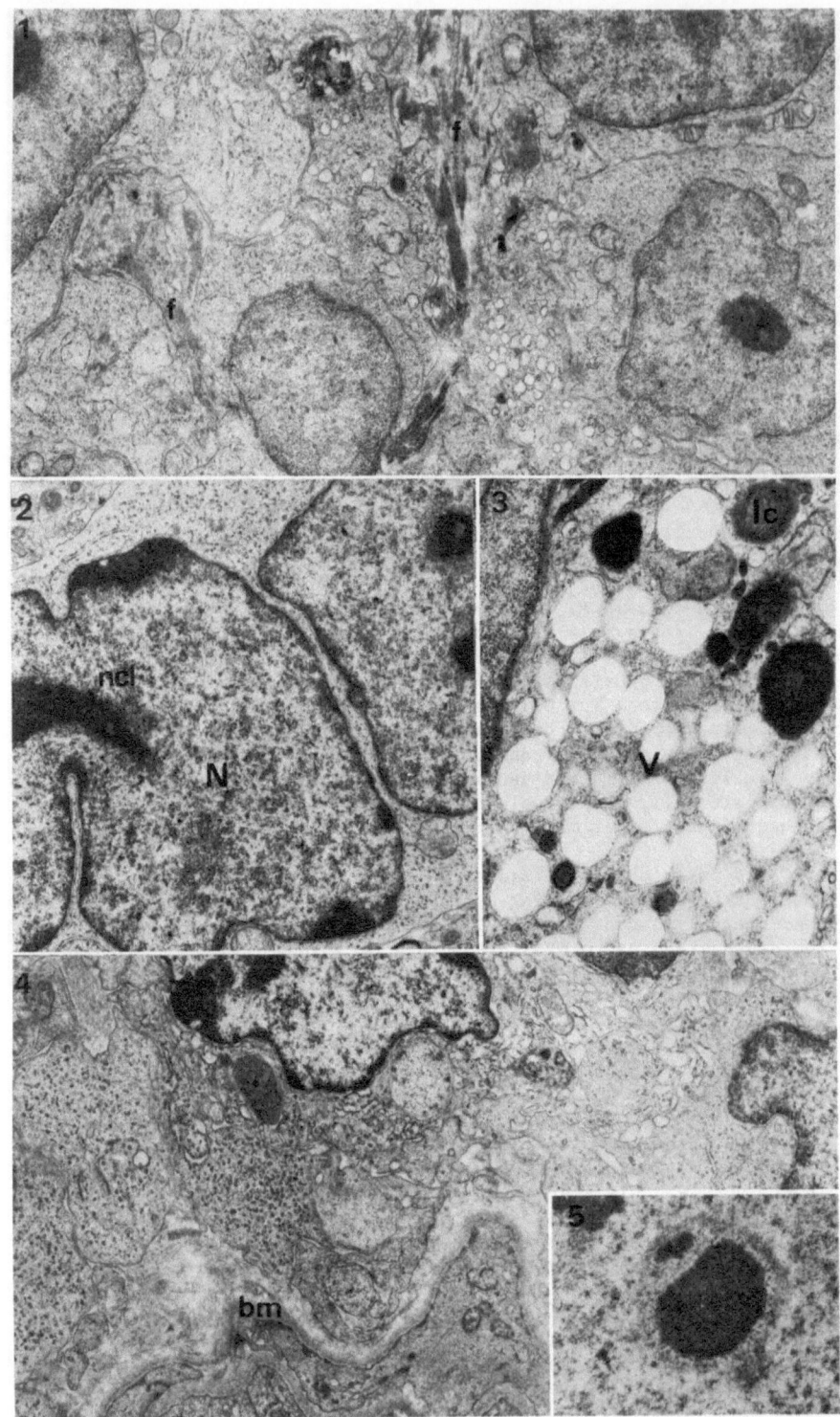

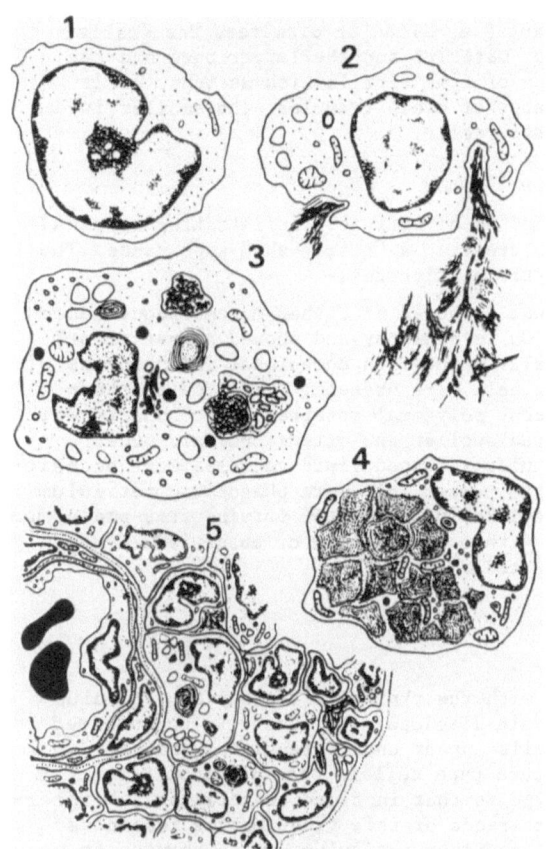

Plate 2: Schematic Representation of Type Cells in Reticulum Cell Sarcoma of the Brain

Fig. 1. Immature or undifferentiated cell type (type 1 cell)

Fig. 2. Reticular cell type (type 2 cell)

Fig. 3. Phagocytic cell type (type 3 cell)

Fig. 4. Type 4 cell

Fig. 5. Neoplastic cells closely packed in the Virchow-Robin space

---

Plate 1:

Fig. 1. Electron micrograph, showing type 1 and 2 cells, and intercellular fibrillated matrix (f). x 4700

Fig. 2. Electron micrograph, showing type 1 cell. The nucleus (N) has an irregular outline with deep indentations. It contains one or two fairly large nucleoli. The cytoplasmic organelles are few in number. x 4900

Fig. 3. Type 3 cell, showing a multitude of vacuoles (V) and inclusions (Ic) in the cytoplasm. x 7100

Fig. 4. Electron micrograph, showing neoplastic cells in the Virchow-Robin space. bm: vascular basement membrane. x 5700

Fig. 5. Electron micrograph, showing a nuclear body. x 6900

were round or ovoid in shape measuring 0.3 - 1.8μ in diameter. The smaller
bodies were made up of fine fibrillar material and the larger ones had the
structure consisting of outer circles of fine fibrils with an inner clear
zone containing occasionally aggregates of dense granules. The smaller inclusions were found also in the neoplastic cells.

2. *Lymphosarcoma of the spinal epidural space*

Light microscopy: This tumor was composed of diffusely infiltrating atypical
lymphoid cells with scattered areas, creating a "starry-sky" appearance. The
clear areas were occupied by phagocytic histiocytes.

Electron microscopy: This neoplasm was composed of rather monomorphous tumor
cells. Most of them measured about 10μ in diameter and showed almost smooth
cell surface. The nuclei were generally round with occasional indentations of
the nuclear membrane. One or two nucleoli were present. The cytoplasm contained abundant ribosomes with frequent polysomal rosettes. Mitochondria were
seen unevenly scattered. They appeared swollen and often abnormal. Other
organelles were inconspicuous. Irregularly shaped lipid vacuoles were occasionally notices. Interspersed amidst the tumour cell were phagocytic reticulum
cells, which contained many lysosome-like inclusions of varying size and composition. A peculiar banded structure with a periodicity of about 1100 Å was
present in the intercellular fibrillated matrix.

DISCUSSION

Electron microscopy of two biopsies with the typical histology of reticulum
cell sarcoma (microglioma) of the brain discloses the tumour to be composed
of several types of cells. Type 1 cells appear undifferentiated and correspond well to that described as immature type cell in the classical reticulum
cell sarcoma (1). The second cell type is that in close association the intercellular fibrillated matrix. The appearance of this fiber matrix resembles
closely that described by MATSUI (1) as fiber reticulum and is thought to be
equivalent to reticulin fibers in light microscopy. The third cell type bears
a close resemblance to that of the histiocyte. Many of the cytoplasmic inclusions are considered to be of lysosomes, since histochemical studies
demonstrate acid phophatase activity in the neoplastic cells. Diverse internal
structures suggest strongly a phagocytic activity in this type of cell. It is
not clear whether the phagocytic type of cells are all tumour cells or not.
Numerous transitional cell forms are, however, present between immature and
phagocytic type cells. It is noteworthy that a peculiar banded structure was
found in the cytoplasm of the tumour constituents of Case 1 and in the intercellular materials of Case 3 tumour, while MONRO and MONGA (2) found similar
structures in their study of connective tissue in pathological lymph nodes.
The nuclear inclusions in occasional neoplastic cells and reactive astrocytes
have similar structure to that described as "nuclear body" in the normal and
pathological lymph node cells (3). As previously noted by HORVAT and others
(4) in their study of the fine structure of reticulum cell sarcoma of the
brain, it would appear that the predominant cells comprising the reticulum
cell sarcoma of the brain exhibit ultrastructural features of the reticulum
cell and histiocyte and that there is no significant difference in the cellular
ultrastructure between the tumour cells in reticulum cell sarcoma of the brain
and those in the extracerebral form of this malignant lymphoma. A lymphosarcoma
of the spinal epidural space was also examined by electron microscopy. Similarities of the cellular ultrastructure are again striking between the tumour cells
in this neoplasm and those described by MORI and LENNERT (5) in their studies
on lymphosarcoma and Burkitt's tumour.

REFERENCES

1. MATSUI, K.: Ultrastructure of reticulum cell sarcoma. In: Proceedings of the IVth international syposium on RES, p. 84 - 93. Kyoto: Nissha 1965
2. MOLLO, F., MONGA, G.: Banded structures in the connective tissue of lymphomas, lymphoadenitis and thymomas. Virchows Arch. Abt. B. Zellpath. *7*, 356 - 366 (1971)
3. BROOKS, R.E., SEEGEL, B.V.: Nuclear bodies of normal and pathological lymph node cells. An electron microscopic study. Blood *29*, 269 - 275 (1967)
4. HORVAT, B., PENA, C., FISHER, E.R.: Primary reticulum cell sarcoma (microglioma) of brain. An electron microscopic study. Arch. Path. *87*, 609 - 616 (1969)
5. MORI, Y., LENNERT, K.: Electron microscopic atlas of lymph node cytology and pathology. Berlin-Heidelberg-New York: Springer 1969

Y. ISHIDA, M.D.
Dept. of Pathology
Gunma University
School of Medicine
3-39-22 Showa Machi
372 Maebashi-Shi
GUNMA - KEN / Japan

Acta Neuropath. (Berlin), Suppl. VI, 155 - 160 (1975)
©by Springer-Verlag 1975

Ultrastructural Study of Two Central Nervous System Lymphomas[1]

P. C. JOHNSON

Department of Pathology
University of Arizona
Arizona Medical Center
Tucson, Arizona, U.S.A.

Summary: Electron microscopy was performed on two CNS lymphomas, one primary
and the second a skull metastasis from a brain primary lymphoma. The former
revealed a tumor perivascularly arranged, which was composed of rounded cells
having no specialized organellae. Biopsies from the primary and metastasis
of the second case revealed a predominance of rounded cells with scanty cytoplasm, another population of cells with phagocytic activity and a third group
with elongated cytoplasmic processes which stain positively for microglia. By
electron microscopy some of these processes resembled neurites or oligodendroglia, while others suggested an astrocytic appearance.

Key words: Central Nervous System - Lymphoma - Electron Microscopy - Microglia

INTRODUCTION

The ultrastructural appearances of only four cerebral lymphomas have been
reported. One report concerned only nuclear morphology (1), another was described in abstract form (2), while the remaining two were more fully documented (3, 4).
  This report concerns the findings in two lymphomas, and emphasizes that the
cytologic diversity of lymphomas of the central nervous system (CNS) parallels
that of the rest of the body. The ultrastructure of the metallophilic cell with
Penfield's method for microglia is defined. Finally, ultrastructural similarity
of the metallophilic cell to known cell types of the brain is discussed.

REPORT OF CASES

Case One: Following an influenza-like illness, a previously healthy 27 year old
man developed persistent headache then had a seizure. Results of physical and
laboratory examinations were normal, but radiographic studies demonstrated a
right temporal lobe mass. After subtotal resection he received radiotherapy and
has returned to work without evidence of recurrence nineteen months later.

Case Two: A 60 year old man was in good health prior to the abrupt onset of
confusion followed two days later by right hemiparesis. Routine laboratory
studies were normal, but an arteriogram revealed a left fronto-parietal mass
which was partially resected. Radiotherapy was given and he slowly deteriorated
over the next 11 months, when skull x-ray demonstrated numerous "punched-out"
lesions resembling those seen with multiple myeloma. One lesion was biopsied.

[1] Work done at the Department of Neuropathology, Massachusetts General Hospital,
Boston. Supported in part by NINDS fellowship NS 2474-01 NSRB

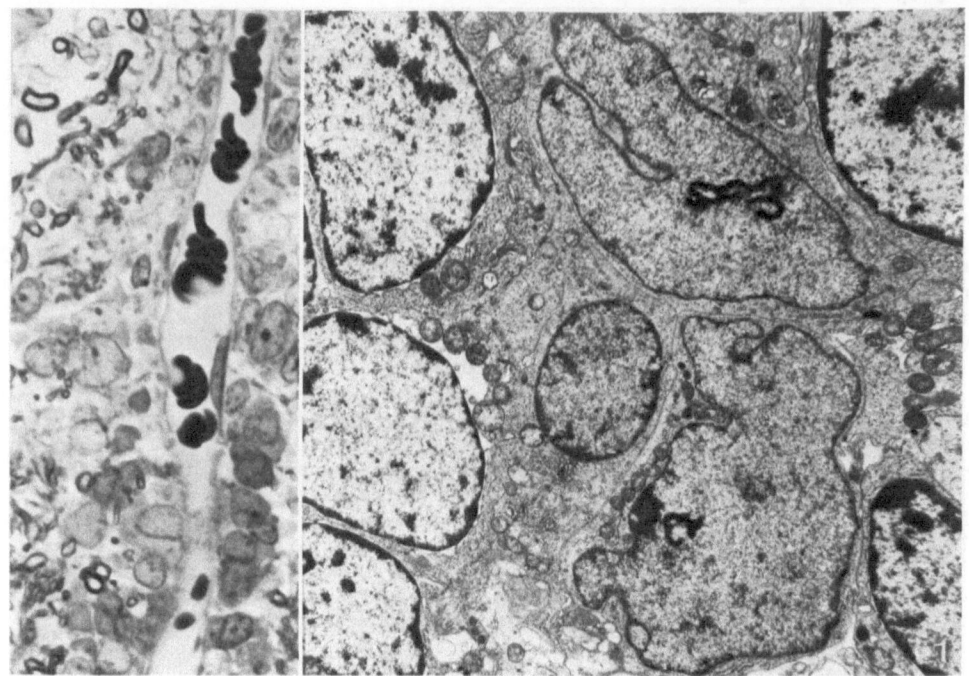

Fig. 1. Case One: A uniform population of tumor cells (insert) encircle a capillary, and invade the immediately adjacent edematous white matter. The nuclei are vesicular and have nucleoli. The cytoplasm is indistinct. Epon semi-thin section, Paragon stain. x 800

Electron micrograph reveals the tumor cells and nuclei to be usually rounded. some have more dense nucleoplasm and nuclear clefts as seen in the upper right. The cytoplasm lacks specialized organelles. Myelinated fibers are evident at the bottom. x 5000

He died three months later. Further dissemination was not documented clinically. Autopsy was not obtained.

MATERIAL AND METHODS

For electron microscopy fresh tissue was briefly fixed in cold phosphate buffered 4 percent glutaraldehyde, dehydrated in alcohol and embedded in Epon 812. Silver-gray thin sections were stained doubly with uranyl acetate and lead citrate.

For light microscopy fresh tissue was fixed in neutral formalin, embedded in paraffin, sectioned and stained with hematoxylin and eosin, cresyl violet, Masson's trichrome, Mallory's phosphotungstic acid hematoxylin, Sweet's reticulin, and Bodian. Portions of wet tissue were frozen sectioned, then stained with Penfield's modification of Hortega's method for microglia.

FINDINGS

Case One: On low magnification the process suggested an encephalitis. Tumor cells had vesicular and somewhat pleomorphic nuclei with inconspicuous cytoplasm (Fig. 1). The reticulin stain and Penfield's method for microglia were negative.

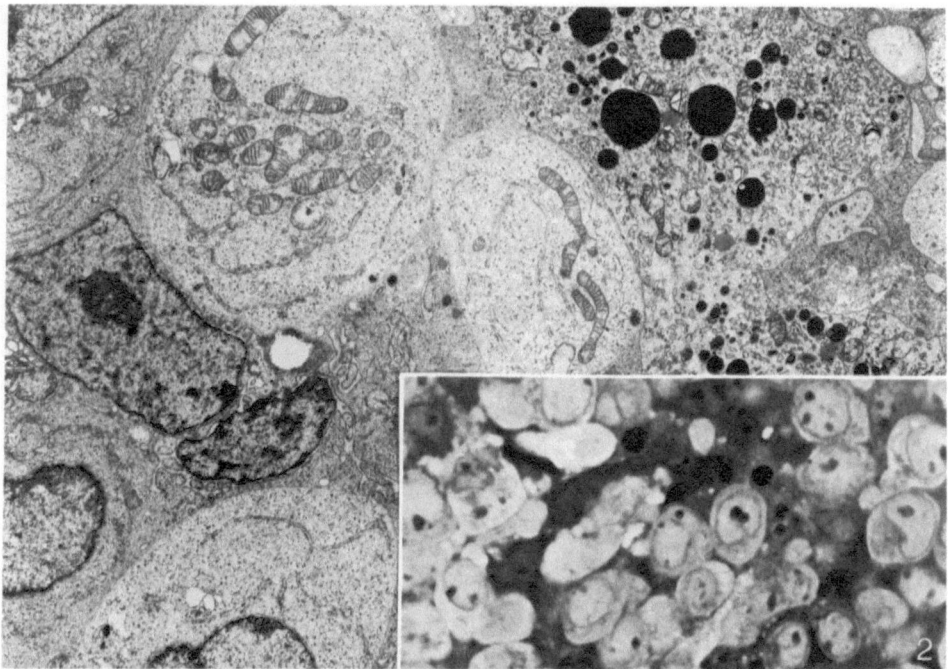

Fig. 2. In semi-thin section (insert), the majority of tumor cells from the
cranial metastasis in Case 2 are undifferentiated and round with vesicular
nuclei and prominent nucleoli. A few cells have cytoplasmic vacuoles and granules, and are classified as phagocytes. A third group of cells have darkly
stained cytoplasm which appears to be ramifying throughout the tumor. Nuclei
are as long and darkly stained. x 800
By electron microscopy three cell types are evident. The undifferentiated type
has lucent cytoplasmic matrix, rounded outline, and contains large plates of
rough ER often arranged concentrically. A. Elongated phagocytic cells are filled
with a variety of organelles including dense bodies, rough ER, and smooth ER.
B. Homogenously of moderate electron density, the branching cells processes
are interspersed throughout. C. An elongated nucleus and dilated rough ER in
the perikaryon are further characteristics of the branched cells at low magnification. x 2450

By electron microscopy (Fig. 1) tumor cells had rounded outlines. Nuclei
were sometimes clefted. Cytoplasmic matrix was moderately dense and embedded
in it were numerous free ribosomes, some rough endoplasmic reticulin (ER) and
scattered microtubules. Many cells were joined by trilaminar tight junctions.
There were not cytoplasmic microfilaments, phagosomes, nor collagen.

Case Two: The primary tumor had a diffuse growth pattern though cells were
concentrated perivascularly. Reticulin stain revealed a lacy perivascular net.
The metastasis had a nodular organization and reticulin was abundant, fine and
fairly diffuse. The two biopsies were cytologically quite similar. Three cell
types were readily distinguished, particularly in semi-thin sectioned material.
The predominant cell was undifferentiated; it was ovoid with clear cytoplasm
and a rounded vesicular nucleus containing prominent and often multiple nucleoli
The second type, phagocytic cells, was marked by abundant cytoplasm containing
granular material. The third group, branching cells, was densely stained with
elongated, arborized processes (Fig. 2). This last group was similar in outline

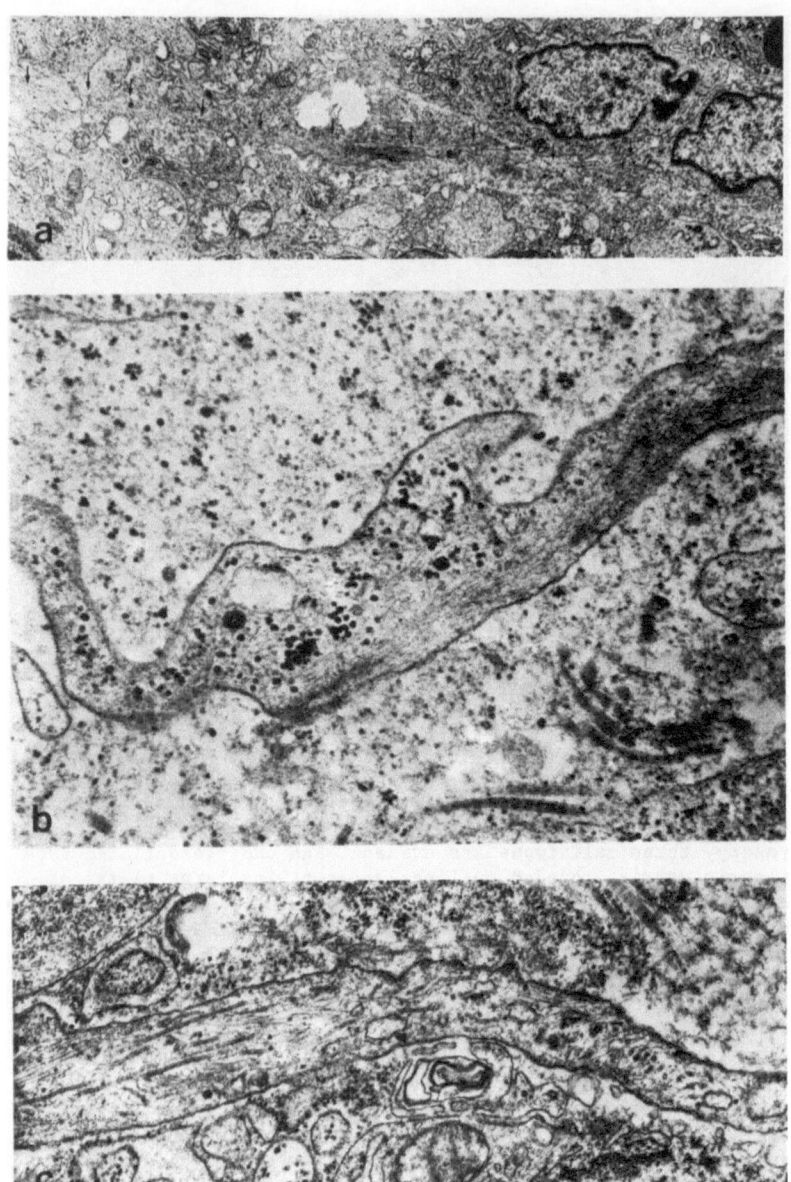

Fig. 3. In **Case** Two (a) the nuclei and two branched cells are on the right. A 35µ thin cytoplasmic process crosses the figure (arrows) giving off short projections. Portions of such processes and collagen are seen in higher magnification in (b) and (c). Filaments and glycogen fill the process in (b), while the one in (c) contains tubules and filaments. Uranyl acetate-lead citrate stain. (a) x 3425, (b) x 26.000, (c) x 28.500

and numbers to cells staining positively with the Penfield method for microglia. Bodian stain impregnated only reticulin fibers.

By electron microscopy the undifferentiated cells had blunt and rounded cytoplasmic processes with lucent matrix containing mitochondria, abundant free ribosomes, and rough ER which was often arranged in concentric circles. The granular material in the phagocytic cells were dense bodies and lysosomes mingled with numerous vesicles of smooth ER, plates of rough ER, and mitochondria. The branching cells were found to have long delicate processes which insinuated themselves throughout the tumor, and were sometimes joined by tight junctions. Their elongated nuclei had large nucleoli and clumped chromatin. The cytoplasmic matrix was variably dense and contained irregular and sometimes dilated cisterns of rough ER, free ribosomes, glycogen, and focal accumulations of microfilaments and tubules. These thin processes (Fig. 3a) resembled those of astrocytes when filaments and glycogen predominated (Fig. 3b). When containing mainly microtubules, the resemblance to unmyelinated axons or oligodendroglial processes was striking (Fig. 3c). Extracellular collagen fibrils were throughout.

DISCUSSION

Two reports (3, 4) have noted cytologically simple cells similar to those of Case One and the undifferentiated cells of Case Two. One point of difference was the presence of tight junctions in Case One, a feature noted to be absent in one case (3), as it was among cells of the undifferentiated group in Case Two. The phagocytic cell of Case Two may be similar to those of a case described but not illustrated (2).

The branched cell in Case Two, impregnated by Penfield's method for microglia, was most likely the extensively branched cell identified by electron microscopy. The resemblance of some processes to those of astrocytes and others to oligodendroglia and unmyelinated axons is noteworthy. One difficulty in ultrastructurally identifying microglia (5) as a distinct cell type in the brain might be explained by their similarity to previously defined cell types. This assumes that the "microglial cell", if it exists, shares ultrastructural features with the metallophilic lymphoma cell. An electron microscopy study of cells stained for microglia (6) revealed no parallel filaments, microtubules or glycogen.

In Case One there appeared to be a diffuse activation or transformation of quite undifferentiated and uniform cells clearly originating around blood vessels. The primary tumor in Case Two seemed to arise from or involve the parenchyma as well as perivascular areas, and was quite pleomorphic. This might imply that the two tumors had different cells of origin, and suggests a perivascular cell of origin for Case One and a parenchymal multipotential cell of origin for Case Two.

REFERENCES

1. TANI, E., AMETANI, T., KAWAMURA, Y., HANDA, H.: Nuclear structures of primary malignant lymphoma in the brain. Cancer 24, 617 - 624 (1969)
2. BLACKBOURNE, B.D., WAGGENER, J.D.: Ultrastructure of a primary cerebral reticuloendothelial sarcoma (microgliomatosis). J. Neuropathol. Exp. Neurol. 26, 141 (1967)
3. HORVAT, B., PENA, C., FISHER, E.R.: Primary reticulum cell sarcoma (microglioma) of brain, an electron microscopic study. Arch. Pathol. 87, 609 - 616 (1969)
4. POON, T.P., HIRANO, A., ZIMMERMAN, H.M.: Electron Microscopic Atlas of Brain Tumors. P. 94 - 97. New York: Grune and Stratton 1971

5. PETERS, A., PALAY, S.L., WEBSTER, H. de F.: The Fine Structure of the
   Nervous System. P. 129 - 130. New York: Harper and Row 1970
6. MORI, S., LE BLOND, C.P.: Identification of microglia in light and electron
   microscopy. J. Comp. Neurol. *135*, 57 - 80 (1969)

P.C. JOHNSON, M.D.
Department of Pathology
University of Arizona
Arizona Medical Center
Tucson, Arizona 85724, U.S.A.

Acta Neuropath. (Berlin), Suppl. VI, 161 - 166 (1975)

Primary Cerebral Reticulosis and Plasma Cell Differentiation

O. VUIA

Institute of Neuropathology
Justus Liebig University
Giessen, F.R.G.

Summary: Cerebral proliferative and tumour forming reticulosis are primary pathologic processes of the brain originating in the perivascular adventitial cell.
   In these conditions this cell can transform into a histiocyte or microglial cell with characters of a macrophage. A reactive cell with endoplasmic reticulum, basement membrane and fibril forming properties, is also present (fibril forming reticular cell). The malignant tumours of the perivascular spaces (cerebral reticulosarcoma) are characterized by the presence of the dedifferentiated cells originating from the intraadventitial cell.
   Under both proliferative and tumour forming conditions this cell may transform into a cell rich in endoplasmic reticulum, sometimes charged with Russell bodies and corresponds morphologically to the protein-forming plasma cell.
   The properties of the intracerebral periadventitial cells are identical with those of the reticulo-histiocytic system described by ASCHOFF. As its structure and the elements into which it differentiates sharply differ from those of the cells belonging to the lymphocyte series the term malignant lymphoma of the brain given to these processes does not correspond to the fundamental characters of these pathological process.

Key words: Reticulosis - Reticulosarcoma - Brain Tumour - Electron Microscopy - Plasmacyte - Russell bodies

Primary, proliferative and tumour forming reticuloses of the brain are pathological processes which start in the cerebral perivascular adventitial cell.
   The ultrastructure study of this perivascular, intra-adventitial cell of the brain, under pathological, reactive, proliferative and tumour forming conditions is the subject of this paper.

MATERIAL AND METHODS

The material consisted of 1 case of primary, proliferative reticulosis, 2 of tumour forming reticulosis (reticulosarcoma) and 12 of perivascular reactive processes of the brain.
   In all cases the material was fixed in glutaraldehyde, postfixed in osmium tetroxide, contrasted with uranyl acetate, and embedded in Epon. Thin and semithin sections were cut in a Reichert mictrotome, the latter sections being stained with paraphenylendiamine.

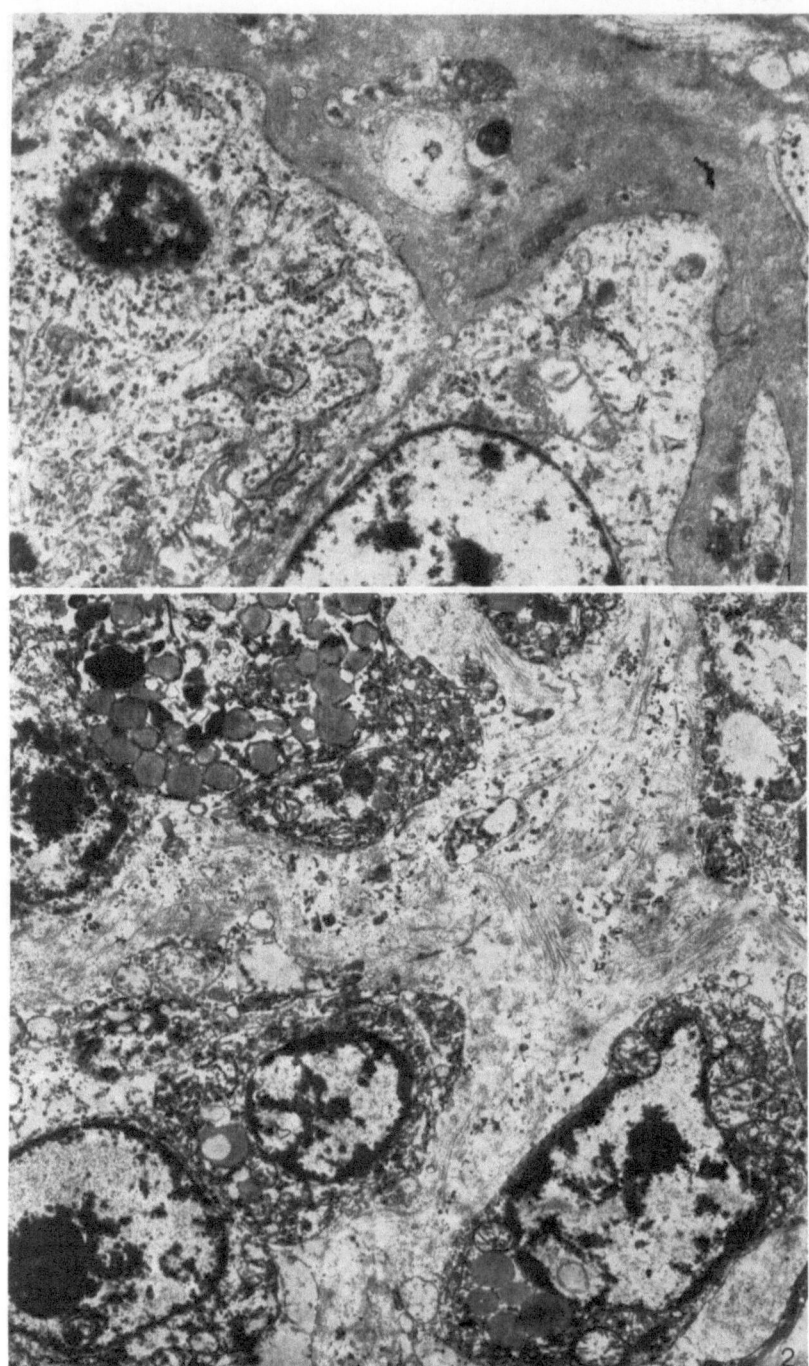

RESULTS

The perivascular cell has an oval nucleus, rich in peripherally arranged
chromatin and cytoplasm containing vesicles, osmiophilic granules, ribosomes
and numerous lipofuscin granules. A particular intraadventitial reactive cell
appears rich in endoplasmic reticulum, in the cisternae of which can be seen
amorphous material of the basement membrane type and sometimes of the microfibrillary type. The relationship of this cell with the basement membrane is
obvious: it secretes the material of the basement membrane that delimits the
outer perivascular space, as well as fibrils of the reticulin type (Fig. 1).
Structurally, this cell resembles the endothelial cell and the fibroblast
(having the same secretory properties), but differs in its cellular characters.
The ultrastructural aspect corresponds to the fibril-forming reticular cell (1).
    In malignant tumour processes of perivascular origin this periadventitial
cell is dedifferentiated:
    its cytoplasm is rich in ribosomes and mitochondria. This cell corresponds
in the light microscope to the cell with a clear nucleus and one or more
nucleoli.
    Under both proliferative and tumour forming conditions (cerebral reticulo-
sarcoma) the perivascular, intraadventitial cell shows a tendency to undergo
transformation into a histiocyte, a cell whose cytoplasm is rich in vesicles
and lysosomes and has macrophage activity (Fig. 2). Some elongated cells with
fine processes correspond to the microglia with a macrophage activity.
    A particular feature is the transformation into a cell rich in endoplasmic
reticulum in whose dilated cisternae osmiophil bodies of the Russell body type
appear, and corresponds to the protein-forming plasma cell and sometimes to
the Mott cell. These features were observed both in the proliferative and in
the tumour forming processes (Fig. 3 - 5).
    In the proliferative processes, the plasma cell character and development
into the Mott type of cell, cannot be questioned. In tumour forming processes
this type of cell exhibits undifferentiated features, which correspond to the
plasma cell (2).
    The bone marrow and blood forming organs in our cases did not reveal any
pathological proliferation or the presence of plasma cells.

DISCUSSION

The perivascular, intraadventitial cell which MARCHAND (3) considered as an
element of the embryonic mesenchyma, appears to be a cell with active cytoplasmic properties, corresponding in the light microscope to an elongated,
histioid cell described in normal histology.
    The non-metallophil cell with a clear nucleus and one or more nucleoli,
observed in the light microscope, does not correspond to the normal reticulo-
histiocytic cell of the brain, but represents the dedifferentiated cell of
this system in perivascular malignant tumours.
    This is of particular importance, since this cell is considered as a normal
component of the brain, and the primary malignant reticulosarcomas of the
brain were for a long time interpreted as encephalitic processes.

Fig. 1. An intraadventitial cell of the perivascular space is delimited by an
outer basement membrane and presents a nucleus poor in chromatin and cytoplasm
with a well developed endoplasmic reticulum. x 9.000

Fig. 2. Malignant, proliferated cells showing a tendency towards macrophagia.
In the extracellular space dense microfibrillary proliferation is present.
x 9.000

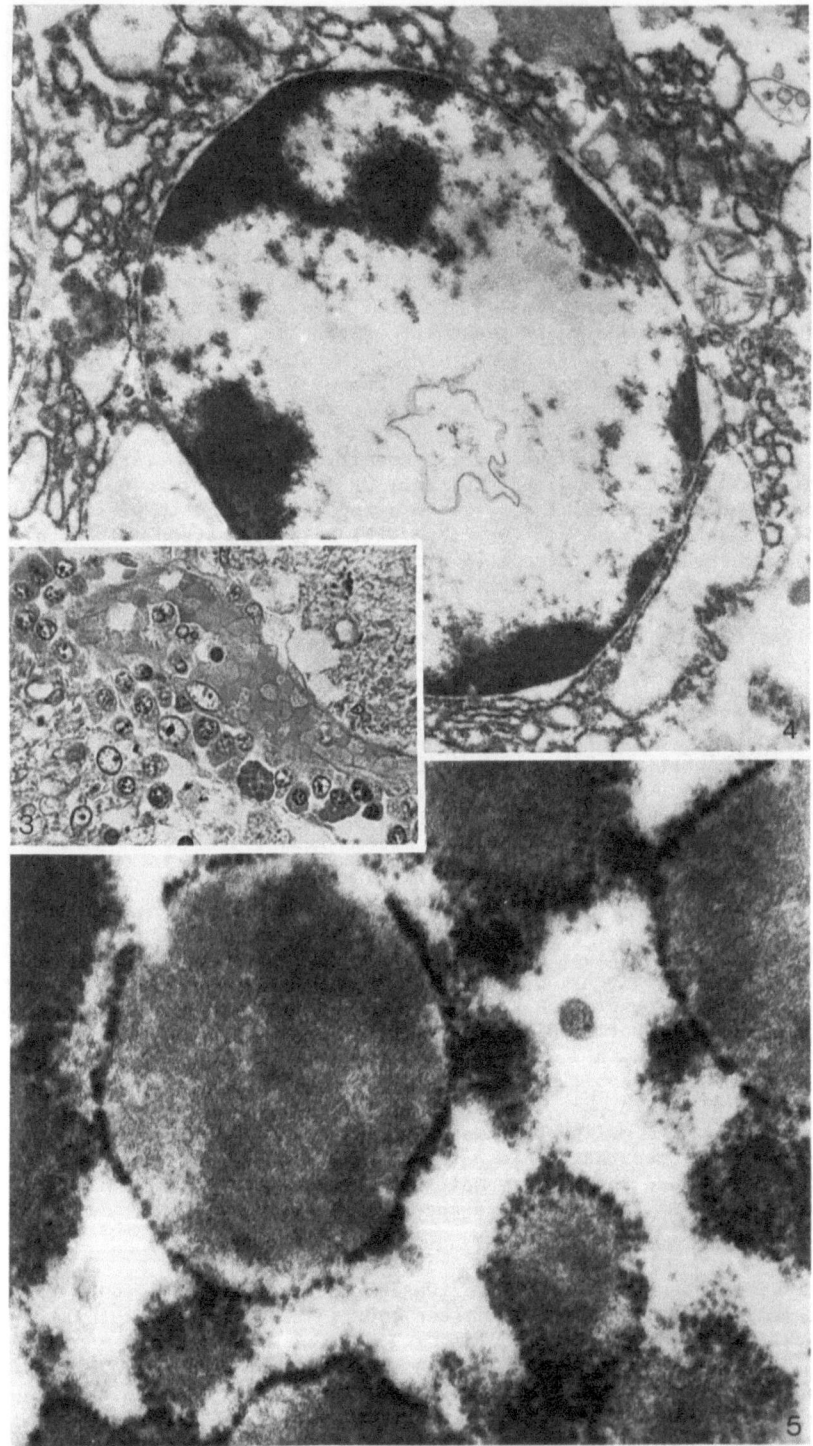

Under pathological conditions differentiation of the perivascular adventitial cell toward a cell with characters of a plasma cell lends support to the protein-forming property that may be exhibited by proliferative or tumour products originating perivascularly and has been reported by several authors (4, 5, 6, 7).

Our findings are consistent with the data published by various authors (8, 9) who describe the existence of the primary intracerebral plasmacytoma and therefore the possible production of plasma cells under local, intracerebral pathological conditions (10). Electrophoretic studies (11, 12) demonstrated the existence of pathological proteins in the cerebrospinal fluid that do not exist in the serum, suggesting that these proteins are a local product in the central nervous system.

In summary the perivascular, intraadventitial cell of the brain, appears to be cell-forming (histiocyte, microglia), defensive (macrophage) and protein-forming; the characteristics of the reticulohistiocyte system described by ASCHOFF (13). The primary pathological products of this system may be designated as reticuloses (14, 15) reticulosarcomas (16), or reticulohistiomicrogliomatoses (17, 18).

From the study of the cells that are responsible for this pathological production, cells which differ sharply from cells of the lymphocytic series, we consider that the term primary malignant lymphomas of the brain (19) does not correspond to the fundamental character of this disease, which starts in the perivascular adventitial mesenchyme cells.

REFERENCES

1. DAVID, H.: Elektronenmikroskopische Organpathologie, p. 423. Berlin: VEB-Verlag, 1967
2. VUIA, O., HAGER, H.: Primary Cerebral Blastomatous Reticulosis. Clinical, Pathological and Ultrastructural Study. J. neurol. Sci. *19*, 407 - 423 (1973)
3. MARCHAND, F.: Referat über die Herkunft der Lymphozyten und ihre Schicksale bei der Entzündung. Verh. dtsch. path. Ges. *16*, 5 - 81 (1953)
4. DRAGANESCU, St., VUIA, O.: Neuroreticuloses. Acta Neuropath. (Berl.) *4*, 669 - 682 (1965)
5. HORVAT, B., PENA, C., FISHER, E.R.: Primary Reticulum cell Sarcoma (Microglioma) of the brain. Arch. Path. *87*, 609 - 616 (1969)
6. CONSTANTINIDIS, J., ESCOUROLLE, R.: Réticulose pallido-pedonculaire bilatérale et nécrosante. Arch. Suisse Neurol. Neurochir. Psychiat. *106*, 223 (1970)
7. VUIA, O., MEHRAIEN, P.: Cerebral reticuloplasmacytosis with hyperglobulinemia. Europ. Neurol. *7*, 155 - 168 (1972)
8. FRENCH, J.D.: Plasmacytoma of the Hypothalamus. J. Neuropath. Exp. Neurol. *6*, 265 - 270 (1947)

Fig. 3. The perivascular cells consists almost entirely of plasma cells, whose cytoplasm is filled with numerous small acidophilic globules (Russell bodies) (Phase contrast x 100)

Fig. 4. A plasma cell from the perivascular cell shows well developed rough endoplasmic reticulum and marginal nuclear chromatin; a central intranuclear vacuole can be seen. x 9.000

Fig. 5. In the dilated cisternae of the endoplasmic reticulum of a plasma cell osmiophil bodies may be seen (Russell bodies)(Case: cerebral reticulosis with plasma cell differentiation) x 18.000

9. MOOSY, J., WILSON, C.L.B.: Solitary Intracranial Plasmacytoma. Arch. Neurol. *16*, 212 - 216 (1967)
10. HAGER, H.: Ultrastrukturelle Befunde zur Zytopathologie der Entzündung im Zentralnervensystem. Z. allg. Path. 115, 619 (1970)
11. WEINER, L.P., ANDERSON, P.N., ALLEN, J.C.: Cerebral plasmacytoma with myeloma protein in the cerebrospinal fluid. Neurology (Minneap.) *16*, 615 - 618 (1966)
12. CUTLER, R.W., TOURTELOTTE, W.W.: Synthesis of gammaglobulin inside the blood-brain barrier in subacute sclerosing panencephalitis. Riv. pat. nerv. ment. *92*, 163 - 170 (1971)
13. ASCHOFF, L.: Morphologie des retikulo-endothelialen Systems. In Schittenhelm: Handbuch der Krankheiten des Blutes und der blutbildenden Organe. Bd. 2, p. 473, Berlin: Springer 1925
14. RUSSEL, D.S., MARSHALL, A.H.E., SMITH, F.B.: Microgliomatosis Brain *71*, 1 - 16 (1948)
15. VUIA, O., MEHRAIEN, P.: Primary Reticulosis of the Central Nervous System. J. neurol. Sci. *14*, 469 - 482 (1971)
16. KERNOHAN, J.W., UIHLEIN, A.: Sarcomas of the Brain. Springfield, Ill.: Thomas 1962
17. PAPILIAN, V.V., VUIA, O., SERBAN, M., NAGY, I.: Primary Reticulo-histio- microglioblastomas of the Central Nervous System. Stud. Cerc. Neurol. *7*, 183 - 192 (1962)
18. VUIA, O.: Das solitäre und multifokale polymorphe Granulom im Nervensystem. Arch. Psychiat. Neurol. *208*, 309 - 325 (1966)
19. POON, P.S., HIRANO, A., ZIMMERMAN, H.M.: Electron Microscopic Atlas of the brain Tumours, p. 94. New York, London: Grune & Stratton 1971

O. VUIA, M.D.
Institute of Neuropathology
Justus Liebig University
Arndtstraße 16
D - 63 Gießen, BRD

Acta Neuropath. (Berlin), Suppl. VI, 167 - 171 (1975)
© by Springer-Verlag 1975

Nuclear Characteristics of Malignant Lymphoma in the Brain

EIICHI TANI and TOSHIO AMETANI

Department of Neurosurgery
Hyogo College of Medicine
Nishinomiya, Hyogo, Japan

Summary: In addition to chromatin and nucleoli, various classes of structures were often seen in nuclei of malignant lymphoma, when compared with other brain tumours. Interchromatin, perichromatin, and atypical dense granules could be ribonucleoprotein in nature on basis of their behaviours in enzymatic extraction and EDTA stain. The perichromatin fibrils became visible at the border of the condensed chromatin only after EDTA stain and might contain substrate for HnRNA. Nuclear bodies and intranuclear fibrillar rodlets also were evident.

Key words: Interchromatin Granules - Perichromatin Granules - Atypical Dense Granules - Perichromatin Fibrils

Intranuclear ribonucleoprotein structures are still poorly understood except the nucleolus. The malignant lymphoma characteristically demonstrated various extranucleolar ribonucleoprotein structures (1). In addition to the classical double fixation and double staining, enzymatic extraction and chelating agent were used to define extranucleolar ribonucleoprotein components in nuclei.

MATERIALS AND METHODS

Specimen was taken at surgery from an intracerebral tumour in the left parieto-temporal region and histologically a malignant lymphoma (1). No treatment with irradiation or anticancer drugs was performed. The surgical specimens were examined with HU-11 A electron microscope after a conventional procedure for thin sectioning (1).

For enzyme studies, 10 - 15 μ thick frozen sections of formalin-fixed specimen were extracted in RNAase, DNAase, or pepsin solution at 37°C for 1 hour, rinsed in cold 5% trichloroacetic acid for 5 minutes and fixed in 1% OsO_4 (pH 7.4) for 1 hour (1).

For EDTA staining (2), the formalin-fixed specimens were embedded in Epon. The section was floated for 1 minute on a 5% aqueous solution of uranyl acetate; rinsed with distilled water; floated on 0.2 M EDTA solution, pH 7.4, for 20 - 30 minutes; rinsed, then poststained with lead citrate for 1 minute.

RESULTS

The nuclei of malignant lymphoma were usually irregularly round or ovoid in shape. The chromatin was often marginated along the nuclear membrane and sometimes irregularly distributed as condensed chromatin throughout the karyoplasm.

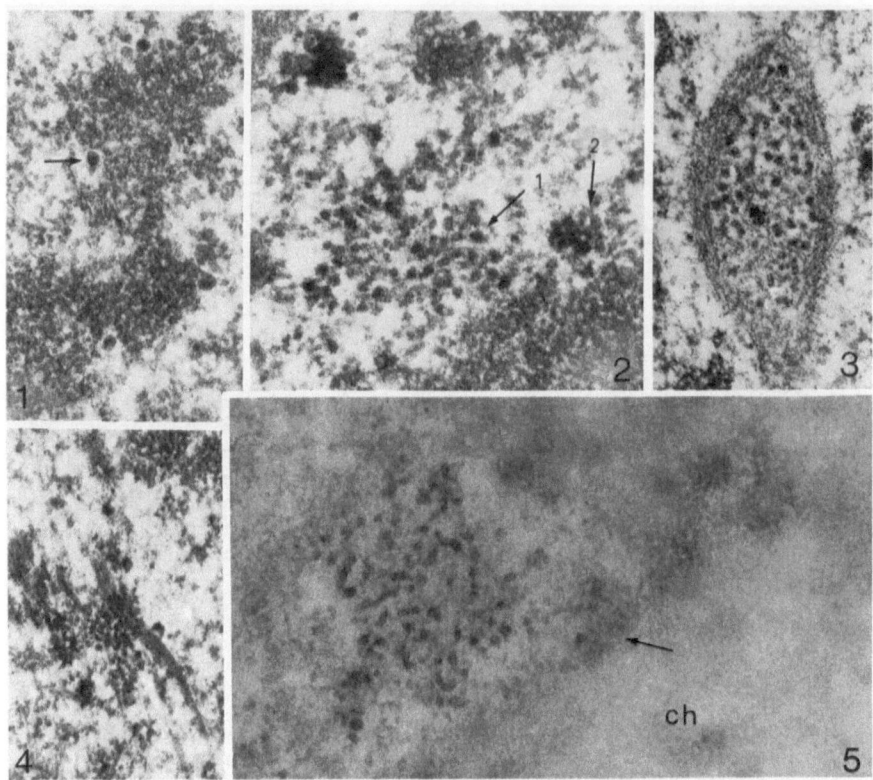

Fig. 1. Four perichromatin granules (arrow) are visible at the periphery of the chromatin clumps and separated from the chromatin by a clear halo. x 57.000

Fig. 2. In addition to a cluster of interchromatin granules (arrow 1), two atypical dense granules (arrow 2) are visible in the interchromatin area near the condensed chromatin and composed of a close aggregation of dense spherical granules. x 59.000

Fig. 3. A nuclear body is characterized by microfibrillar cortex surrounding cluster of interchromatin granules. x 35.000

Fig. 4. Intranuclear fibrillar rodlets are composed of closely packed and parallel fibrils. x 43.000

Fig. 5. EDTA stain. Chromatin (ch) is bleached, whereas interchromatin granules keep their density. In addition, perichromatin fibrils (arrow) are seen as narrow fringe at the border of chromatin. x 66.000

The matrix of interchromatin area was mainly formed by fine fibrillar substances of low contrast, which were distributed diffusely or scatteredly (Figs. 1 - 2). A small number of perichromatin granules (Fig. 1) were found at the periphery of the chromatin clumps, and sometimes isolated in the interchromatin area. They appeared mostly as single dense spherical granules of about 400 - 500 A in diameter, clearly separated from the chromatin by a regular halo of about 200 A in thickness.

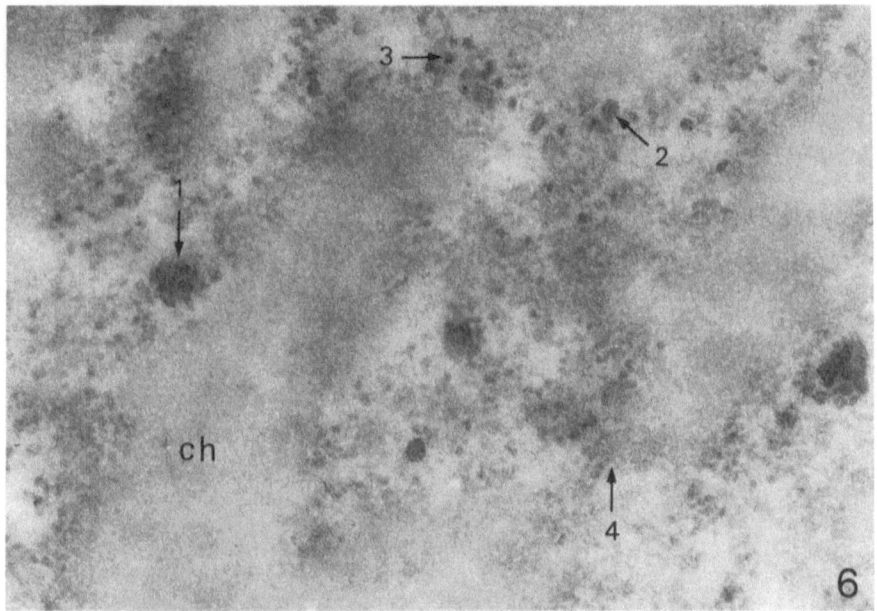

Fig. 6. Chromatin (ch) is faintly stained with EDTA treatment. Atypical dense
granules (arrow 1), perichromatin granules (arrow 2), interchromatin granules
(arrow 3), and perichromatin fibrils (arrow 4) are still clearly evident with
dense contrast. x 61.000

The interchromatin granules were most conspicuous and often formed single
or multiple clusters, about 0.2 - 1.0 μ in size per section (Fig. 2). The
individual granules were about 200 - 300 A in diameter and often round, ovoid,
or sometimes angular or rod in shape, up to about 500 A in length. Some of
them were extremely dense and others moderately dense. They were often inter-
connected with fibrils of low density, thus appearing as chains which in turn
formed a loose network. There was no clear evidence of any limiting membranes
around the dense granules. Atypical dense granules occasionally appeared in
the interchromatin area (Fig. 2). They were about 600 - 2000 A in diameter and
appeared as irregularly round granules, and larger atypical dense granules
(Fig. 2) were often composed of a close aggregation of dense spherical granules,
about 150 - 200 A in diameter, resembling a segregated granular area of the
nucleoli.

Nuclear bodies (Fig. 3) were about 0.5 - 1.5 μ in size and characterized by
a microfibrillar cortex surrounding dense osmiophilic granules. The central
dense granules were not seen in some nuclear bodies. Intranuclear fibrillar
rodlets (Fig. 4) were sometimes found in the interchromatin area and consisted
of filaments, about 50 - 70 A in diameter, which were closely packed and
oriented parallel to each other.

Enzyme extraction was attempted to examine chemical nature of the interchromatin granules (1). After enzyme extraction with either RNAase, DNAase,
or pepsin, the interchromatin granules were still clearly evident. If pepsin
and RNAase were combined, the interchromatin granules appeared to decrease
their electron density or could not become visible.

When EDTA staining was used, the condensed chromatin was faintly stained,
whereas the nucleoli as well as the perichromatin, interchromatin, and atypical
dense granules were exhibited with a dense contrast (Figs. 5 and 6). The inter-

chromatin granules often showed a central less dense core. In addition, the bleaching of the chromatin rendered visible a surrounding narrow fringe of moderately dense fibrils and granules (Figs. 5 and 6), which was called perichromatin fibrils (3). Some fibrillar connection might be found between the perichromatin fibrils and the interchromatin granules on one hand and between the perichromatin fibrils and the perichromatin granules on the other.

DISCUSSION

The perichromatin, interchromatin, and atypical dense granules were not bleached with EDTA stain. In addition, the perichromatin granules were decreased in density only by the combined action of pronase and RNAase (3). Their biological function was supposed to be a transport of information from the genes towards the cytoplasm (3). The interchromatin granules might be a complex of RNA and acidic protein on basis of the present study (1). Their biological significance is still poorly known. The perichromatin fibrils were readily destroyed by RNAase as if they were only protected by protein and probably a heterogeneous mixture of biochemically defined RNA species of known or unknown function, wrapped into a protein carrier (4, 5, 6).

FAKAN and BERNHARD (7) demonstrated extranucleoler RNA synthesis by the rapid incorporation of ^{3}H-uridine at the border of condensed chromatin and by the slow incorporation in the RNP containing interchromatin area. The presence of RNA polymerase in the interchromatin area and at the border of the chromatin was suggested on the basis of visualized inorganic cation accumulation (8). It is suggested, therefore, that the perichromatin fibrils might contain the morphological substrate for the rapidly labeled DNA-like RNA or HnRNA as found in biochemical studies.

It is well known that the nucleoli are main site of RNA synthesis in nuclei, but the present study suggests that extranucleolar RNA synthesis evidently occurs in malignant lymphoma. In addition, the interchromatin and the atypical dense granules also were often evident in malignant lymphoma outside the central nervous system (9, 10, 11, 12). In this regard, the extranucleolar RNA morphology in malignant lymphoma seems to be unique and to represent a characteristic extranucleolar RNA synthesis as compared with other brain tumours.

REFERENCES

1. TANI, E., AMETANI, T., KAWAMURA, Y., HANDA, H.: Nuclear structures of primary malignant lymphoma in the brain. Cancer 24, 617 - 624 (1969)
2. BERNHARD, W.: A new staining procedure for electron microscopical cytology. J. Ultrastruct. Res. 27, 250 - 265 (1969)
3. MONNERON, A., BERNHARD, W.: Fine structural organization of the interphase nucleus in some mammalian cells. J. Ultrastruct. Res. 27, 266 - 288 (1969)
4. DARNELL, J.E.: Ribonucleic acids from animal cells. Bacteriol. Rev. 32, 262 - 290 (1968)
5. PENMAN, S., VESCO, C., PENMAN, M.: Localization and kinetics of formation of nuclear heterodisperse RNA, cytoplasmic heterodisperse RNA and polyribosome-associated messenger RNA in HeLa cells. J. mol. Biol. 34, 49 - 70 (1968)
6. SOEIRO, R., VAUGHAN, M.H., WARNER, J.R., DARNELL, J.E.: The turnover of nuclear DNA-like RNA in HeLa cells. J. Cell Biol. 39. 112 - 118 (1968)
7. FAKAN, S., BERNHARD, W.: Localization of rapidly and slowly labelled nuclear RNA as visualized by high resolution autoradiography. Exp. Cell Res. 67, 129 - 141 (1971)

8. KIERSZENBAUM, A.L., TRES, L.L.: Nucleolar and perichromosomal RNA synthesis during meiotic prophase in the mouse testis. J. Cell Biol. *60*, 39 - 53 (1974)
9. LEPLUS, R., DEBRAY, J., PINET, J., BERNHARD, W.: Lésions nucleaires décelées au microscope électronique dans les cellules de lymphomes malins chez l'homme. Compt. Rend. Acad. Sci. *253*, 2788 - 2790 (1961)
10. BESSIS, M., THIERY, P.: Etude au microscope électronique des hémosarcomes humains. Nouv. Rev. Franç. Hématol. *2*, 577 - 601 (1962)
11. BERNHARD, W., LEPLUS, R.: "Fine Structure of the Normal and Malignant Lymph Node." Oxford: Pergamon Press 1964
12. KRISHAN, A., UZMAN, B.G., HEDLEY-WHYTE, E.T.: Nuclear bodies: a component of cell nuclei in hamster tissues and human tumors. J. Ultrastruct. Res. *19*, 563 - 572 (1967)

EIICHI TANI, M.D.
Department of Neurosurgery
Hyogo College of Medicine
Nishinomiya, Hyogo
Japan

Acta Neuropath. (Berlin), Suppl. VI, 173 - 176 (1975)

The Ultrastructure of Reticulin

J. CERVOS-NAVARRO AND F. MATAKAS

Institut für Neuropathologie
Klinikum Steglitz, F.U. Berlin

Summary: The electron microscopic examination of various organs and tumours of different species proved that the ultrastructural equivalent of reticulin fibres is not a uniform substance. Reticulin fibres are either basement membranes or an amorphous mass which appears as argyrophil fibres under the light microscope. Microfibrils may in some cases produce an argyrophilic reticulum. The claimed identity of reticulin and collagen can partly be explained by the chemical similarity of collagen and basement membranes. It seems possible, moreover, that the amorphous mass and microfibrils, which may be an ultrastructural substrate of reticulin, are composed of a material essentially similar to that of collagen.

Key words: Reticulin Fibres - Electron Microscopy - Collagen - Basement Membranes - Microfibrils

Since KUPFFER (7) in 1876 first described reticulin, the nature of this structure has been controversial. Reticulin has been identified with collagen (3) or with precursors of collagen (12). Other authors stressed the essential difference between both substances (1, 5, 6). However, all authors assumed that reticulin is a fibrillar substance the main characteristic of which is its argentophil nature. In some publications the occurence of reticulin was regarded as an indication of the non-mesenchymal nature of the tissue (2, 4). Until our first publication in 1972 there had been no examination of the ultrastructure of reticulin fibres in tissue sections.

MATERIAL AND METHODS

We examined lymph nodes, muscle, kidney, spleen, subcutaneous connective tissue, brain and peripheral nerves of man, cat, rabbit, rat, guinea pig. Tissue specimens of human sarcomas, angioblastomas, medulloblastomas, gliomas, neurinomas, meningiomas, plasmocytomas, adenomas of the adrenal glands, pheochromocytomas were also examined. The tissues were fixed in 5% glutaraldehyde for 5 hours immediately after excision. In a few cases the material was prepared for electron microscopy after formalin fixation. The material was embedded in micropal or epon. Formalin-fixed specimens were impregnated according to the techniques of GOMORI, POLAK and MOVAT.

RESULTS

After silver impregnation reticulin fibres appear as black slender fibres. They are of different length, in some tissues stretched, in others spiral. In most cases the fibres seem to have branches. In many tissues the reticulin is

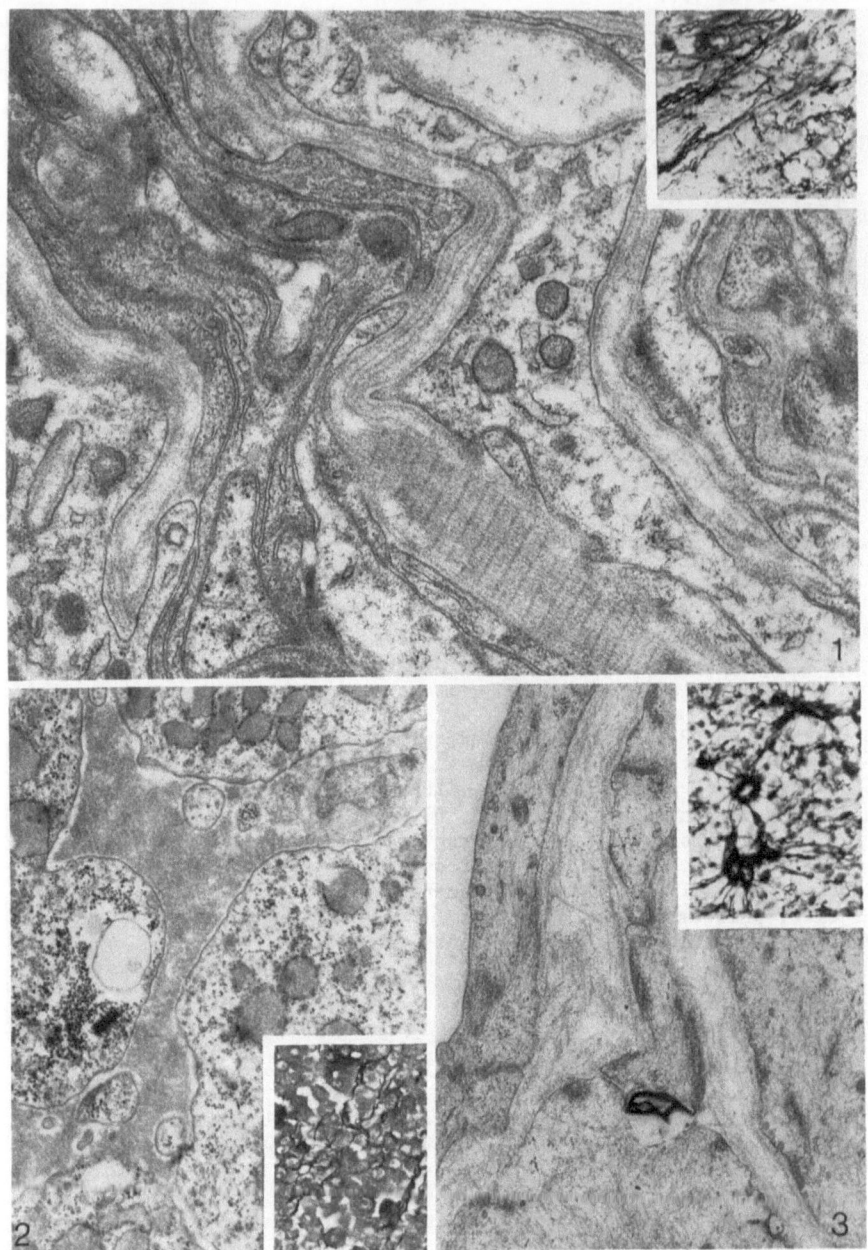

Fig. 1. Neurinoma. The small cytoplasmic lamellae of the tumor cells are surrounded by basement membranes. x 6,000. Gomori x 160

Fig. 2. Plasmocytoma. The intercellular space is filled with an amorphous material. x 10,000. Gomori x 100

Fig. 3. Haemangiopericytoma. In the perivascular space numerous microfibril which is some areas form a basement membrane. x 8,000. Gomori x 100

formed as a meshwork. In all tissues containing reticulin fibres collagen ·is
also found. Collagen fibres can easily be identified by their diameter and by
the periodicity of 64 nm. The amount of collagen combined with reticulin however, is extremely different.

.The substrate of reticulin under the electron microscope has no uniform
structure. In our material the reticulin had three different ultrastructural
forms. There was a predominance of one type in each tissue specimen but no
specific correlation between tissue and reticulin fibre type.

1. In many organs and tissues the substrate of reticulin is basement membrane.
An outstandig example of this is seen in neurinomas. In fibrillar areas of
this tumour the cells are surrounded by one, two or more basement membranes
(Fig. 1). This corresponds well with the light microscopical observation that
reticulin fibres surround all tumour cells. The perivascular reticulin of
cerebral small vessels corresponds to the basement membranes. The situation
is similar in the kidney. Haemangioblastomas of the cerebellum and spinal cord
are very rich in basement membranes and contain many reticulin fibres. Basement membranes in these tissues are usually combined with collagen fibres.
However, the relation between the amount of collagen and basement membranes in
the perivascular space of the brain, in muscle, spleen and neurinomas is such
that the collagen fibres cannot be the substrate of reticulin.

2. In a number of tumours, e.g. lymphosarcomas, plasmocytomas (Fig. 2),
medulloblastomas, pheochromocytomas, tumours of the adrenal glands, gliomas
and in the reticular endothelial tissue, i.e. spleen and lymph nodes the
ultrastructural substrate of reticulin is an amorphous mass. The intercellular space in these tissues is of different extension but is almost completely
filled by amorphous material. The electron density of this material is greater
than that of basement membranes. It never displays a laminar structure. In
lymphosarcoma and the spleen the amorphous material contains collagen fibres,
the number of which, however, is very small. In some cases the amorphous
material is intermingled with microfibrils which are a third possible substrate
of reticulin.

3. Microfibrils are in a few tissues the main intercellular structure which
appears as reticulin after impregnation. The fibrils have a diameter of 5 to
12 nm. They are not located in the periphery of amorphous material as elastic.
fibres. The microfibrils are found in muscle where they are mixed with basement membranes and in meningiomas. In haemangiopericytomas which contain many
reticulin fibres they were the main component of the intercellular material
(Fig. 3.). In this tumour they had a tight connection to basement membranes.

DISCUSSION

In most of the publications which refer to reticulin fibres it has been
neglected that the reticular appearance of reticulin under light microscope
has no significance for its fine structure. In fact, reticulin may be either
basement membranes, an amorphous or a filamentous material. The different
forms of the ultrastructural substrate correspond well with reticulin as it
appears after impregnation under the light microscope. The reticulin in the
spleen, in lymphnodes, in lymphosarcomas and medulloblastomas consists of
small fibres which are independent from the perivascular spaces. The fibres
may be very long, they are branched and surround single cells or cell groups.
There is little or no collagen. The reticulin fibres which are basement
membranes, e.g. in neurinomas, in the perivascular space, in muscle, appear much
greater, due to the fact that multilayers of basement membranes may be rather
thick. The correspondance between basement membranes and reticulin was first
mentioned by ROBB-SMITH (11).

The fibrillar form of reticulin as it appears after impregnation seems to be
a mere light microscopical phenomenon. Occasionally, it seems to be caused by
shrinkage of the material during formalin fixation. If the intercellular
material is condensed and uniformly impregnated it may display a fibrillar
structure if the intercellular space is small.

We therefore think that there is a distinct morphological difference between
reticulin and collagen. It seems possible, however, that there is some correlation between both structures. The chemical nature of collagen and basement
membranes is similar (13). PIERCE *et al.* (10) have claimed an essential difference between reticulin and basement membranes since they found different
immunological qualities of both substances. This is not convincing, however,
since a different immunological quality is also found in basement membranes
of different organs (9). The chemical relation between basement membranes and
the reticulin which consists of an amorphous material was reported by the
above mentioned authors. The reticulin which appears as a filamentous material
seems to be of similar nature as basement membranes since they are both found
in combination.

REFERENCES

1. ENGHUSEN, E.: Über Reticulin, Kollagen und die Intercellularsubstanz des
   Bindegewebes. Acta anat. (Basel) *31*, 46 - 61 (1957)
2. GULLOTTA, F.: Das sogenannte Medulloblastom. Berlin-Heidelberg-New York:
   Springer 1967
3. ISHII, T.: Das Silberbild der Retikulinfasern des Lymphknotens (mit
   besonderer Berücksichtigung des Übergangs in die kollagenen Fasern).
   Verh. anat. Ges. (Jena) *62*, 353 - 359 (1967)
4. KERNOHAN, J.W., UIHLEIN, A.: Sarcomas of the brain, Springfield: CH.C.
   Thomas 1962
5. KRAMER, H., WINDRUN, G.M.: Metachromasia after treating tissue sections
   with sulfuric acid. J. clin. Path. *6*, 239 - 240 (1953)
6. KRAMER, H., WINDRUN, G.M.: Sulfuration techniques in histochemistry with
   special reference to metachromasia. J. Histochem. Cytochem. *2*, 196 -
   208 (1954)
7. KUPFFER, C.W.: Über Sternzellen der Leber: Briefliche Mitteilung an Prof.
   Waldeyer. Arch. mikr. Anat. *12*, 353 - 358 (1876)
8. MATAKAS, F., CERVOS-NAVARRO, J.: Die Ultrastruktur des Retikulins. Virchows
   Arch. Abt. B. Zellpath. *10*, 67 - 82 (1972)
9. PIERCE, G.B.: Epithelial basement membrane: Origin, development and role
   in disease. In: Chemistry and molecular biology of the intercellular
   matrix (ed. E.A. Balasz), p. 471 - 506
10. PIERCE, G.B., MIDGLEY, A.R., SRI RAM, J.: The histogenesis of basement
    membranes. J. exp. Med. *117*, 339 - 348 (1963)
11. ROBB-SMITH, A.H.T.: The functional significance of connective tissue. In:
    General pathology (ed. Florey), p. 457. London: Lloyd-Luke 1970
12. ROSS, R., BENDITT, E.P.: In vivo, extracellular, collagen fibrillogenesis.
    Nature (Lond.) *197*, 395 - 396 (1963)
13. VELICAN, C., VELICAN, D.: Studies on the reticulin network of human liver.
    Virchows Arch. Abt. B Zellpath. *1*, 297 - 316 (1968)

Prof. Dr. J. CERVOS-NAVARRO
Klinikum Steglitz der Freien Universität Berlin
Institut für Neuropathologie
Hindenburgdamm 30
D - 1000 Berlin 45

Acta Neuropath. (Berlin), Suppl. VI, 177 - 180 (1975)
© by Springer-Verlag 1975

Certain Notable Clinical Attributes of the Histiocytic Sarcomas of the Central Nervous System

R. D. ADAMS

Neurology Service
Massachusetts General Hospital
Boston, Mass., U.S.A.

Summary: By the term reticulum cell sarcoma we denote any tumor composed predominantly of undifferentiated cells, some of which have the qualities of histiocytes. The origin of such CNS tumors may be traced to circulating monocytes,
perithelial or meningeal histiocytes or microgliocytes. The ubiquity of cells
of the monocyte-histiocyte series allows six possibilities of CNS involvement:
a) primary in the brain:
b) secondarily involve the brain or spinal cord by extending from a cranial
   bone or vertebra to the epidural space
c) rarely to involve extraneuronal tissues (lymph nodes, bone, viscera) and
   then later to localize to the brain substance
d) to spread from brain outside the nervous system
e) to evoke any one or several of· the paraneoplastic diseases (polymyositis,
   polyneuritis, cerebellar degeneration,
f) to permit widespread infections of the nervous system such as multifocal
   leucoencephalitis.
Clinical attributes to be emphasized are the relative rarity of hematogenous
metastases (2 of 121 cases), the relatively high incidence of such tumors
in immunologically suppressed individuals (12 of 5000 cases), the frequency
of primary tumors of CNS (23 of 144 cases), the high incidence of epidural
and dural involvement from osseous lesions (13 of 121 cases); the rapid
evolution of clinical phenomena; the rarity of paraneoplastic syndromes; the
occasional spontaneous and frequent therapeutic regression upon x-radiation.
   The common invasion of pia and ependyma by the tumor cells and their natural
tendency to phagocytosis opens unrealized possibilities of clinical diagnosis
by cytological examination and culture of CSF. Early diagnosis by these
methods permits avoidance of surgery and the use of radiation and possibly
chemotherapy, which may be rewarded by symptomatic regression and potential
cure.

Key words: ·CNS Lymphomas - Histiocytic Sarcoma - Clinical Conditions -
Neurologic Syndromes

In view of the emphasis given in this Symposium to the morphologic features
of the lymphomas, and more particularly the reticulum cell sarcoma (RCS) of
the nervous system, my remarks will be restricted largely to the clinical
features of the histiocytic sarcomas.
   The opinions of our neuropathology laboratory at the MGH concerning the
histogenesis and identification of the so-called reticulum cell sarcoma are
generally known. Since the first descriptions of a primary tumor of the brain
having all the characteristic features of the reticulum cell sarcoma (6),
its histiocytic - microglial - origin has been widely acknowledged.

I must add that our refusal to introduce the 'term microglioma was based not on our unawareness that many of the component cells were microgliacytes but in adherence to histogenetic theory we could not determine whether the cells were derived from adventitial and meningeal histiocytes, blood monocytes or microgliacytes. The interesting perivascular pattern suggested more a derivation from adventitial cells than microglial. Argentophilia we thought not to be a criterion of microglial since as HORTEGA showed, Kupffer cells, reticulum cells of lymph nodes and spleen manifest a similar reaction.

The unusual stroma derived, we believed, from adventitial fibroblasts of vessels for which the tumor is named, expresses the curiously intimate relationships between tumor cell and collagenic connective tissue. We were also impressed with the phagocytic properties of adventitial histocytes. And, finally it seemed that a close and harmonious relationship of tumor cells to the vasculature of the brain rarely permits the tumor cells to outgrow their blood supply.

We were not inclined then, nor am I now convinced that the lymphocytic infiltrates are part of the tumor or that they should confer on the tumor the designation lymphoma, unless qualified by the adjective histiocytic or reticulum cell.

Noteworthy is the fact that of all the lymphomas only the histiocytic sarcoma, by which I would include not only the RCS but also many of the Hodgkin's sarcomas (HS), has the unique quality of being able to originate in the brain. Thus there are now many examples of primary RCS and HS in the nervous system and only rare and somewhat controversial cases of pure lymphocytoma, lymphoblastoma (lymphosarcoma) and plasmacytoma that are limited to the nervous system. The obvious explanation is that the histiocyte and microgliacyte are normal cellular inhabitants of the CNS whereas the lymphocyte, lymphoblast and plasmacyte are not.

The group of tumors referred to as the histiocytic sarcomas exhibit a number of unusual clinical features which doubtless reflect biological attributes of the cell type.

Firstly, it is of interest that certain general clinical conditions of the body appear to favor the ultimate development of RCS of the brain. Chronic uveo-cyclitis and chronic parotitis (inflammatory form of Mikulicz syndrome) have been followed by a peculiarly high incidence of RCS of the brain. Renal transplantation also has favored the later development of RCS, and of the cases collected by PENN (3) an extraordinarily high proportion (23 of 29) were restricted to the central nervous system. Immunosuppressive therapy, which is essential for the survival of organ transplants, is postulated as the factor which favors the tumor growth. And, the brain as a favored site may be related to its known isolation from the natural protection given by the immune mechanisms of the body. Infectious mononucleosis and chronic, relapsing multiple sclerosis have also been followed by RCS of the brain, but this may be only a fortuitous association. The apparent increase in the incidence of RCS of the brain in our own neuropathological material may be a reflection of the increasing use of antiimmune drugs and prolonged survival in chronic diseases in which there is impairment of the immune processes.

Clinical data are in accord with the pathological observations that the tumor possesses special growth characteristics and modes of dissemination. RCS of lymph nodes, bone, skin, and viscera rarely set up independent foci in the brain. SPARLING, PARKER and the author (4) found not a single case in the large series of lymphomas from the Mallory Institute of Pathology and SCHAUMBERG et.al. (5) uncovered only 2 cases in 121 autopsied cases of RCS's over a 30 year period in the files of the Homer Wright Institute of Pathology of the Massachusetts General Hospital (25.200 autopsies). At same time there were 23 primary RCS and 11 cases where extraneural tumor extended to epidural tissues.

Indeed a mass lesion occuring in the brain of a patient with lymphogenous or visceral RCS, in the absence of cranial or spinal bone involvement, is

statistically more likely to be a second tumor of another cell type than a
RCS metastasis.

Primary reticulum cell sarcomas tend to behave like gliomas, spreading to
other parts of the nervous system (often via CSF channels) but not to extraneural tissues.

This brings us to another interesting feature of RCS, namely its tendency
to originate in bone, due presumably to neoplastic conversion of marrow histiocytes or monocytes. Thus in one respect it behaves towards the nervous system
like a bone-metastasizing carcinoma, except that the focus is usually solitary
(only 1 multiple in our series). The neurological syndromes to which they give
rise are related to the osseous lesion and spread through the foramens of exit
of cranial nerves, as follows (5):

a) Epidural compression of spinal cord and roots from lesions of vertebras
b) Parasellar syndromes (hypothalamic-ocular palsies-optic nerves) of sphenoid
   bone,
c) Petrous-occipital cranial nerve syndromes from lesions of base of skull and
   posterior fossa.

In our original reports of primary RCS of brain we had the impression that the
temporal lobe was a favored site, but later experience was brought to light
cases in which the frontal lobe, periventricules zones, fornices, corpus callosum and cingulum, other parts of the cerebrum, brainstem and cerebellum have
been involved. Many instances of multiple unconnected tumor foci have also
been observed.

We have not succeeded in defining a diencephalic-hypothalamic syndrome as
would be suggested by the frequent involvement of the wall of the III. ventricle.
A Korsakoff syndrome was a feature of one case with hippocampal lesion.

The growth characteristics of RCS have approximated that of the more malignant
gliomas for which they have clinically been mistaken. Contiguity to pia-arach-
noid, a common pathological feature, accounts for a higher incidence of tumor
cells shed into CSF (and identifiable in cytological preparations) than in
glioma.

We have not been able to identify the sclerosing form of reticulum sarcoma
(of URIBE-ROSAS and RAPPAPORT) or to confirm a more benign form of highly
fibrous tumors.

In one of our own cases and at least one other in the published accounts of
primary RCS of brain there had been an earlier (several years before the
terminal illness) spontaneously regressing neurological syndrome. In our case
the original lesion could not be identified at autopsy; in another it proved
to be multiple sclerosis. One can appreciate the diagnostic problem posed by
such cases.

In contrast to many other tumors the incidence of paraneoplastic diseases,
infective and other, has been singularly low. We have seen no cases of multifocal leucoencephalitis in conjunction with RCS, nor have CURRIE et al. (3)
found instances of polyneuropathy, polymyositis, cerebellar degeneration, viral,
mycotic, tuberculous and parasitic meningitis and encephalitis.

Extraordinary sensitivity to diagnostic and therapeutic x-ray exposure is the
noteworthy attribute of the cell type, to which I would call attention. In this
respect it contrasts to gliomas and metastatic carcinomas of the brain (5). In
one of our cases, diagnosed by surgical biopsy (glioblastoma had been suspected), X-ray therapy literally eradicated the tumor, and only one small nodule
was found in the brain at autopsy 6 years later. Another patient returned
to work with nearly complete regression of symptoms after X-ray of what had
been clinically diagnosed as a glioma of speech areas (no operation was performed at the time). Symptoms recurred and proved fatal 18 months later. In
our opinion data regarding newer classifications of the histiocyte-lymphoma
series and subdivisions in terms of nodularity or diffuseness of growth have
been predictive of prognosis.

Finally I would suggest that the interesting phenomenon of phagocytosis of many of the more mature cells of the RCS offers unrealized possibilities of therapeusis. Radioactive or antineoplastic particulate material might be selectively assimulated by the tumor tissue, with beneficial clinical effect.

REFERENCES

1. CURRIE, S., HENSON, R.A., MORGAN, H.G., POOLE, A.T.: The incidence of non-metastatic neurological syndromes of obscure origin in the reticuloses. Brain *93*, 629 - 640, (1970)
2. KINNEY, T.D., ADAMS, R.D.: Reticulum cell sarcoma of the brain. Arch. Neurol. Psychiat. *50*, 522 - 564 (1943)
3. PENN, I.: Malignant tumors in organ transplant recipients. Berlin, Heidelberg, New York: Springer, 1970
4. SPARLING, H.J., ADAMS, R.D., PARKER, F.: Involvement of the nervous system by malignant lymphomas. Medicine *26*, 285 - 332 (1947)
5. SCHAUMBERG, H.H., PLANK, C.R., ADAMS, R.D.: The reticulum cell sarcoma-microglioma group of brain tumors. A consideration of their clinical features and therapy. Brain *95*, 199 - 213 (1972)
6. YUILE, C.L.: Case of primary reticulum sarcoma of brain. Arch. Path. *26*, 1036 - 1044 (1938)

Dr. R.D. ADAMS
Neurology Service
Massachusetts General Hospital
Boston, Mass. 02114

Acta Neuropath. (Berlin), Suppl. VI, 181 - 186 (1975)

Differential Diagnostic Aspects in Malignant Lymphomas Involving the Central Nervous System

O.J. KOLAR

Dept. of Neurology
Indiana Univ. School of Med.
Indianapolis, Ind., USA

Summary: Neoplastic cells were found in the cerebrospinal fluid (CSF) cytograms in 57% of patients with lymphocytic leukemia and reticulum cell sarcoma.
Tumor cells may be observed in CSF specimens showing normal cell count and
total proteins. Quantitative and/or qualitative changes in CSF proteins in
absence of corresponding abnormalities in serum may indicate a malignant
lymphoproliferative process involving the central nervous system even in absence of neoplastic cells.

Key words: Lymphomas - CSF cytology - CSF electrophoresis - CSF immunoelectrophoresis

Intra vitam diagnosis of a malignant lymphoma (ML) involving the central
nervous system (CNS) is very difficult, particularly in absence of extracranial manifestations of the neoplasia.
    The clinical neurologist is primarily interested in the following aspects:

1. to obtain the diagnosis of CNS involvement by ML in the earliest stage of
the disease,
2. to establish the histiopathological features of the ML indicating the
probable prognosis of the CNS involvement
3. to introduce the most appropriate treatment and
4. to receive laboratory data reflecting the effect of the therapeutical
program.

    It should be emphasized that for the pathogenetic point of view, CNS involve-
ment in ML can be carried out by

1. direct and
2. indirect mechanisms (Table 1).

    The purpose of this paper is to emphasize abnormal cerebrospinal fluid (CSF)
findings indicating CNS affliction by ML.

MATERIALS AND METHODS

CSF and serum from 35 patients with ML, in whom the diagnosis was confirmed by
autopsy, spleen, lymph node and/or brain biopsy or during neurosurgical inter-
vention were examined. In the series studied, there were three instances of
lymphocytic lymphosarcoma, four patients with primary CNS reticulum cell sarcoma (RCS), six cases of primary extraneural and CNS manifestations of RCS,
four instances of lymphocytic leukemia (LL), six patients with Hodgkin's

Table 1. *CNS Involvement in Malignant Lymphomas*

I. Direct Mechanisms: 1) <u>Mechanical</u> (compression, obstruction
by the tumorous tissue--secondary
ischemic or hemorrhagic intraparenchymal lesions)

                      2) <u>Biochemical</u>
                      Paraproteinemic encephalopathy
                                    mononeuropathy
                                    polyneuropathy
                      Hyperviscosity syndrome

II. Indirect Mechanisms Secondary to: Blood dyscrasias
                                            Hypercalcemia
                                          Immunosuppressive therapy
                                          Kidney failure
                                            Recurrent infections . . . .

disease, five cases of unclassified ML, five instances of myeloma, one patient
with granulocytic leukemia and one case of neoplastic endotheliosis.

Cytomorphology (1), protein electrophoresis and immunoelectrophoresis (2),
concentration of IgG, IgA, IgM and IgD[1] and kappa/lambda light polypeptide
chain ratio (3) were determined in CSF and in the corresponding serum specimens. The results obtained were compared with CSF cytomorphology and protein
electrophoresis and immunoelectrophoresis in 3,179 patients with various
neurological disorders.

RESULTS

CSF Cytomorphology

In our material, CSF cytomorphology in multiple myeloma did not reveal abnormalities suggestive of neoplasia. In the remaining 30 patients studied,
30% showed in CSF cytograms definite neoplastic cells (Fig. 1) diagnostic of
ML. In cases of RCS and LL associated with neurological symptomatology, tumor
cells were found in 57% of the patients. In subjects with clinical signs of
meningeal involvement, neoplastic cells were detected in all instances. CSF
cytology revealed tumor cells in two patients with CSF specimens displaying
normal cell count and total protein concentration. Indirect indication of
CNS invasion by ML were established in two cases showing over 70% reticulo-
monocytes in the CSF cytograms. In our series, manifestations of pathological
bleeding, glial cells, clumps of cells, eosinophils and/or plasma cells in
CSF cytograms of patients with extraneural manifestations of ML were associated
with CNS metastases in 16 patients.

Regarding the survival time, patients with malignant reticulohistiocytic
cells in CSF cytograms showed the worst prognosis.

CSF Electrophoresis

One M-component of identical electrophoretic mobility in the CSF and serum
electropherograms was seen in all patients with multiple myeloma (Fig. 2 A).
Additional M-component was demonstrated in the CSF electropherogram in one

---

[1] By means of electroimmunodiffusion and radial immunodiffusion techniques.

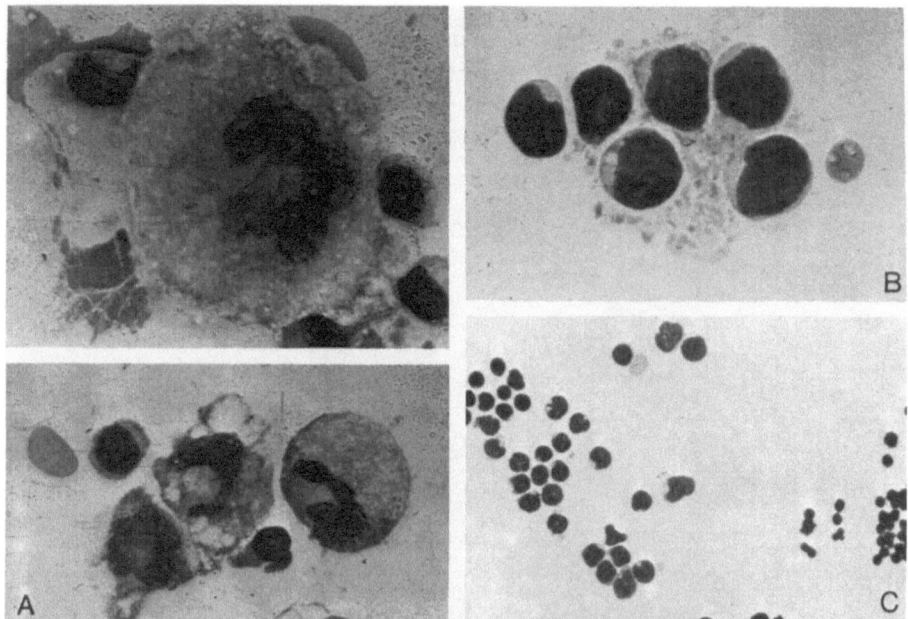

Fig. 1 A - C. A) Multinucleated giant cell with ill-defined cellular outlines
showing resemblence to a Reed-Sternberg cell (upper picture) and neoplastic
histiocytic cells with conspicuous variations in nuclear shapes. CSF cytograms
in a 32 year old female with an unclassified malignant lymphoma primarily involving CNS. May-Grünwald, 1,000 x
B) Clump of immature lymphocytes with scanty cytoplasm in the CSF cytogram of
a 6 year old male with acute lymphocytic leukemia. May-Grünwald, 1,000 x
C) Marked variations in the cellular and nuclear diameter and immature lymphocytic cells in the CSF cytograms of a 48 year old male with intracranial malignant lymphoma, presumably lymphocytic lymphosarcoma. May-Grünwald, 400 x

case of multiple myeloma. More than two bands in the CSF gamma-globulin field
suggest multiple sclerosis or a chronic inflammatory process. Presence of
monoclonal gammopathy in CSF electropherogram in absence of corresponding serum
abnormalities in a patient with extraneural manifestations of ML indicates
CNS metastases (Fig. 2 B). More than four M-components and/or their cathodal
position in the CSF electropherogram is diagnostic for subacute sclerosing
panencephalitis (Fig. 2 C). Abnormal density of bands in the beta globulin
field should be immunoelectrophoretically investigated for immunoglobulin
G (IgG), A (IgA), M (IgM) and D (IgD) paraproteins.

CSF Immunoelectrophoresis

Paraproteins were demonstrated in CSF immunoelectropherograms (IE) of all
patients with multiple myeloma and in four other patients studied (Fig. 3).
Increased concentration of CSF glycoproteins with electrophoretic mobility
of gamma and/or alpha globulins in absence of corresponding serum abnormalities was present in five patients. Prominent precipitates of light polypeptide
chains in CSF IE (Fig. 3 B) were noticed in eight instances. Immunoglobulin A
precipitation arc was demonstrated in the CSF IE in a patient with an epidural

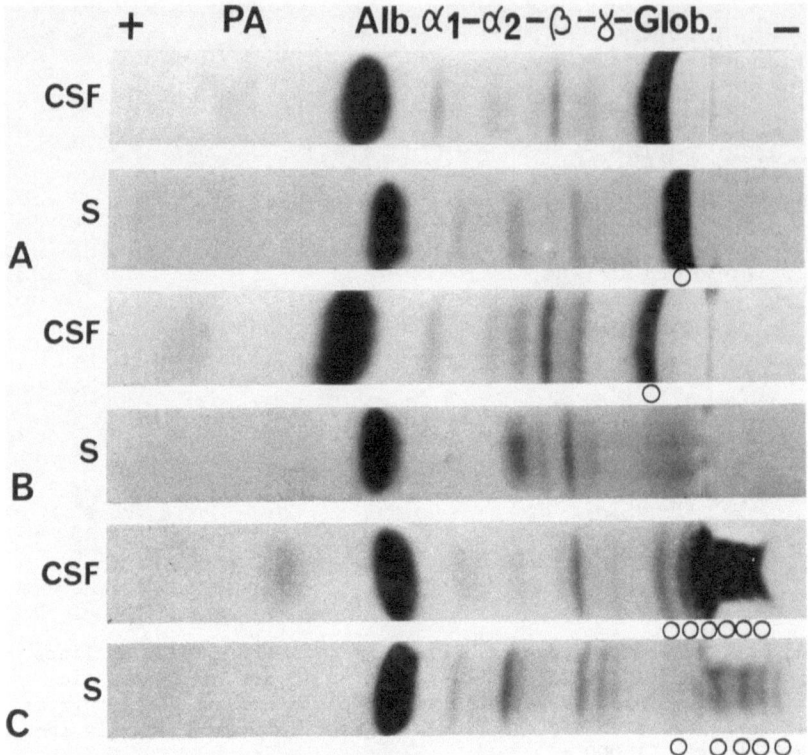

Fig. 2 A - C. Cellulose polyacetate serum (S) and CSF electrophoresis. M-components are indicated by circles.
A) Monoclonal gammopathy in the serum and CSF electropherograms in a 65 year old male with multiple myeloma, neurologically manifested by disorientation, confusion and hallucinations.
B) Monoclonal gammopathy in the CSF electropherogram in a 57 year old male with a primarily extraneural lymphosarcoma and no localizing neurological signs.
C) M-Components of slow electrophoretic mobility in the serum and CSF electropherograms of a 12 year old male with subacute sclerosing panencephalitis

unclassified ML (Fig. 4 B) associated with serum IgA concentration below 30 mg/100 ml in absence of tumor cells in the CSF cytogram.

Concentration of immunoglobulins

60% of patients in our series showed quantitative abnormalities in serum immunoglobulins. Increased concentration of CSF IgG and IgA and/or presence of IgM in the CSF specimen in absence of abnormalities indicating blood-brain barrier disturbances was established in 14 instances. Alteration in the CSF ratio of Kappa/Lambda polypeptide chains was noticed in eight instances.

In a patient with neoplastic endotheliosis (4) (Fig. 4 C), presenting clinical signs of multiple brain infarctions, dramatic improvement in the neurologi-

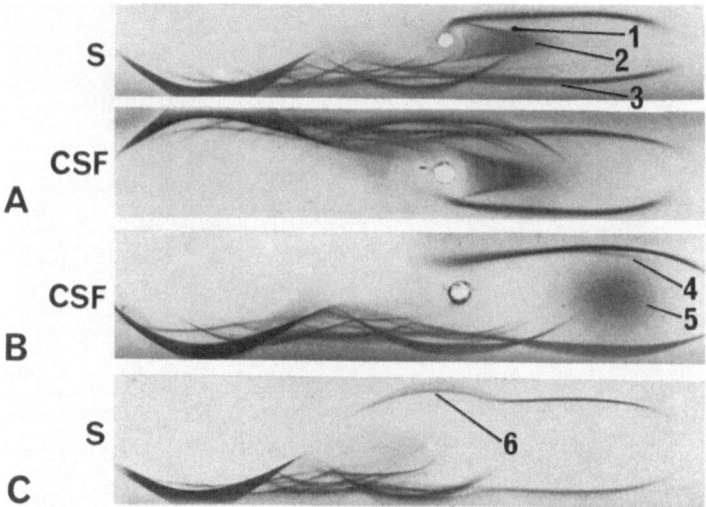

Fig. 3 A - C. Serum (S) and CSF immunoelectrophoresis.
A) Serum and CSF immunoelectropherograms in a 53 year old male with multiple myeloma. In the middle groove, rabbit antiserum to human serum and in the marginal grooves, rabbit antiserum to Fab fragments of IgG (Hoechst, Kansas City, Mo.) were used. Paraprotein (1), abnormal glycoproteins (2) and abnormal deconfiguration of the IgG precipitation line (3) is demonstrated in both, the serum and the CSF immunoelectropherograms.
B) CSF immunoelectropherogram in a 19 year old female with reticulum cell sarcoma predominantly involving leptomeninges. In the proximal groove, rabbit antiserum to Fab fragments of IgG and in the distal groove, rabbit antiserum to human serum were applied. Prominent precipitate of the light polypeptide chains (4) and markedly increased concentration of glycoproteins with electropho retic mobility of gamma globulins (5) is demonstrated.
C) Serum immunoelectropherogram in a 67 year old male with generalized weakness and early manifestations of hyperviscosity syndrome. In the proximal groove, rabbit antiserum to IgG (Hoechst, Kansas City, Mo.) and in the distal groove, rabbit antiserum to human serum were used. Marked deconfiguration in the anodal segment of the IgG precipitate (6) indicates IgG paraproteinemia

cal and EEG (Fig. 5) symptomatology was obtained on intravenous application of Decadron.

DISCUSSION

ML is evidently not one disease but represents many diseases with different pathogenetic mechanisms. In their classification and early diagnosis, manifestations of abnormal protein metabolism including disturbed synthesis of immunoglobulins appear to be equally important as the classical cytomorphology of ML.

In ML involving CNS, CSF studies performed synchronously with exploration of extraneural tissues are particularly suitable to assist to a clinical neurologist in his diagnostic and therapeutic effort.

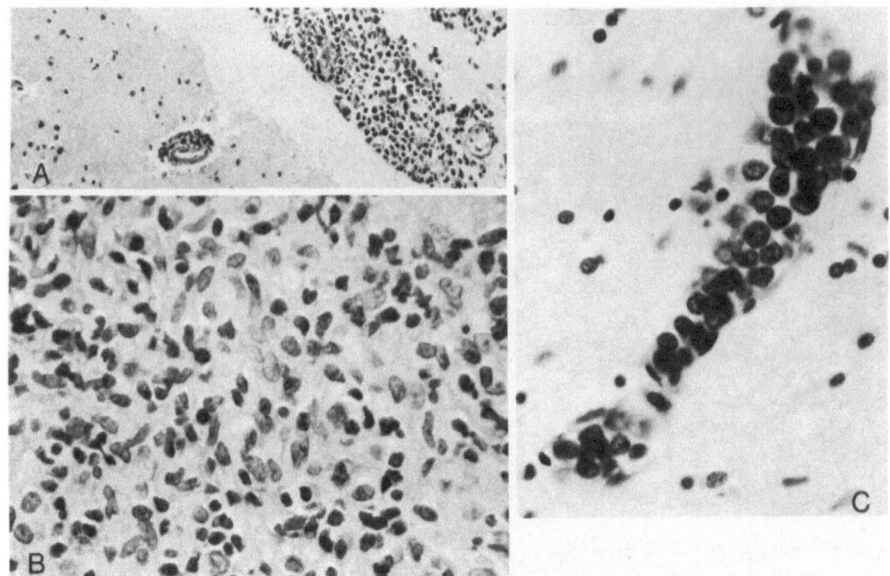

Fig. 4 A - C. A) Diffuse infiltration of leptomeninges with tumor cells in the patient with immunoelectrophoretic CSF abnormalities presented on Fig. 3 B, H & E, 90 x
B) Biopsy specimen obtained during explorative neurosurgery from the epidural space at the level Th10-L2 in a 65 year old male. Unclassified malignant lymphoma. H & E, 425 x
C) Section of the brain obtained at the time of autopsy in a 58 year old female with neoplastic angioendotheliosis. Small vessel packed with neoplastic cells is demonstrated. Nissl, 425 x

REFERENCES

1. KOLAR, O., ZEMAN, W.: Spinal fluid cytomorphology. Arch. Neurol. *18*, 44 - 51, (1968)
2. KOLAR, O.J., ROSS, A.T., HERMAN, J.T.: Serum and cerebrospinal fluid immunoglobulins in multiple sclerosis. Neurology (Minneap.) *20*, 1052 - 1061, (1970)
3. KOLAR, O., ANTHONY, E.: Cerebrospinal fluid and serum light polypeptide chains in 160 patients with various nervous system disorders. Z. Neurol. *202*, 1 - 12, (1972)
4. STROUTH, J.C., DONAHUE, S., ROSS, A., ALDRED, A.: Neoplastic angioendotheliosis. Neurology (Minneap.) *15*, 644 - 658, (1965)

O.J. KOLAR, M.D.
Dept. of Neurology
Indiana Univ. Med. Center
1100 West Michigan Street
Indianapolis, Indiana 46202 USA

Acta Neuropath. (Berlin), Suppl. VI, 187 - 191 (1975)
© by Springer-Verlag 1975

Cytology of the Cerebrospinal Fluid in Patients with Hodgkin's Disease or Malignant Lymphoma[1]

D.G. RAWLINSON, M.E. BILLINGHAM, P.F. BERRY, R.L. KEMPSON

Stanford Univeristy Medical School and the University of
Southern California School of Medicine, U.S.A.

Summary: The cerebrospinal fluids (CSF) of 18 patients with Hodgkin's disease
and 33 patients with malignant lymphoma were evaluated for the presence of
malignant cells. The CSF cytology was correlated with the neuropathologic
findings at surgery or autopsy. In the 51 patients included in the study there
were seven false-negative CSF cytodiagnoses. Methods to improve detection in
the false-negatives will be discussed. There were two false-positives. Expla-
nations for the two false-positive cytodiagnoses will be presented. It is
concluded that cytological examination of the CSF in patients with Hodgkin's
disease and malignant lymphoma is a useful and reliable diagnostic tool.

Key words: Cerebrospinal fluid - cytology - Hodgkin's disease - lymphoma

INTRODUCTION

The purpose of this paper is to document the reliability of CSF cytodiagnosis
in the detection of Hodgkin's disease or malignant lymphoma involving the
central nervous system (CNS). Between 1951 and 1973 in 15 publications (1-15)
there have been approximately 44 reports of positive CSF cytology in patients
with Hodgkin's disease or malignant lymphoma. Thirty-four of these cases have
been correlated with neuropathologic findings at subsequent surgery or autopsy
(1, 2, 4, 5, 7, 8, 10, 14). We will discuss 51 patients with Hodgkin's disease
or malignant lymphoma whose CSF cytodiagnoses were correlated with histologic
findings at surgery or autopsy.

MATERIAL AND METHODS

Fifty-one patients were included in this study. Eighteen patients had Hodgkin's
disease and 33 patients had malignant lymphoma (16). All patients had been investigated and treated at Stanford University Hospital. The investigation of
each of the selected patients had included cerebrospinal fluid cytology. Only
specimens obtained in the six-month period prior to surgery or autopsy were
considered in this correlative study. Cytologic preparations had to exhibit
unequivocal evidence of malignancy before they were considered positive.
Preparations which might otherwise have been considered atypical or suspicious
were classed as negative. The justification for eliminating the categories of
atypical and suspicious is based on the fact that clinicians must consider
equivocal diagnose tantamount to negative.
The cytology specimens were prepared by filtration using a Nucleopore[2]

---

[1] Supported in part by Graduate Neuropathology Training Grant (5 TO1 NS 5500 -
08) of the National Institute of Neurological Diseases and Stroke, U.S. Public
Health Service
[2] General Electric Company, Irradiation Processing Plant, Pleasanton, Cal.

Table 1. *Correlation of CSF cytology with CNS histology in patients with Hodgkin's disease and malignant lymphoma*

	Hodgkin's	Lymphoma
Number patients	18	33
Pos. cytology/pos. histology	1/3	8/12
Neg. cytology/neg. histology	17/15	25/21
False pos.	0	2
False neg.	2	6
Correct correlation	16/18 (89%)	25/33 (76%)

filter and the method described by REYNAUD and KING (17). The filters were stained by the Papanicolaou technique. In two patients tissue was obtained at surgery. In the remaining 49 autopsies were performed, and the dura, brain, and spinal cord were examined histologically.

RESULTS

1. Hodgkin's disease

The CSF cytology of 18 patients with Hodgkin's disease was studied (Table 1). At surgery or autopsy only three patients had histologic evidence of involvement of the CNS by Hodgkin's disease. The CSF contained cells of Hodgkin's disease (Fig. 1) in only one of these three cases. The CSF of the other two cases did not contain unequivocally malignant cells. There were, therefore, two false negatives. There were no false positives, i.e. malignant cells were not found in the CSF of any of the 15 patients whose CNS was histologically free of Hodgkin's disease.

2. Malignant lymphoma

The CSF cytology of 33 patients with malignant lymphoma was studied (Table 1). At autopsy the CNS was involved by malignant lymphoma in twelve patients. Six of these patients had cells of malignant lymphoma in their CSF (Fig. 2). The other six patients had negative CSF cytology. There were, therefore, six false-negatives. Two patients had cells of malignant lymphoma in their cerebrospinal fluid and no histologic evidence of malignant lymphoma involving the CNS at autopsy. These two must be considered false-positives.

DISCUSSION

The detection of cells of Hodgkin's disease or malignant lymphoma in the CSF is an important and reliable laboratory examination enabling the clinician to diagnose and treat Hodgkin's disease and malignant lymphoma of the CNS. The reliability of the test is directly proportional to the number of false-nega-

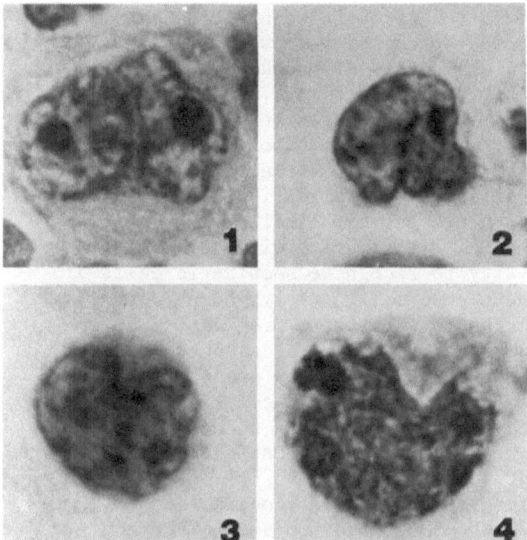

Fig. 1. Hodgkin's disease. A cerebrospinal fluid Nucleopore filter preparation demonstrating a Reed-Sternberg cell. The cell is binunucleate with prominent nucleoli, one of which is surrounded by a clear zone. Papanicolaou stain. x 1920

Fig. 2. Malignant lymphoma, undifferentiated. A cerebrospinal fluid Nucleopore filter preparation demonstrating a primitive cell without histiocytic or lymphocytic differentiation. The cell has nuclear indentations, a single small nucleolus and scanty, palely staining cytoplasm. Papanicolaou stain. x 2160

Fig. 3. Malignant lymphoma, poorly differentiated lymphocytic. A cerebrospinal fluid Nucleopore filter preparation demonstrating a cell which is larger than a mature lymphocyte, has scanty cytoplasm, a nucleus with an irregular outline, deep indentations and coarsely clumped chromatin. Papanicolaou stain. x 2160

Fig. 4. Malignant lymphoma, histiocytic. A cerebrospinal fluid Nucleopore filter preparation demonstrating a neoplastic histiocyte. This cell has a large nucleus with a jagged outline, several large nucleoli and abundant cytoplasm. Papanicolaou stain. x 2160

tive and false-positive cytodiagnoses in a histologically controlled study such as this one. In this study of 51 patients there were eight false-negative and two false-positive cytodiagnoses.

Cell detection will depend upon the number of cells exfoliated into the CSF, the number examined and the cytodiagnostician's ability to identify them as cells of Hodgkin's disease or malignant lymphoma.

Exfoliation of malignant cells into the CSF will depend upon their cohesiveness and their proximity to the subarachnoid space or ventricular system. Tumor within the dura or deep within the brain substance is not likely to be detected cytologically. Thus, two patients in this series, each having malignant lymphoma involving the dura alone, did not have malignant cells in the CSF and were considered false-negatives.

The number of exfoliated cells available for examination will depend upon the number and volume of specimens obtained and the method of collection and demonstration of the exfoliated cells. In the eight false-negative cytodiagnoses in this series nor more than two CSF specimens were submitted from each patient; while in the seven patients in whom cells of Hodgkin's disease or malignant lymphoma were correctly identified five had more than four CSF specimens examined. Methods commonly employed in the preparation of CSF for cytological evaluation include centrifugation, sedimentation, flocculation or filtration. Filtration using the Nucleopore filter has the theoretic advantage of making all cells in the specimen available for examination.

The ability of the cytodiagnostician to recognize the cells of Hodgkin's disease or malignant lymphoma depends on his familiarity with cells native to the normal or reactive CSF, his ability to recognize neoplastic cells in general and the cells of Hodgkin's disease and malignant lymphoma in particular. Unfortunately, this clear distinction of neoplastic from native or reactive cells is not always possible and diagnoses of atypical or suspicious must occasionally be made. In this series two CSF cytology preparations from a patient with Hodgkin's disease involving the brain were considered suspicious and one preparation from a patient with lymphoma involving the brain was considered atypical. Under the protocol the specimens were considered negative and appear in this study as false-negatives.

The two false-positives in this series require special consideration. The first was a patient with histiocytic lymphoma who had two suspicious and two positive cerebrospinal fluid cytology specimens in the six months prior to death. At autopsy he had massive extradural lymphoma, but in the microscopic sections of spinal cord examined there was no histologic evidence of lymphoma. We are confident this represents inadequate histologic examination of the spinal cord. The second patient had mixed histiocytic-lymphocytic lymphoma and one positive CSF cytology. Two days after the lumbar puncture for cytodiagnosis she received 25 mgm. of intrathecal methotrexate. At autopsy eleven days after treatment there was no microscopic evidence of lymphoma involving the CNS. This might represent either inadequate histologic evaluation or response to therapy.

From this series it appears that CSF cytology is a useful and reliable diagnostic tool in determining the involvement of the CNS by Hodgkin's disease or malignant lymphoma. We suggest that CSF cytology be considered an important procedure in the investigation, staging and follow-up of any patient with Hodgkin's disease or malignant lymphoma.

REFERENCES

1. PLATT, W.R.: Exfoliative-cell diagnosis of central nervous system lesions. Arch. Neurol. Psychiat. (Chic.) 66, 119 - 144 (1951)
2. SPRIGGS, A.I.: Malignant cells in cerebrospinal fluid. J. Clin. Path. 7, 122 - 130 (1954)
3. McCORMACK, L.J., HAZARD, J.B., BELOVICH, D., GARDNER, W.J.: Identification of neoplastic cells in cerebrospinal fluid by a wet-film method. Cancer, (Philad.) 10, 1293 - 1299 (1957)
4. MILLER, A.A., RAMSDEN, F.: Primary reticulosis of the central nervous system. "Microgliomatosis". Acta neurochir. (Wien) 11, 439 - 478 (1963)
5. JANOTA, I.: Malignant lymphoma-cells in the cerebrospinal fluid. Lancet 2, 677 - 678 (1964)
6. NAYLOR, B.: The cytologic diagnosis of cerebrospinal fluid. Acta cytol. (Philad.) 8, 141 - 149 (1964)
7. DEN HARTOG JAGER, W.A.: Cytopathology of the cerebrospinal fluid examined with the sedimentation technique after Sayk. J. neurol. Sci. 9, 155 - 177 (1969)

8. GRIFFIN, J.W., THOMPSON, R.W., MITCHINSON, M.J., DE KIEWIET, J.C.,
   WELLAND, F.H.: Lymphomatous leptomeningitis. Amer. J. Med. *51*, 200 -
   208 (1971)
9. RICH, J.R.: A membrane filter technique for cerebrospinal fluid cytology.
   J. Neurosurg. *36*, 661 - 666 (1972)
10. SCHAUMBURG, H.H., PLANK, C.R., ADAMS, R.D.: The reticulum cell sarcoma-
    microglioma group of brain tumours. Brain, *95*, 199 - 212 (1972)
11. WERTLAKE, P.T., MARKOVITS, B.A., STELLAR, S.: Cytologic evaluation of
    cerebrospinal fluid with clinical and histologic correlation. Acta cytol.
    (Philad.) *16*, 224 - 239 (1972)
12. DREWINKO, B., SULLIVAN, M.P., MARTIN, T.: Use of the cytocentrifuge in the
    diagnosis of meningeal leukemia. Cancer (Philad.) *31*, 1331 - 1336 (1973)
13. IIVANAINEN, M., TASHKINEN, E.: Cytological examination of the cerebrospi-
    nal fluid. Ann. Clin. Res. *5*, 80 - 86 (1973)
14. JELLINGER, K., WRCHOVSZKY, A.: Liquorzytologische Befunde bei malignen
    Lymphomen des Zentralnervensystems. Wien. klin. Wschr. *85*, 522 - 525 (1973)
15. WOODRUFF, K.H.: Cerebrospinal fluid cytomorphology using cytocentrifuga-
    tion. Amer. J. clin. Path. *60*, 621 - 627 (1973)
16. RAPPAPORT, H.: Tumors of the Hematopoietic System. Washington, D.C.:
    Armed Forces Institute of Pathology, 1966
17. REYNAUD, A.J., KING, E.B.: A new filter for diagnostic cytology. Acta
    cytol. (Philad.) *11*, 289 - 294 (1967)

D.G. RAWLINSON, M.D.
Cajal Laboratory of Neuropathology
Los Angeles County - University of
Southern California Medical Center
1200 North State Street
Los Angeles, California 90033

Acta Neuropath. (Berlin), Suppl. VI, 193 - 198 (1975)

Light- and Electron Microscopic Studies in Hemoblastosis with CNS-Disorder

W. MÖBIUS[1], C. STANG-VOSS, H.H. HENNEKEUSER[2]

Medizinische Universitätsklinik Freiburg
Anatomisches Institut der Universität Freiburg, BRD

Summary: Some cases of hemoblastosis with CNS-involvement were investigated by methods of light microscopy, cytochemistry and electronmicroscopy. The unique cell picture, as observed by light microscopy could not be proven by electronmicroscopic results. This fact was supported by comparative investigations of inflammation processes. Typical structures are described and discussed.

Key words: Meningosis leukaemica - Hemoblastosis - Cytochemistry - Ultrastructure

Meningosis leukaemica (meningosis blastomatosa in malignant lymphoma) is always a serious complication during the course of hemoblastosis (1, 5, 6, 9). Neurological symptoms, which are variable or can even be missed, are dependent on the localisation of blast infiltration (1, 7). Differentiation of CSF-cells is the most relevant diagnostic feature, because cell count, protein content and glucose level in spinal fluid are not specific.

We report about light- and electronmicroscopic findings in CSF-cells of different hemoblastoses. These results are compared with lymphocytic meningitis.

MATERIAL AND METHODS

The material comprised 3 cases of acute lymphoblastic leukemia (ALL), 3 cases of acute myelogenous leukemia (AML), 1 reticulum cell sarcoma and 1 case of lymphocytic meningitis. For cell concentration we used the sedimentation chamber (9) and Shandon cytocentrifuge (2). Cytochemical stainings: peroxydase, chloro-acetate-esterase, non-specific esterase, PAS, acid phosphatase and β-glucuronidase (see 3).

For electronmicroscopic investigation all specimens were fixed in OsO_4, glutaraldehyde and uranyl acetate after the method of HIRSCH and FEDORKO (4), embedded in Epon-812 and sectioned with the LKB 4902/A ultrotome. The thin sections are stained with uranyl acetate and lead citrate (8), Electronmicroscope ZEISS EM/9S.

---

[1] Prof. Dr. W. SCHEID to his 65. birthday

[2] Supported by a Grant from the "Schutzkommission beim Bundesministerium des Inneren"

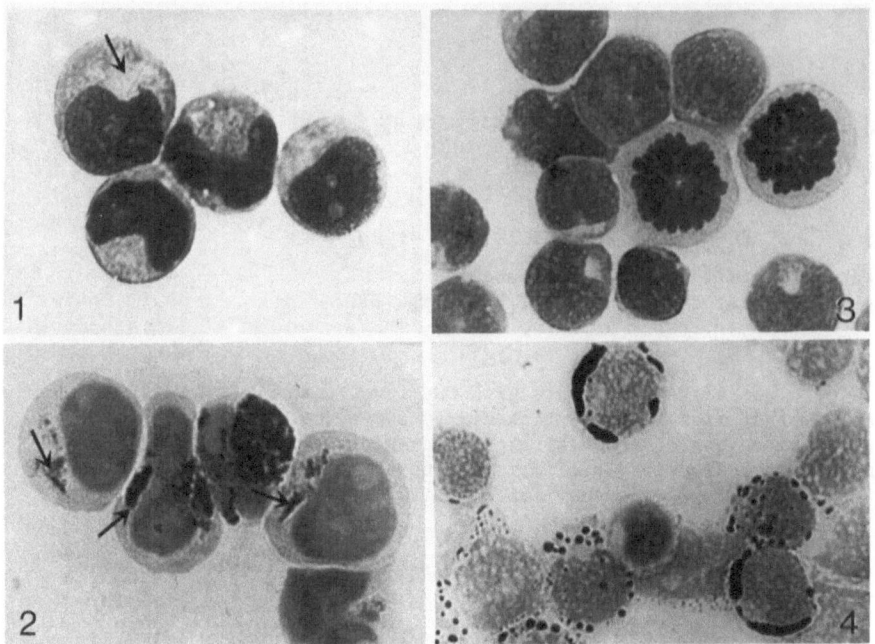

Fig. 1. Myeloblasts in CSF. Pappenheim-Staining; (/) = Auer body. 1200 x

Fig. 2. Peroxydase positive granules and Auer bodies in myeloblasts of the same case. (/) = Auer bodies. 1200 x

Fig. 3. ALL; leukemic cells in CSF. Two cells in mitosis. Pappenheim-Staining; 1200 x

Fig. 4. ALL; PAS-Staining with coarse granules and blocks. 1200 x

RESULTS

Light microscopy:

Cell differentiation of CSF showed a uniform picture of blast cells, (Fig. 1). Mitoses were frequently observed, (Fig. 3, 9). Compared with the cells of peripheral blood and bone marrow the CSF-cells showed similar reactions. In cases of AML so-called Auer bodies could be detected (Fig. 1, 2), which were particulary evident with peroxydase staining, (Fig. 2). In all cases of ALL and lymphosarcoma we found in a part of the leukemic cells coarse granules or blocks with PAS-staining, (Fig. 4). Some of these cases revealed a negativ PAS-reaction while β-glucuronidase activity was striking in form of a granular reaction.

Fig. 7. ALL; Blast-like cell with a deep nuclear invagination. (/) = Golgizone; N = nucleus. 12 000 x

Fig. 8. ALL; Cell with polymorphous nucleus forming nuclear pockets (/). The cytoplasm contains numerous mitochondria and cytofilaments. N = nucleus; 13 800 x

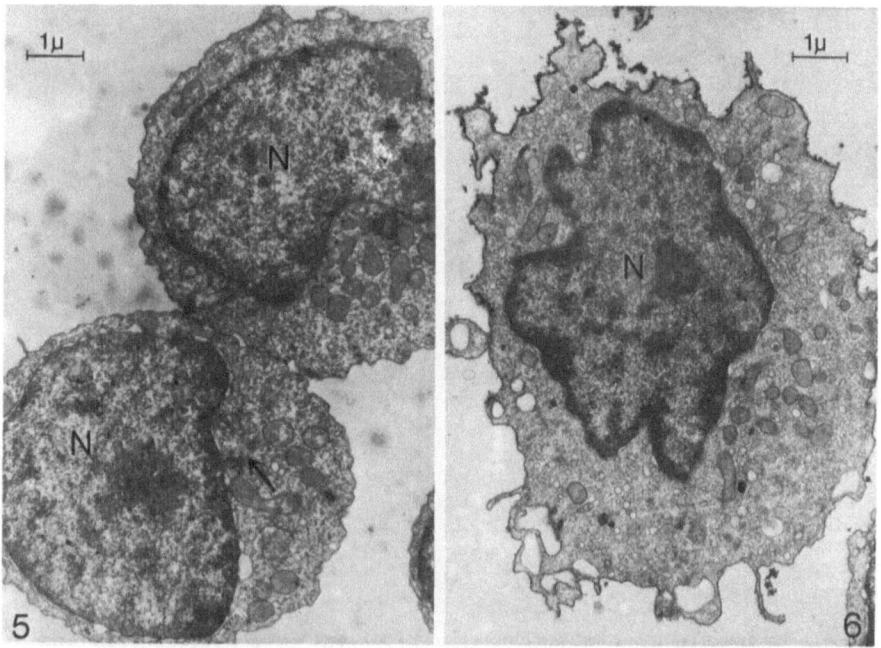

Fig. 5. ALL; Blast-like cells in close contact. The cytoplasm contains numerous mitochondria. N = nucleus" (/) = Centriole. 10 000 x

Fig. 6. ALL; Cell showing pinocytotic activity. N = nucleus. 10 000 x

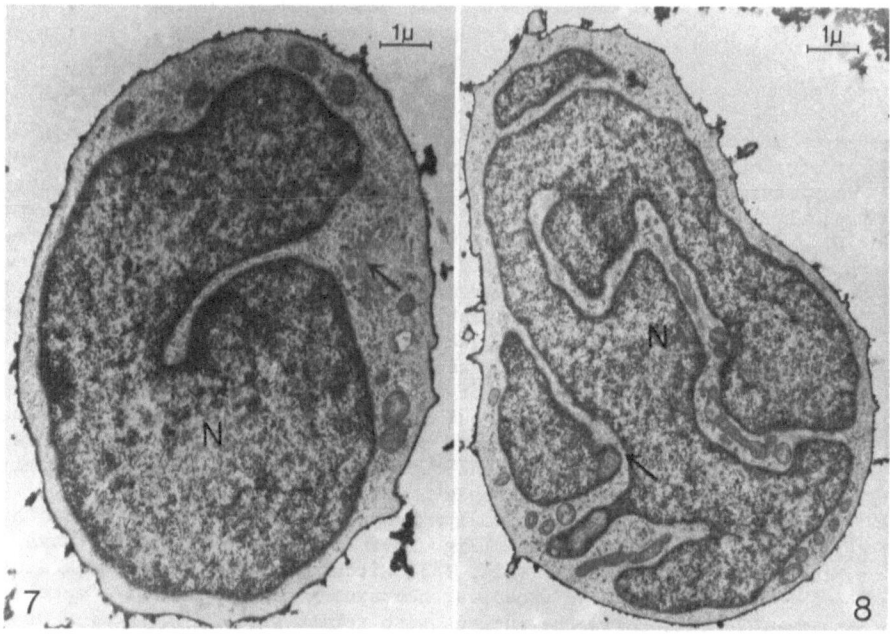

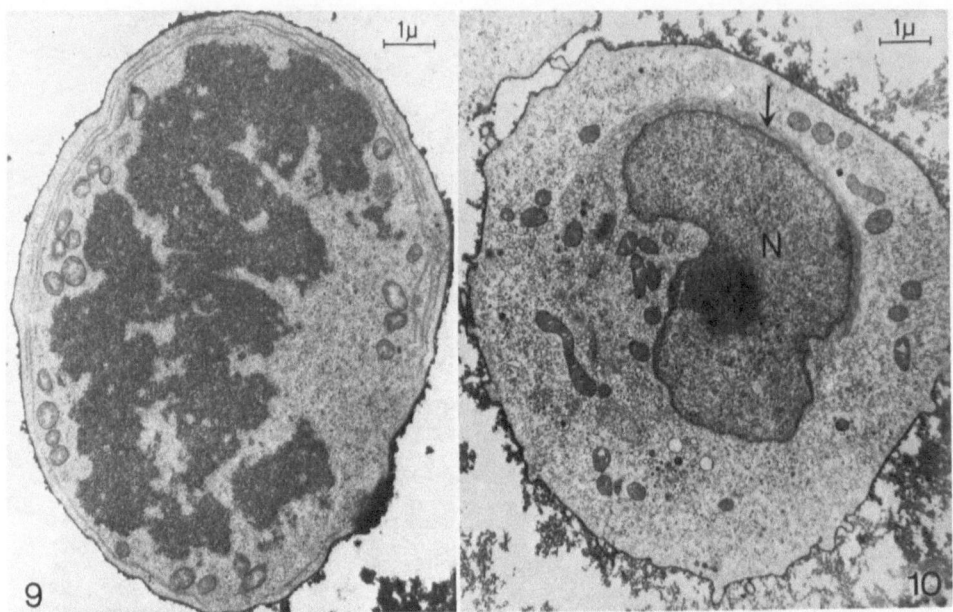

Fig. 9. ALL; Cell division stage. In the peripheral area mitochondria and membrane profiles are located. Ch = Condensed chromatin. 14 000 x

Fig. 10. AML; Cytofilaments arranged in a bundle near the nucleus (∫). In the cytoplasma Golgizones, mitochondria and numerous vesicles can be observed. N = nucleus. 6 600 x

Electron microscopy:

By electron microscope we found an undifferentiated cell type which had a diameter of about 7 μ, (Fig. 5). The nucleus was oval or kidney shaped. Sometimes deep invaginations were detected (Fig. 7). Electron dense chromocenters were randomly localized, (Fig. 6). The cytoplasma contained numerous mitochondria, centriols with satellites and Golgi zones. Ribosomes were scattered free in the cytoplasma. The endoplasmic reticulum was reduced to sparse, smooth vesicles. The cell membrane showed few micropinocytotic vesicles, (Fig. 6). Sometimes we found pseudopodes. Frequently the cells formed small groupes and the cell membranes were in direct contact. Furthermore, large cells could be observed with numerous empty vacuols, and some which contained phagocytised material, (Fig. 11, 12). In one case of AML formation of cytoplasmic filaments was the striking feature, (Fig. 10). One cell type of a case of ALL was especially impressive with a very polymorphous nucleus, forming nuclear bridges and pockets. ER was reduced only to the perinuclear cisterna. Polysomes, mitochondria, cytofilaments and lipid troplets were abundant (Fig. 8).

The investigation of CSF-cells of a lymphocytic meningitis demonstrated a less differentiated cell type, too, (Fig. 13). In cytoplasma ER was always detectable in more mature cells, (Fig. 14). Mitochondria and Golgi apparatus were regulary developed. Large vacuoles, containing an electrondense material were observed. In this cells the nucleus also formed nuclear pockets.

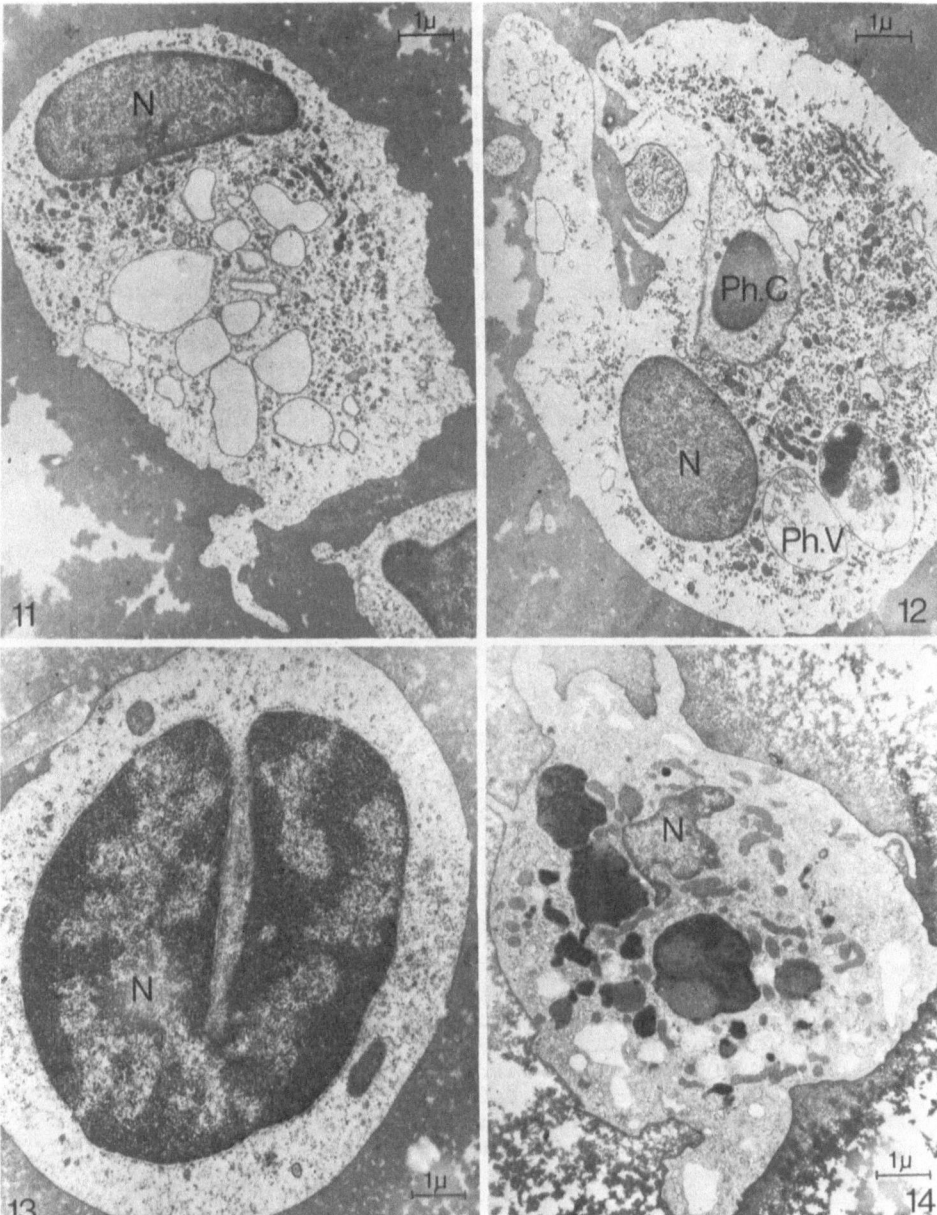

Fig. 11. Reticulum cell sarcoma: Vacuolated cell. N = nucleus. 6 000 x

Fig. 12. Reticulum cell sarcoma; Phagocyting cell. N = nucleus; Ph.V.=
Phagocytotic vacuole; Ph. C = Ingested cell with nucleus. 6 000 x

Fig. 13. Meningitis; Blast-like cell with deep nuclear invagination. N =
nucleus. 14 000 x

Fig. 14. Meningitis; Pinocyting cell. In the cytoplasm phagocytotic vacuoles
containg an electrondense material are located. The nucleus is polymorphous.
N = nucleus. 7 600 x

DISCUSSION

The light microscopical results show that the majority of the cells consists of blasts, which is in agreement to other authors (2, 6, 7, 10). Due to cyto-chemical stainings the leukemic origin of this cell type can be demonstrated and allows the classification of hemoblastosis. The reactions of CSF-cells are identical to those of peripheral blood and bone marrow. So viral or chronic meningitis can be distinguished from meningosis leukaemica.

Analysis of ultrastructure revealed no uniform cell picture. This technic should not be used for diagnosis. In some instances there was evidence of similar structures like in inflammation processes. On the other hand, completely different cells occurred. In hemoblastosis as well as in meningitis the occurrence of a blast-like cell type was a common feature. Occasionally mitoses and pseudopodes could be seen. The other cells were variable in respect to their structure. The anomaly of nucleus, formation of bridges and pockets may be regarded as a sign of a division's defect. Centriol alternations may be interpreted in the same way. The excess of mitochondria in the increased cyto-plasmic filaments suggest increase of metabolic activity and migration ability. Both phaenomena can be interpreted as an expression of the invasive growth of these cells.

We wish to thank Mrs. O. CAESAR for her skilful help.

REFERENCES

1. BEARD, M.E., FAIRLEY, G.H.: Acute leukemia in adults. Semin. Hematol. *11*, 5 - 24 (1974)
2. DREWINKO, B., SULLIVAN, M.P., MARTIN, T.: Use of the cytocentrifuge in the diagnosis of meningeal leukemia. Cancer *31*, 1331 - 1336 (1973)
3. HENNEKEUSER, H.H.: Untersuchungen zur Klassifizierung akuter Leukämien. Ergebn. inn. Med. *33*, 69 - 112 (1972)
4. HIRSCH, H.G., FEDORKO, M.J.: Ultrastructure of human leukocytes after simultaneous fixation with glutaraldehyde and osmium tetroxide and "post-fixation" in uranyl acetate. J. Cell Biol. *38*, 615 - 627 (1968)
5. MÖBIUS, W., HELLRIEGEL, K.P., TERHEGGEN, H.G.: Liquorcytologie bei unreif-zelligen Leukosen. Verh. dtsch. Ges. inn. Med. *77*, 91 - 93 (1971)
6. MOORE, E.W., THOMAS, L.B., SHAW, R.K., FREIREICH, E.J.: The central nervous system in acute leukemia. Arch. intern. Med. *105*, 451 - 468 (1960)
7. PRICE, R.A., JOHNSON, W.W.: The central nervous system in childhood leukemia: I. The arachnoid. Cancer *31*, 520 - 533 (1973)
8. REYNOLDS, E.S.: The use of lead citrate at high pH as an electron-opaque stain in electron microscopy. J. Cell Biol. *17*, 208 - 211 (1963)
9. SAYK, J.: Cytologie der Cerebrospinalflüssigkeit. Jena: Fischer 1960
10. SIMONE, J.: Acute lymphocytic leukemia in childhood. Semin. Hematol. *11*, 25 - 39 (1974)

Dr. W. MÖBIUS
Med. Universitätsklinik Freiburg
Hugstetter Straße 55
D-7800 Freiburg

Acta Neuropath. (Berlin), Suppl. VI, 199 - 203 (1975)
© by Springer-Verlag 1975

Electron Microscopy of Lymphocytic Leukaemia Cells in the Cerebrospinal Fluid

A. GUSEO

Department of Neurology and Psychiatry
University Medical School Pécs, Hungary

Summary: The ultrastructure of cells in the CSF are reported in 2 cases of
lymphocytic leukaemia of the CNS. Unusual nuclear pockets, margination of
the nuclear chromatin and fragmentation of the nuclei were frequent in the
first case, whereas in the second nuclear pockets were rare and deep indentations of the nuclei frequent.

Key words: Ultrastructure - CSF Cells - CNS Leukaemia - Nuclear Pockets -
Indirect Fragmentation

Cytoplasmic material filling nuclear pockets - sometimes referred to as nuclear
loops or blebs - as well as margination of the nuclear chromatin showing a
triple-membered structure due to infolding of the nuclear envelope, were observed in human and animal lymphosarcoma and leukaemies, and in human retino-
blastoma (1, 2, 3, 4, 5, 6, 7, 8, 13, 9). The nature of these phenomena is
obscure.
   We studied cerebrospinal fluid (CSF) cells from two patients with lymphocytic leukaemia of the central nervous system (CNS) for special ultrastructural alterations.

MATERIAL AND METHODS

CSF cells were collected from the patients in 1% OsO_4 or 2,5% glutaraldehyde,
centrifuged, embedded in fibrin, dehydrated and embedded in Durcupan ACM
resin. Ultrathin sections were contrasted with uranyl acetate and lead citrate (10).
   In *Case 1,* a boy of 11 years, lymphocytic leukaemia had begun 2 1/2 years
before admission. Cranial irradiation (1000 rads) given for meningeal prophylaxis on admission was unsuccessful, and severe leukopaenia developed. Thir-
teen month after the onset of lymphocytic leukaemia, leukaemia of the CNS was
diagnosed. Despite close observation and treatment with Prednisolon and Vincristine and intrathecal treatment with Methotrexate, six meningeal relapses
have been observed during the past fifteen months.
   In *Case 2,* a boy of 12 years, leukaemia of the CNS developed eight months
after lymphocytic leukaemia had been detected. After admission he was given
regular Prednisolon, Vincristine and intrathecal Methotrexate for three
months, at the end of which subarachnoid haemorrhage developed, and the
patient died of increasing intracranial pressure.

RESULTS

Case 1: The cells measured 12 - 17 µ, the scanty cytoplasm was packed with
ribosomes and mitochondria were sparse and no endoplasmic reticulum or Golgi

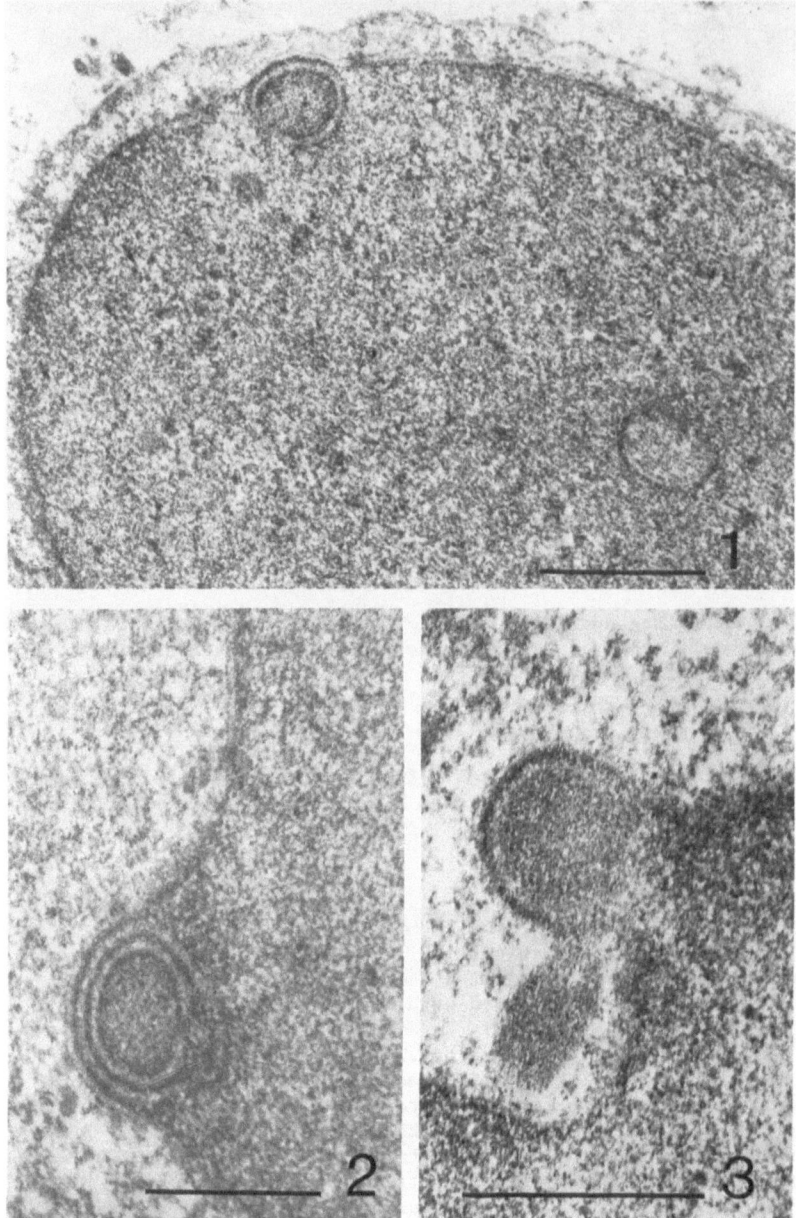

Case 1.

Fig. 1. Nuclear pockets are seen under the nuclear envelope and deep in the nucleus

Fig. 2. Nuclear pocket with six layers

Fig. 3. Finger-like extensions with margination of the chromatin becoming detached

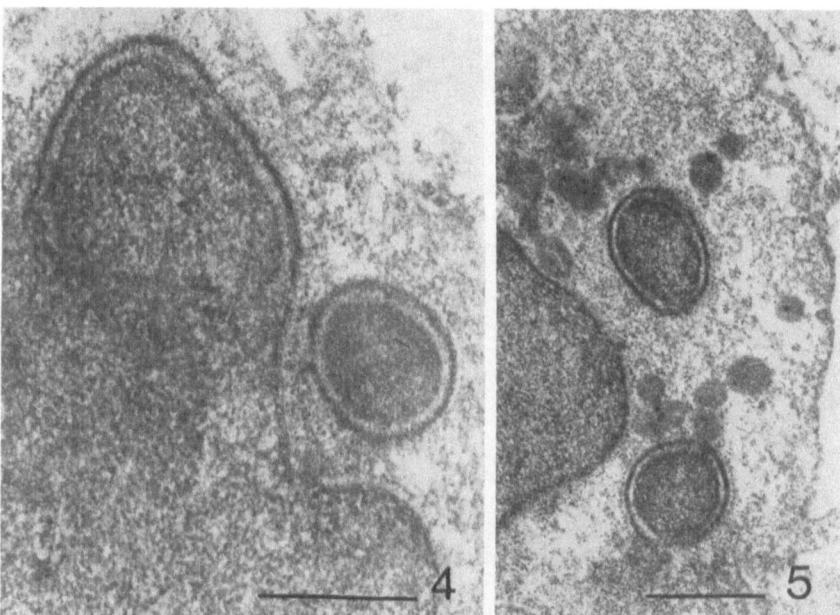

Fig. 4. Protrusions of the nucleus covered with double-layered chromatin;
in the cytoplasm is a ring-shaped projection without apparent nuclear attache-
ment

Fig. 5. Two ring-shaped projections in the cytoplasm

complexes were observed. Most nuclei were round or kidney-shaped and sometimes
irregularly lobed by indentations. In at least 10% of the cells there were
unusual nuclear pockets under the nuclear membrane and also deep in the nucleus,
which contained material similar to the nuclear chromatin (Fig. 1). Multi-
layering, 3 sometimes 6 layers of marginal chromatin was also seen (Figs. 4
and 2). The osmiophilic inner layer measured 300-500 Å and on each side of it
an electron lucent layer measuring 400-600 Å was seen. Parts of the nucleus
containing nuclear pockets were demarcated and occasionally detached (Fig. 3).
Ring shaped projections with no visible nuclear attachment were seen here and
there in the cytoplasm (Fig. 5).

Case 2: The cells had more cytoplasm and were larger and less uniform than in
case 1 measuring 14-20 µ. The cell surface was irregular and presented frequent
microvilli (Fig. 6). The cytoplasm was packed with ribosomes; mitochondria
were grouped at one pole and lipid bodies and a few annulate lamellae were
seen. The nuclei were of irregular shape, with many deep indentations (Fig. 7)
and the chromatin was evenly distributed. Some nuclear pockets were found,
which contained homogenous material similar to that seen in the cytoplasm
(Fig. 7).

DISCUSSION

The phenomenon of nuclear pockets and the alteration of the nuclear envelope
to form layered structure in CSF cells have not been previously reported. We

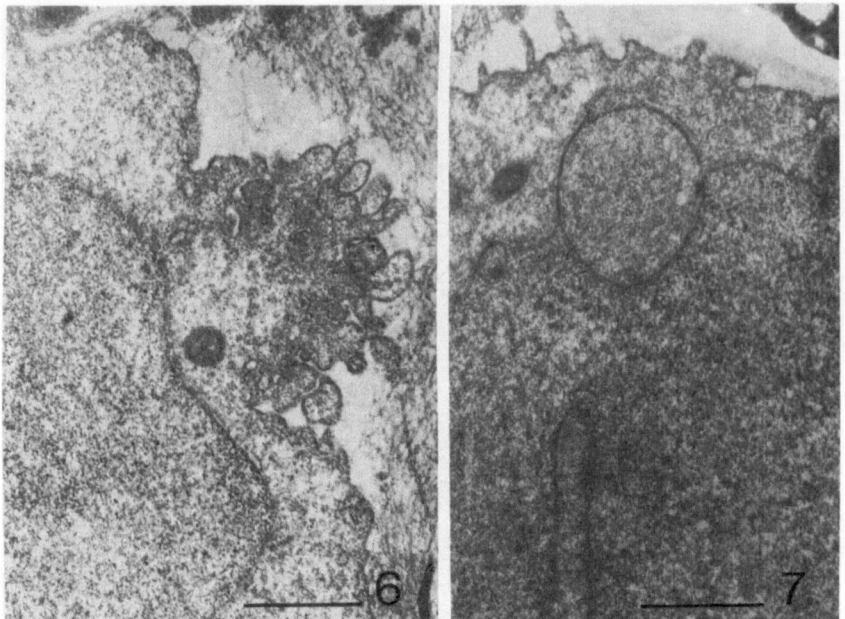

Case 2.

Fig. 6. Microvilli are seen on the edge of a pseudopodium, which contains an increased number of ribosomes

Fig. 7. Nuclear pocket, deep identation of the nucleus. (The scale on each Fig. indicates 1 μ.)

failed to find similar nuclear alterations in lymphocytic cells of the CSF in aseptic pleocytoses (10). Inside the nuclear pockets, which were atypical in Case 1, no cytoplasmic organelles were found.

The ring shaped nuclear projections might have been cross sections of finger-like nuclear extrusions (see Figs. 2 and 3). The globules were seen also by light microscopy in these two cases but also in cells in the CSF of a patient with primary lymphoma of the midbrain. The globules appeared to be "indirect nuclear fragmentation" which may be the result of disturbed mitotic activity and was first described by ARNOLD (11). Since it is known that some viruses (12), may cause nuclear fragmentation, the role of a specific viral agent causing nuclear fragmentation in leukaemia and lymphoma cells should be considered.

In view of their presence in normal as well as in pathological cells, the nuclear pockets and the alterations of the nuclear envelope cannot be regarded as a sign of leukemia or any other disease; their frequency, however, might be of diagnostic importance. These phenomena have been related to enhanced nucleo-cytoplasmic interactions (13). We assume that malignant cells in particular those that are of mesenchymal origin and synthesize a considerable amount of protein, might frequently develope nuclear pockets and alterations of the nuclear envelope.

REFERENCES

1. EPSTEIN, M.A., ACHONG, B.G.: Fine structural organization of human lympho-
    blasts of a tissue culture strain (EB 1) from Burkitt's lymphoma. J. nat.
    Cancer Inst. *34*, 241 - 254 (1965)
2. EPSTEIN, M.A., BARR, Y.M., ACHONG, B.G.: The behaviour and morphology of
    a second tissue culture strain (EB 2) of lymphoblasts from Burkitt's
    lymphoma. Brit. J. Cancer. *19*, 108 - 115 (1965)
3. DORFMAN, R.F.: The fine structure of malignent lymphoma in a child from
    St. Louis Missouri. J. nat. Cancer Inst. *38*, 491 - 505 (1967)
4. MC DUFFIE, N.G.: Nuclear blebs in human leukemic cells. Nature (London)
    214, 1341 - 1342 (1967)
5. SCHRECK, R.: Ultrastructure of blood lymphocytes from chronic lymphocytic
    and lymphosarcoma cell leukemia. J. nat. Cancer Inst. *48*, 51 - 64 (1972)
6. SMITH, C.F., O'Hara, P.T.: Structure of nuclear pockets in human leukocytes.
    J. Ultrastruct. Res. *21*, 415 - 423 (1968)
7. DAVIES, H.G.: Electron microscope observation on the organization of hetero-
    chromatin in certain cells. J. Cell Sci. *3*, 129 - 150 (1968)
8. MILLER, J.M., MILLER, L.D., GILETTE, K.G., OLSON, C.: Incidence of lympho-
    cytic nuclear projections in bovine lymphosarcoma. J. nat. Cancer Inst.
    43, 719 - 728 (1969)
9. POPOFF, N., ELLSWORTH, R.M.: The fine structure of nuclear alterations in
    retinoblastoma and in developing human retina. In vitro and in vivo ob-
    servations. J. Ultrastruct. Res. *29*, 535 - 549 (1969)
10. GUSEO, A.: Über die Makrophagen des Liquor cerebrospinalis. Z. Neurol. *200*,
    136 - 147 (1971)
11. ARNOLD, J.: Beobachtungen über Kerne und Kernteilungen in den Zellen des
    Knochenmarkes. Virchows Arch. path. Anat. *93*, 1 - 39 (1883)
12. LEVINSON, W.: Fragmentation of the nucleus in Roux sarcoma virus infected
    chick embryo cells. J. nat. Cancer Inst. *44*, 151 - 158 (1970)
13. MOLLO, F., PRATO, V.: Nuclear projections in eosinophils. Lancet, II.
    924 - 925 (1968)

A. GUSEO, M.D.
7623 Pécs, Rét u. 2. Hungary

Acta Neuropath. (Berlin), Suppl. VI, 205 - 208 (1975)

Family Studies in Cases with Malignant Lymphomas

TH. HARDMEIER AND H. RELLSTAB

Department of Pathology
Thurgauisches Kantonsspital
Münsterlingen / Switzerland

Summary: A short review of the genetic aspects of tumors of the reticulo-endothelial system is given. Of special interest is the observation of a "familial lymphohistiocytosis of the nervous system" published by PRICE *et al.* in 1971. Important are also our own observations with different types of malignant lymphoma in the same family. In addition to the possibilities of classical mendelian inheritance and the possibility of multifactorial inheritance preexisting immunological deficiency syndromes and chromosomal aberrations have to be considered as causal factors.

Key words: Heredofamilial Disease - Tumors of the Reticuloendothelial System - Malignant Lymphoma - Nervous System

The greatest part of tumors of the nervous system do not appear to be of genetic origin. Genetically predisposed tumors are here interesting exceptions rather than the rule (2). On the other side, the role of genetic and host factors seems to be important for malignancies of the reticuloendothelial system. Since VIRCHOW (quoted 13) numerous reports of leukemia in 2 or even more members of individual families have appeared in the literature. In 1947 VIDEBAEK (13) collected 26 observations of familial leukemia in the literature for a careful study together with 11 of his own. The study of twins yields a concordance rate of about 25% for leukemia in monozygous twin sets (8). The results of the different familial studies in the field of leukemia show a great difference. Several authors think that there is no significance at all (6). For VIDEBAEK (13) an *irregular dominance* seemed most likely. HEATH and MOLONEY (8) discussed a *dominant trait with incomplete penetrance* and a "vertical" viral transmission in three successive generations of the same family. GUNZ *et al.* (7) came to a similar conclusion. McKUSICK (9) in the third edition of his "Catalogs of autosomal dominant, autosomal recessive, and X-linked phenotypes" accepts an autosomal dominant inheritance for some familial occurences of chronic lymphatic leukemia.

Familial concentration of any given disease may occur as a mere coincidence. Therefore, epidemiologic studies of statistical significance have been made for instance in cases of Hodgkin's disease. RAZIS *et al.* (12) came to the conclusion, that the probability that the immediate relatives of a patient with Hodgkin's disease will also develop it is three times as great as the corresponding probability for the immediate relatives of a person without the disease. Hodgkin's disease apparently does not have a simple inheritance. Familial observations of multiple myeloma and macroglobulinemia are also known. For some observations of familial multiple myeloma suggestions of an autosomal recessive inheritance are strong enough (9).

Table 1. *Heredity and Malignancies of the Reticuloendothelial System*

1. cases following mendelian inheritance in man: rare
    a) autosomal dominant : chronic lymphatic leukemia
    b) autosomal recessive : multiple myeloma
                              hemophagocytic reticulosis
2. possibility of multifactorial inheritance : probably the most important
   group
3. observations on the basis of a preexisting immunological deficiency
   syndrome

    a) autosomal recessive : Ataxia teleangiectasia (LOUIS-BAR)
    b) X-linked recessive   : WISKOTT-ALDRICH syndrome
4. observations on the basis of chromosomal aberrations (not discussed here).

In other more heterogenous groups of diseases we find a proliferation of
reticuloendothelial cells. Familial occurences of these histiocytic disorders,
also known as reticuloendotheliosis or familial hemophagocytic reticulosis
have been published since the first observation (5). Despite differences the
familial observations have in common an unknown etiology, similar clinical
courses and pathological findings, occasionally with central nervous system
infiltration. In 1971 PRICE *et al*. (11) published paper on *"familial lymphohistiocytosis of the nervous system"*. Four of 12 children showed an unusual
neurological disease with multiple lesions of the central nervous system
characterized by foci of necrosis and diffuse infiltration of lymphocytes and
histiocytes mainly in the white matter of the cerebral hemispheres and cerebellum. In one case they found also significant lymphohistiocytic infiltrates
in organs outside the central nervous system. PRICE *et al*. (11) came to the
conclusion that a genetically-determined atypical response to an undisclosed
infection is possible. Earlier, NELSON *et al*. (1) discussed transmission as a
mendelian recessive trait in a similar familial observation.
Our idea to look for families with different types of the above mentioned
diseases, is based on the knowledge that all cells producing these tumorous
lesions go back to pluripotential stem cells (4).
In this family from a mountainous part of our country we could find hitherto
11 cases with clinically and morphologically proved malignant neoplastic diseases (Fig. 1). There were 5 patients with *myelocytic leukemia,* 4 cases with
HODGKIN's disease, 1 observation of *reticulosarcoma* and finally one member
with *malignant melanoma*. Important is the observation of *consanguinity* in
7 couples of the family. We hope to prove an autosomal recessive inheritance
by statistical methods, but a multifactorial inheritance cannot be excluded.
Up to now in our study of over 100 families, we have found not one observation with lesions of the nervous system. Another example of a careful genetic study is that of a Swiss family published by CLEMENCON (3). Beside one
patient with leukemia and several cases of carcinomas, 5 observations of
malignant lymphoma of different types are of interest. A 4 year old boy (case
3 of CLEMENCON) died of a lymphoma localized in the basal ganglia of the
brain. Also the brother and the grandfather had malignant lymphoma but without lesions of the nervous system. Of more interest are two other brothers of
the same family with malignant lymphoma and an agammaglobulinemia of the X-
linked recessive BRUTON type. We know that several other primary immunologic
deficiency syndromes are hereditary and can be associated with the frequent
development of malignant lymphomas (1). Therefore we think that more of these
disorders and the mentioned malignant neoplastic diseases have to be taken
into consideration for genealogical studies.

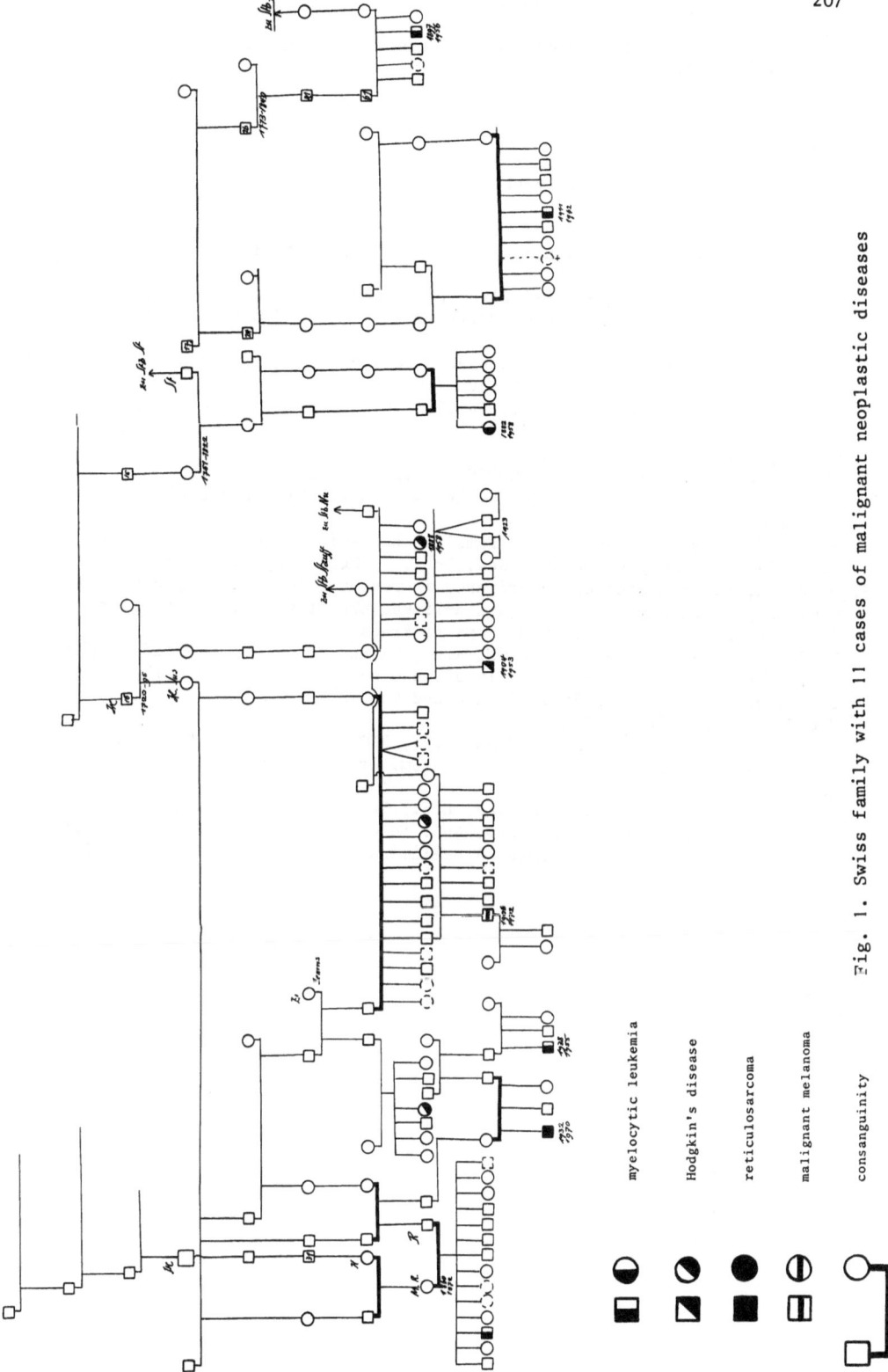

myelocytic leukemia

Hodgkin's disease

reticulosarcoma

malignant melanoma

consanguinity

Fig. 1. Swiss family with 11 cases of malignant neoplastic diseases

A summary of our actual knowledge and interpretation of facts and fancies is given in Table 1.

REFERENCES

1. AISENBERG, A.C.: Malignant lymphoma. New Engl. J. Med. *288*, 883 - 890 and 935 - 941 (1973)
2. AITA, J.A.: Genetic aspects of tumors of the nervous system. *In:* Lynch, H.T.: Hereditary factors in carcinoma. P. 86 - 110. Berlin, Heidelberg, New York: Springer 1967
3. Clémencon, J.-C.: Rencontre simultanée, dans une famille, de lymphomes malins, d'agammaglobulinémie et d'hémophilie. A. J. Génét. hum. *21*, 85 - 138 (1973)
4. CLINE, M.J., GOLDE, D.W.: A review and reevaluation of the histiocytic disorders. Amer. J. Med. *55*, 49 - 60 (1973)
5. FARQUHAR, J.W., GLAIREAUX, A.E.: Familial haemophagocytic reticulosis. Arch. Dis. Child. *27*, 519 - 525 (1952)
6. GUASCH, J.: Hérédité des leucémies. Sang *25*, 384 - 421 (1954)
7. GUNZ, F.W., FITZGERALD, P.H., CROSSEN, P.E., MACKENZIE, I.S., POWLES, C.P., JENSEN, G.R.: Multiple cases of leukemia in a sibship. Blood *27*, 482 - 489 (1965)
8. HEATH, C.W. jr., MOLONEY, W.C.: Familial Leukemia. Five cases of acute leukemia in three generations. New. Engl. J. Med. *272*, 882 - 887 (1965)
9. McKUSICK, V.A.: Mendelian inheritance in man. Catalogs of autosomal dominant, autosomal recessive, and X-linked phenotypes. Third edition. Baltimore and London: The Johns Hopkins Press 1971
10. NELSON, P., SANTAMARIA, A., OLSON, R.L., NAYAK, N.C.: Generalized lympho-histiocytic infiltration. A family disease not previously described and different from Letterer-Siwe disease and Chediak-Higashi syndrome. Pediatrics *27*, 931 - 950 (1961)
11. PRICE, D.L., WOOLSEY, J.E., ROSMAN, N.P., RICHARDSON, E.P.: Familial lymphohistiocytosis of the nervous system. Arch. Neurol. *24*, 270 - 283 (1971)
12. RAZIS, D.V., DIAMOND, H.D., CRAVER, L.F.: Familial Hodgkin's disease: its significance and implications. Ann. intern. Med. *51*, 933 - 971 (1959)
13. VIDEBAEK, A.: Familial leukemia. A preliminary report. Acta med. scand. *127*, 26 - 52 (1947)

T. HARDMEIER, M.D.
Department of Pathology
Thurgauisches Kantonsspital
CH - 8596 Münsterlingen
Switzerland

Acta Neuropath. (Berlin), Suppl. VI, 209 - 212 (1975)
© by Springer-Verlag 1975

Clinical and Pathological Studies in a Case of Reticulum Cell Sarcoma

T. INOSE AND J. KINOSHITA

The Department of Neurology & Psychiatry
Yokohama City University School of Medicine, Japan

Summary: A case of reticulum cell sarcoma associated with involvement of the central nervous system was presented. This seems to be an atypical case of reticulum cell sarcoma for the following reasons.
1. Hepatosplenomegaly and enlarged lymph nodes were not observed through the entire clinical course. The main abnormalities were psycho-neurological.

2. These cells did not form a tumour mass, but infiltrated diffucely into the central nervous system and extraneural sites, and the primary focus could not be determined. Four cases of reticulum cell sarcoma in Japan, in which the initial symptoms were of neurological involvement, are reviewed.

Key words: Reticulum Cell Sarcoma – Neuropsychiatric Manifestation – Cerebral Lesion without Tumour Formation

INTRODUCTION

Involvement of the nervous system is a well-recognized complication of malignant lymphoma, but it is unusual for the main manifestations of malignant lymphoma to be psycho-neurological and for any other somatic signs and symptoms indicating malignant lymphoma to be clinically unsignificant. In the so-called malignant lymphoma group, reticulum cell sarcoma (RCS), in which the origin of the tumour cell is the histiocyte, monocyte or clasmatocyte, can be to be divided into two types; lymph node-visceral, systemic type and primary RCS of the brain (1).
   The case presented here was one of the systemic type of RCS at autopsy, but hepatosplenomegaly and enlarged lymph nodes were not observed throughout the entire clinical course, and the most obvious manifestations were marked changes of the level of consciousness.

CLINICAL HISTORY

A 42 year-old Japanese female initially showed unsteadiness of gait of the left in August 1970, but several months later it disappeared. However, she appeared slovenly and indolent. In January 1971, she stumbled easily and was readily provoked to laughter. One month later, the patient was admitted to hospital in a delirious state with visual hallucinations, delusions, fever and urinary incontinence which subsided a few days later. Thereafter, the level of consciousness fluctuated.
   Examination showed nuchal rigidity and absent knee and ankle jerks and a positive Babinski sign on the left side. Hepatosplenomegaly and enlarged lymph nodes were not found. Routine laboratory studies revealed; LDH 710 units,

CRP (+++), total protein 5.8 g/dl, blood sugar 77 mg/dl, total cholesterol
133 mg/dl, GOT 23 units, GPT 12 units, A/G 1.1, albumin 34.0%, $\alpha_1$globulin
8.5%, $\alpha_2$globulin 17.o%, β globulin 16.0%, γ globulin 24.5%. Urinalysis was
normal. The blood count and the radiological examination of the chest were
normal. Blood pressure was 120/75 mmHg. A lumbar puncture revealed clear fluid
with a pressure of 180 mm. 5 mononuclear leukocytes /cmm; protein 290 mg/dl.
A carotid angiogram and a pneumoencephalogram were normal and electroencephalo-
grams showed a non-focal generalized slow wave pattern.

On April 1, the patient became restless and delirious. Blood examination at
this time showed; Hb 10.7 g/dl, Ht 33%, RBC 3,870,000/mm^3, WBC 11,500/mm^3,
polymorphs 84.5%, lymphocytes 2.5%, monocytes 4.5%, basophils 0.5%, and atypical
lymphocyte-like cells 8% (Fig. 1). Concurrently, thrombocytopenia (42,000/mm^3)
occurred. Atypical lymphocyte-like cells and thrombocytopenia were still present
in peripheral blood smears.

On April 9, she became unconscious with dyspnoea and cyanosis and ventricular
fibrillation of the heart. Death occurred on May 14 with deep coma, status
epilepticus and high fever. The entire clinical course lasted eight months.
The tentative clinical diagnosis was that of a subacute viral encephalitis.

POSTMORTEM EXAMINATION

The brain weighed 1,460 g. There was moderate cerebral oedema and the meninges
were slightly thickened and cloudy. Atypical abnormal cells were spread diffusely through the leptomeninges, being more numerous over the temporal lobes and
at the base of the brain. There was scattered involvement of the choroid
plexuses. Where the meninges were extensively infiltrated, vascular invasion
spread along the Virchow-Robin spaces (Fig. 2). The lumina of many vessels were
filled with tumour cells and the walls infiltrated by tumour cells (Fig. 3).
The tumour cells were almost limited to the perivascular spaces. Bordering the
margins of the infiltrations were pleomorphic cells, resembling activated
microglia (Fig. 4).

The tumour cells had a moderate amount of ill-defined cytoplasm and round
or oval nuclei, and measured 10 to 15 µ in diameter. Multinucleated cells
could be seen but not true tumour giant cells. The chromatin content was
variable, but in general it was moderate. There were many mitotic figures
(Fig. 5). Some of the cells contained phagocytosed cellular material. A reticulin stain showed the vessels surrounded by rings of fibres between which
lay tumour cells, and a silver carbonate preparation (Hortega) showed plump
argentophilic processes of some of the tumour cells (Fig. 6).

There were multiple foci of softening and perivascular hemorrhages scattered
in the cortex and the white matter of the cerebrum, cerebellum and pons. This
seems to correspond with the clinical course in which there were fluctuations
in the level of consciousness.

In the other organs, many small grayish nodules composed of tumour cells
were found. They merged with the surrounding tissue, a localized tumour mass
was not seen, and the normal architecture of the organs was preserved. In the
liver, portal areas were occasionally expanded by dense infiltrates of tumour
cells. The kidneys were swollen as a result of diffuse invasion by tumour
cells. The tumour cells were present in the interstitium and led to separation
of tubules with slight destruction of epithelium (Fig. 7). In the heart the
tumour cells strikingly infiltrated from the perivascular areas into the interstitial tissues of the myocardium, and the network of reticulin fibres surrounding groups of tumour cells and individual cells was illustrated by means
of the reticulin stain (Fig. 8). Cervical and mesenteric lymph nodes were not
involved. Bone marrow was not destroyed. In addition cytomegalovirus were
found in the lung and pancreas.

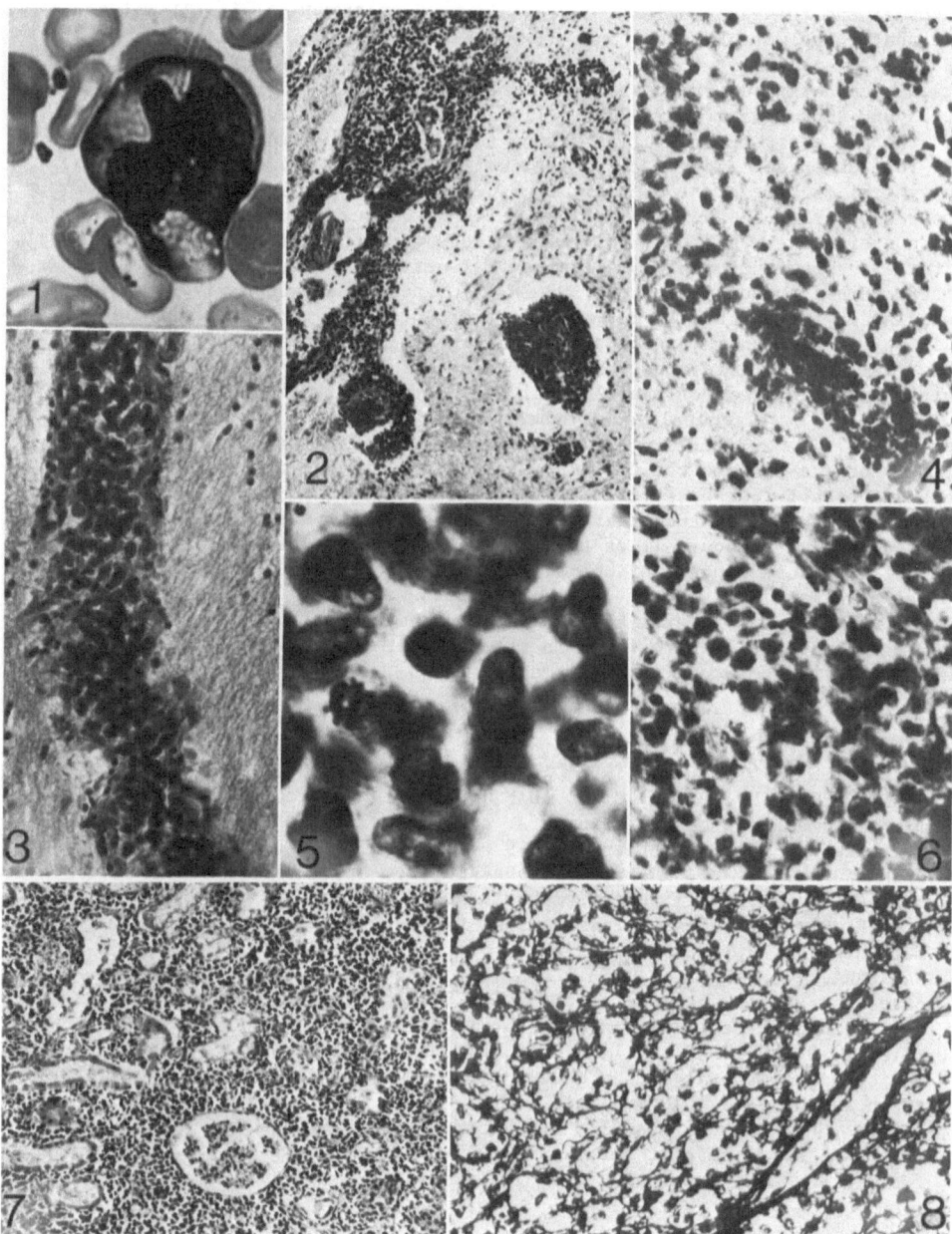

Figs. 1 - 8

DISCUSSION

The clinical picture in this case was characterized by neurological and
psychiatric symptoms without other somatic manifestations. In spite of intensive clinical and laboratory investigations, there was no evidence of any
systemic disease.

Concerning the pathological findings in RCS, SPARLING *et al.* (2) pointed out that there was often evidence of ameboid activity as shown by irregular pseudopodal processes to the tumour cells. They also emphasized that silver stains demonstrated irregular fibrils of reticulin passing between groups of cells and surrounding individual cells and that silver carbonate stains brought out the processes of the cells proving their close kinship to the histiocyte, the reticulum cell and the microglial cell. This case was essentially similar to typical microscopical pictures of RCS. However, in the great majority of previously observed cases, single or multiple circumscribed tumour masses of various sizes were present. Only a few cases were found to have extensive diffuse involvement, including the central nervous system, without any large circumscribed tumour formation. SORGER (3) reported a case of systemic RCS associated with diffuse involvement of the central nervous system in which it was the initial and major focus of a multicentric malignant lymphoma.

In the Japanese literature only four cases of RCS have been reported where initial symptoms were of neurological and mental invilvement.

In the 1st case generalized lymphadenopathy occurred with a progressive course (4). The 2nd and 3rd cases had diffuse infiltrative involvement of many organs through the entire course of the disease (5, 6). It was characteristic of all four cases that diffuse infiltrations of tumour cells were found in the meninges and other reticuloendothelial systems and the course of the disease was subacute (less than 10 months). In two cases a high protein and a low glucose content of spinal fluid were found and in three cases the spinal cord was involved. In the authors' case atypical lymphocyte-like cells were observed in peripheral blood smears, and also in the case of MIYOSHI *et al.* (5), the tumour cells were found in the peripheral blood and a diagnosis of leukemic reticulosarcomatosis was made.

REFERENCES

1. SCHAUMBURG, H.H., PLANK, C.R., ADAMS, R.D.: The reticulum cell sarcoma - microglioma group of brain tumours. A consideration of their clinical features and therapy. Brain *95*, 199 - 212 (1972)
2. SPARLING, H.J., Jr., ADAMS, R.D., PARKER, F., Jr.: Involvement of the nervous system by malignant lymphoma. Medicine *26*, 285 - 332 (1947)
3. SORGER, K.: Reticulum cell sarcoma of the central nervous system. Can. med. Ass. J. *89*, 503 - 507 (1963)
4. NAGASAWA, T., TAKUMA, T., SHIOZAWA, R., KINUGASA, K., TOYOKURA, Y.: A case of reticulum cell sarcoma showing variegated neurological symptoms. Japanese Medicine *8*, 981 - 986 (1961)
5. MIYOSHI, S., SHIRABE, T., TANIMOTO, F.: An autopsy case of leukemic reticulosarcomatosis with abducens nerve palsy and transverse myelopathy. Brain and Nerve *22*, 1209 - 1217 (1970)
6. ITO, K., MIHARA, S., ADACHI, S., SENDA, A., MASUYA, S., YASUDA, S., TAKAHARA, K.: A case of reticulum cell sarcoma forming multiple softening foci in the CNS. Japanese Clinical Neurology *11*, 739 (1971)

T. INOSE and J. KINOSHITA
Department of Neurology & Psychiatry
Yokohama City University School of Medicine
Urafune-cho, Minami-ku
Yokohama, Japan

Acta Neuropath. (Berlin), Suppl. VI, 213 - 215 (1975)

Lymphoblastic Extramedullary Spinal Tumor During Remission of Acute Lymphoblastic Leukaemie

P. KREPLER (St. Anna - Children's Hospital, Vienna)
K. JENTZSCH (Dept. of Radiotherapy, Univ. Vienna)
J. MAYER-OBIDITSCH (Dept. of Pathology, Univ. Vienna)
S. SALAH (Dept. of Neurosurgery, Univ. Vienna)

Summary: An unusual case history of a girl with ALL is presented. The diagnosis
was established at the age of 7. At the age of 11, 5 years and 3 months after
remission due to treatment an extramedullary tumour of a lumbar vertebra produced a transverse lesion of the spinal cord and meningeal leukaemia. The tumour consisted mainly of connective tissue with small foci of lymphoblastic
cells, identical with those originally seen in the peripheral blood stream.
After laminectomy, irradiation and chemotherapy the girl is still in her
first haematological remission, lasting nearly 7 years.

Key words: Acute lymphoblastic leukaemia - transverse lesion of the spinal
cord - leukaemic destruction of vertebra

CASE REPORT

The diagnosis of a typical large cell acute lymphatic leukaemia (ALL) was made
on Oct. 20th, 1967 in a girl aged 7 years and 10 months. She had been treated
previously for rheumatoid arthritis and anaemia for 2 years, conditions associated with a preleukemic stage.

On admission severe anaemia (1,5 mill.), leukopenia (2500) and thrombopenia
(30,000) were noted. The liver and spleen were enlarged (10 cm below the costal
margin). The bone marrow showed 84% blasts, rather large cells with multilobular
nucleoli and dark blue cytoplasm (macrolymphoblastic type). The most striking
findings were a severe osteoporosis and extensive osteolytic lesions, especially
in the proximal metaphysis of the tibia. She complained of severe pain and was
unable to walk. X-rays of the lumbar vertebrae showed osteoporotic changes only.
The thoracic spine seemed free of disease. X-rays revealed a left pleuropneumonic
infiltration while there was a severe septicaemia during the aplastic phase
(only 100 granulocytes) after remission induced with Vincristine. There were
also unusual septic skin lesions (up to 5-7 cm in diameter and 2-3 cm deep)
and areas of necrosis without any inflammatory reaction. A severe infection of
the urinary tract also developed. These complications were controlled with antibiotics and six weeks later a complete remission was achieved. She was kept on
maintenance therapy with methotrexate (MTX) 2,5 - 3,5 mg/kg every 14 days i.v.
and Vincristine (VCR) 1,5 mg/m^2 i.v. every 5-7 weeks. After 4 years this therapy had to be discontinued because of severe MTX stomatitis. Nevertheless the
child remained in complete remission and excellent health without therapy for
about 7 months.

In May 1972 whilst riding a bicycle and passing over a hole in the road she
felt a sudden pain in the lumbar region. X-rays showed a funnel-shaped indentation of the 2nd lumbar vertebra. This was interpreted as a traumatic lesion
associated with general osteoporosis. At this time the thoracic spine was

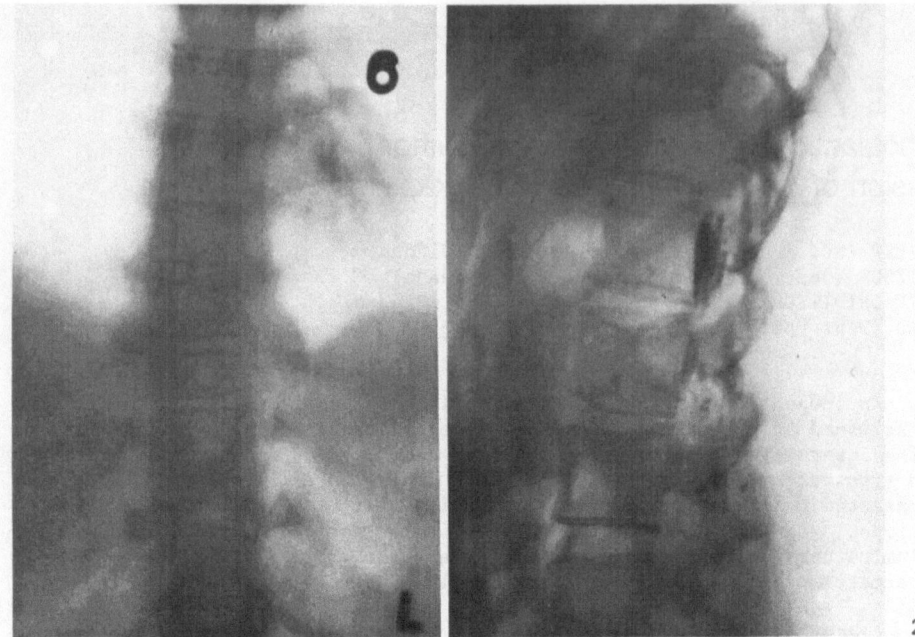

Fig. 1. Tomogram of the thoracic spine. Compression of the 9th vertebra, with a spindle-shaped soft tissue shadow on the left side

Fig. 2. Myelographie with arrest at the 2nd lumbar vertebra, funnel-shaped depression of the upper and lower surfaces of this vertebra

normal. Aspiration of bone marrow and spinal fluid gave normal values. The patient felt better after immobilisation of the spine.

Some weeks later during a church service there was dramatic, loss of consciousness: this lasted several hours. Arteriography excluded haemorrhage or other space occupying lesions in the brain. Examination of the spinal fluid revealed a neutrophilic pleocytosis and pneumococci. Intensive care following of respiratory arrest and treatment with Chloramphenicol brought rapid relief and clearance of the cerebro-spinal fluid. Unfortunately retrobulbar neuritis of the right eye developed which led, despite treatment with cortisone, to optic atrophy and complete unilateral blindness.

During convalescence the girl complained again of severe pain, now in the thoracic spine. X-rays revealed reduction in size of the 9th thoracic vertebra with a spindleshaped paravertebral soft tissue shadow (Fig. 1). There was no haematological relapse and meningeal leukaemia was excluded by a normal CSF. The lesion was therefore interpreted as steroid osteoporosis. At the beginning of Jan. 1973 the onset of paraplegia and disturbed micturation indicated a transverse lesion of the spinal cord. Myelography (Fig. 2) revealed complete arrest at the second lumbar vertebra.

Laminectomy showed a protruding dural sac to be under increased tension. The spinal cord was surrounded by tumour masses, extending mainly to the left and anteriorly, which could be removed only in part. Nevertheless most of the symptoms of the transverse lesion regressed. Histological examination showed a tumour, mainly composed of connective tissue, containing small perivascular foci of large cells. these had polymorphic nuclei which were moderately rich in

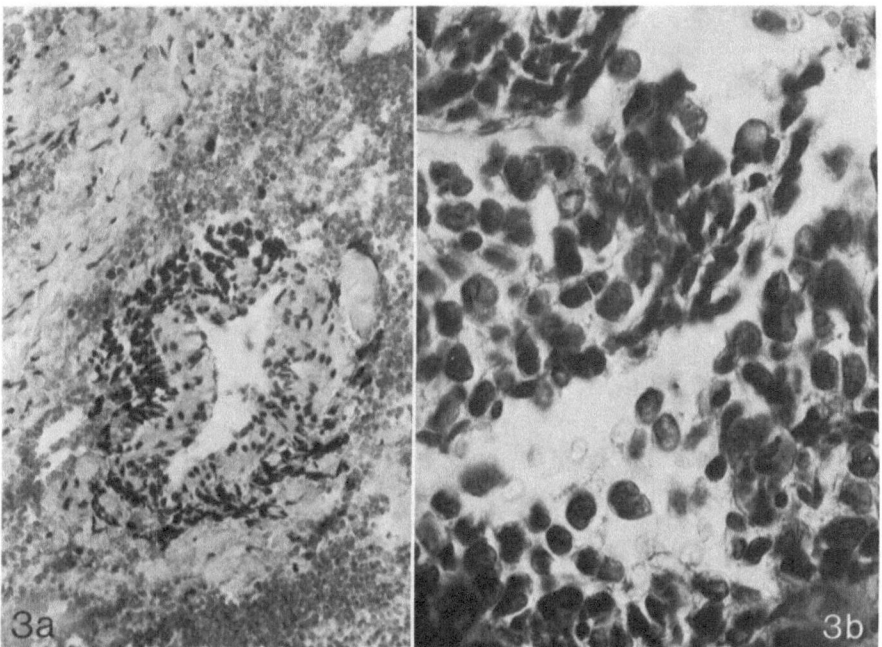

Fig. 3 a and b. *a)* Extradural tumour, arising from the vertebra, mainly consisting of connective tissue and small foci of macrocellular lymphoblasts.
b) Higher magnification of a group of lymphoblastic tumour cells

chromatin, had large nucleoli, and a narrow rim of basophilic cytoplasm (Fig. 3).
The infiltrations corresponded morphologically to a macrolymphoblastic AL. The
preoperative investigation of the spinal fluid revealed 430/3 typical macrocellular leukaemic blast cells with PAS positive granules.

These findings proved that the tumour consisted of leukaemic cells, seemingly
arising from the vertebrae. Extradural tumour growth was the cause of the transverse lesion and the meningeal leukaemic infiltration. Operation was followed
by irradiation of affected vertebrae (up to 2000 rad with Co^{60}) and by subocci-
pital injections of MTX. Concomitantly cytostatic maintenance therapy was
started. After recovery prophylactic irradiation of the skull was given
(2400 rads).

The patient is now 17 years old, has been in haematological remission for
7 years and is free of major symptoms. Minor neurological sequelae remain from
the transverse lesion.

Prof. Dr. P. KREPLER
St. Anna Kinderspital
Kinderspitalgasse 6
A - 1090 W i e n

Acta Neuropath. (Berlin), Suppl. VI, 217 - 220 (1975)

Radiotherapy of Malignant Lymphomas

K.H. KÄRCHER AND K. JENTZSCH

Strahlentherapeutische Klinik und Institut für klinische
Strahlenbiologie der Universität Wien

Summary: Radiotherapy of non-Hodgkin's lymphomas situated in the central nervous
system is basically similar to the treatment applied to any other part of the
body. There are two requirements: the first is the prophylactic irradiation of
the CNS in a systemic disease of the reticuloendothelial system, mainly in acute
lymphatic leukemia; the second is the treatment of solitary tumors in the CNS.
   Radiotherapy can improve dramatically the results obtained with intrathecal
chemotherapy, particularly in leukemic involvement of the CNS in childhood.
The fractionated single radiation dose should be increased slowly and total
doses of 2 500 rd should not be exceeded.
   Prophylactic radiotherapy of the CNS in acute leukemia has to include the
entire subarachnoid space. It is therefore necessary to irradiate the entire
skull and spinal cord. This treatment schedule and its results will be discussed. There is a tendency to use prophylactic radiotherapy in other systemic
diseases of the RES as well. The indications and contraindications for this
will be discussed.
   The methods and results of treatment of focal lesions with regard to the
morphologic tumor pattern are discussed. Rare primary tumors of the CNS which
have the histological features of lymphoma-sarcoma or reticulosarcoma have
the best prognosis as far as radiotherapy is concerned.

Key words: Radiotherapy - Prophylactic Irradiation - Treatment Schedule

In contrast to Hodgkin's disease radiotherapy takes second place in the treatment of malignant lymphomas of the nervous system. In spite of, or because of,
high radiosensitivity lympho-reticular tumors of the CNS are first treated
chemotherapeutically, but as LENA *et al.* (4) mention radiotherapy may be used
for consolidation.
   Reticulosarcoma, lymphosarcoma and germinoblastoma are uncommon and only in
elderly patients are the first two of these likely to be solitary. After neurosurgical exploration to establish the histological diagnosis, there is a fare-
ly good chance of cure with postoperative radiotherapy (6).
   So called non-Hodgkin lymphomas occur more often in children. Involvement of
the central nervous system is common and JENKIN (2) reports about 30 children
out of 102 which had CNS involvement. Lymphocytic and histiocytic lymphoma
also has a poor prognosis compared to Hodgkin's lymphoma. LINDGREN (5) reports
that half of the children died within 3 months of the diagnosis being established. The pattern of lymph node involvement may have an influence on later
conversion into leukemia. There may also be a different response to chemotherapy.
Radiotherapy therefore has to be applied sometimes locally and sometimes systemically to the CNS.
   Modern onco-radiotherapy uses simultaneous combinations of megavoltage radiation and chemotherapy. In addition to systemic and intrathecal chemotherapy,
radiation of the entire CNS may be necessary.

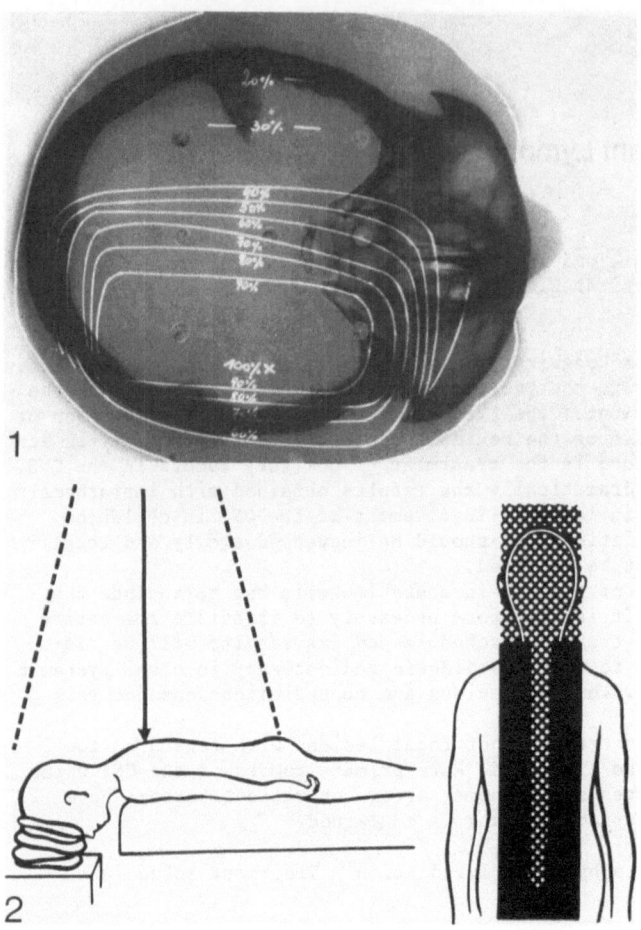

Fig. 1. Isodose curves of 3 field Co^{60}-teletherapy to a localised malignant lymphoma in the right cerebral hemisphere

Fig. 2. The back field needed for entire CNS radiation, showing the area irradiated (6)

Figs. 1 to 5 illustrate some of the possibilities using different types and qualities of ionizing radiation and also different treatment methods.

Solitary lesions can be treated with high energy electrons of variable energy based on the shape and depth of the lesion. Co-60-teletherapy may be used as well as single field or moving beam. Radiation techniques for systemic nodal or other extranervous involvement will not be discussed.

FRANKE *et al.* reported excellent results after treating leukemic infiltrations with systemic radiation of the whole CNS combined with chemotherapy. KREPLER, JENTZSCH *et al.* reported similar successful results with this regime.

Our clinic uses a more individualized course of therapy. Starting with 50 rd daily, the dose is increased slowly up to 200 rd per day. The entire brain including the optic nerves has to be treated, and within 2 - 3 weeks 2400 rd are

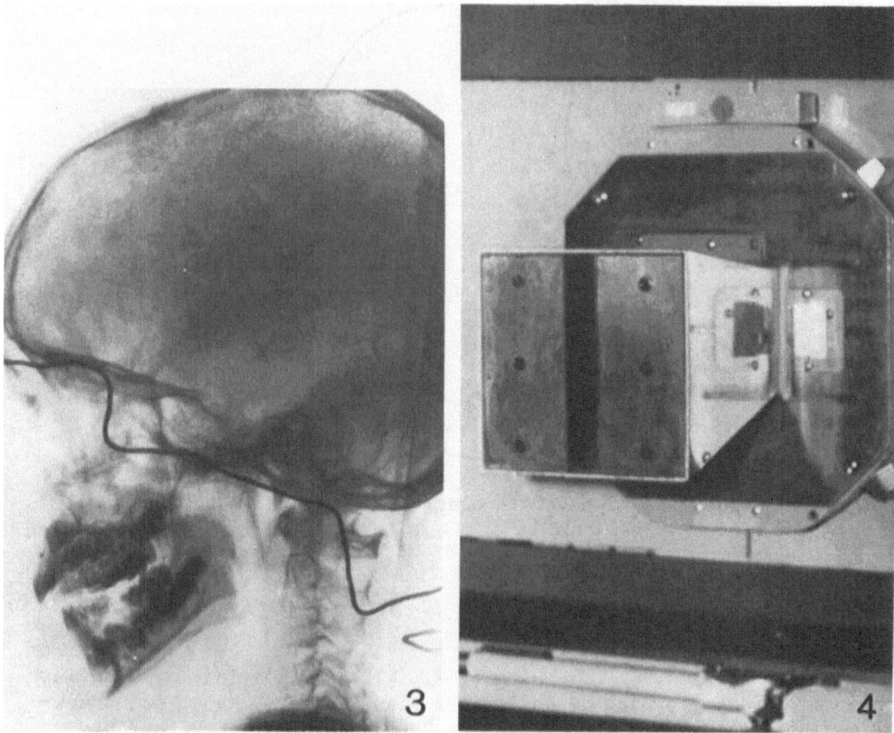

Fig. 3. Field outlined treated with Co⁶⁰-teletherapy in leukemic conversion of malignant lymphoma of CNS

Fig. 4. Field outlined with a combination of plexiglas-lead-absorbers for radiation of the spinal cord

administered. Co-60-teletherapy is most useful for this purpose. To treat the spinal cord fast electrons of 15 - 20 MeV are used, limiting the field borders with a combination of lead and perspex. Higher initial doses and shorter courses of treatment do not seem to be well-tolerated and are rather dangerous.

If single lympho-reticular tumours of the CNS have to be irradiated, we go up to a total dose of 4000 rd. With this type of radiation policy we have obtained excellent palliation or long term remissions. Special considerations and results will be given by KREPLER et al. (see p. 241).

Summarizing the place of onco-radiotherapy in the treatment of malignant non-Hodgkin lymphomas of the CNS, we would conclude, that this form of treatment has a well-defined place and plays an important role as additional or consolidating therapy. The prognosis remains poor especially in children, but could improve markedly as better combinations of therapeutic programs have found. Modern preparations and chemical combinations as well as megavolt radiation are responsible for this improvement. The addition of immunological treatment may be advantageous in the future. We are of the opinion that radiotherapy has not yet been used as frequently as it should be in this field especially in our country. We hope that this will change as the potency of current therapy becomes more widely recognised.

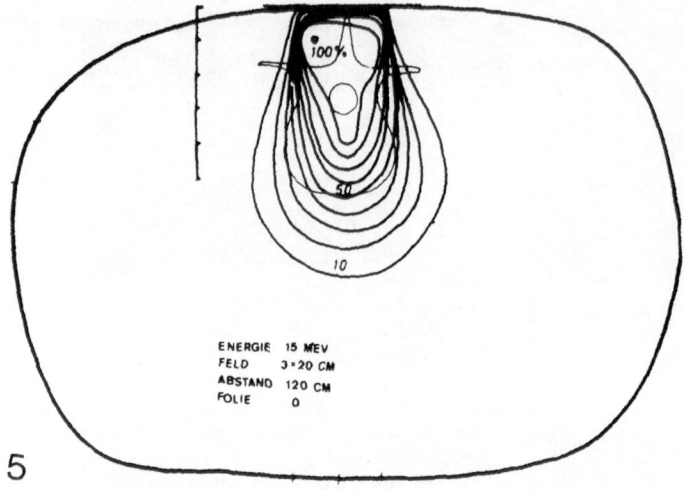

ENERGIE 15 MEV
FELD   3×20 CM
ABSTAND 120 CM
FOLIE   0

5

Fig. 5. Isodose curves with 15 MeV fast electrons, field size 3/20 cm, FSD 120 cm for radiation of spinal cord

REFERENCES

1. FRANKE, H.D., LANDBECK, G., TIMMERMANN, J., WINKLER, K.: Indikationen zur Strahlentherapie bei akuten Leukämien des Kindes unter besonderer Berücksichtigung des klinisch nicht manifesten ZNS-Befalls. Strahlentherapie *147*, 139 (1974)
2. JENKIN, R.D.T.: The Management of Malignant Lymphomas in Childhood. In: Modern Radiotherapy & Oncology - Malignant Diseases in Children, edited by T.J. Deeley. London: Butterworth 1974
3. KHAN, F.R.: Extradural Metastases of the Spinal Cord. In: Modern Radiotherapy & Oncology - Central Nervous System Tumours, edited by T.J. Deeley. London: Butterworth 1974
4. DE LENA, M., MONFARDINI, S., BONADONNA, G.: Intensive Combination Chemotherapy for Malignant Lymphomas. In: Leukämien und maligne Lymphome, Hrsg. A. Stacher. München, Berlin, Wien: Urban & Schwarzenberg 1973
5. LINDGREN, M.: Strahlentherapie der Tumoren im Kindesalter. Strahlentherapie *147*, 109 (1974)
6. PEARSON, D.: Tumours of the Central Nervous System. In: Modern Radiotherapy & Oncology - Malignant Diseases in Children, edited by T.J. Deeley. London: Butterworth 1974

Prof. Dr. K.H. KÄRCHER
Strahlentherapeut. Klinik
Alserstr. 4
A - 1097 Wien/Austria

Acta Neuropath. (Berlin), Suppl. VI, 221 - 225 (1975)
© by Springer-Verlag 1975

Chemotherapy of Malignant Lymphomas

A. STACHER

1st Medical Department and the Ludwig Boltzmann-Institute
for Leukemia Research and Hematology, Hanusch-Krankenhaus,
Vienna, Austria

Summary: In malignant lymphomas generally, radiotherapy is the treatment of
choice. Chemotherapy cannot be very effective in lymphomas of the CNS because
most of the cytostatic drugs in question are not able to pass the blood-brain
barrier. But in cases in which malignant lymphomas are disseminated throughout
the body including the CNS, cytostatic chemotherapy is the only means of prolonging the life of the patient. In such cases one has to distinguish between
Hodgkin's disease and non-Hodgkin lymphomas. Alkylating agents, metaphase inhibitors and antibiotics are used in the treatment of malignant lymphomas.
The best results are achieved with combination schedules. In Hodgkin lymphomas
the so-called MOPP-schedule is the most effective. In non-Hodgkin lymphomas the
same drugs are usually given without procarbacine. After having achieved a
remission, maintenance therapy is very important. Vinblastine and Chlorambuzil
are able to prolonge the remission. When resistance to these drugs occurs
Bleomycin, Adriamycin, CCNU and Peptichemio are effective agents. The results
as well as the side effects of such regimens are described.

Key words: Chemotherapy - Malignant Lymphomas - Induction Therapy - Maintenance
Therapy

In any consideration of the chemotherapy of malignant lymphomas, two main groups
can be distinguished:

1. Hodgkin's disease and
2. the non-Hodgkin lymphomas, which can be subdivided into those of high grade
   malignancy and those of low grade malignancy as well as leukemic and non-
   leukemic types.

We have already heard from LENNERT (8) that the main difficulties are encountered
in the classification of non-Hodgkin lymphomas, in which group the sarcomas and
leukemias overlap. The new classification also makes one question Waldenström's
macroglobulinaemia as an entity. But from the point of view of therapy, we still
have to use the older classification, since we have very little experience of
the value of diverse chemotherapeutic agents in the types of lymphoma identified in the new classification.

Difficulties also arise when the chemotherapy of malignant lymphomas in the
central nervous system is considered separately. Most of the cytostatic drugs
in question are not able to pass the blood-brain barrier if it is intact, and
cannot be administered intrathecally. Therefore, most cytostatics can only be
effective if this barrier is disturbed by the tumor. On the other hand, primary
malignant lymphomas of the central nervous system are rare, most cases of CNS
lymphoma or meningeal leukemia being part of a generalised disease. In such
cases the only way of prolonging the life of the patient is the use of systemic
chemotherapy.

Table 1

	DRUG	DOSAGE	TOXICITY
alky- lating agents	NITROGEN MUSTARD	0,4mg/kg once weekly 3 - 4 weeks	leukopenia, thrombocytopenia nausea, vomitus
	CYCLOPHOSPHAMIDE	40mg/kg once every 3 - 4 weeks 15mg/kg weekly	leukopenia, hemorrhagic cystitis, alopecia
	CHLORAMBUCIL	0,2 - 0,1mg/kg daily, oral	leukopenia, thrombocytopenia
	PROCARBACINE	3 - 5mg/kg daily oral	leukopenia, nausea, allergy
	BCNU	200mg/m^2 every 6 weeks	leukopenia, thrombocytopenia
	CCNU	100mg/m^2 every 6 weeks	leukopenia, thrombocytopenia
	PEPTICHEMIO	25mg/m^2 for 4 days every 3 weeks	leukopenia, venous fibrosis
plant alkaloids	VINBLASTINE	0,1 - 0,3mg/kg weekly	leukopenia, thrombocytopenia myalgia
	VINCRISTINE	0,025 - 0,05mg/kg weekly	neuropathy, obstipation, alopecia, myalgia
anti- biotics	ADRIAMYCIN	0,4 - 0,6mg/kg 3 days daily every 3 weeks	leukopenia, thrombocytopenia, stomatitis, alopecia
	BLEOMYCIN	15mg daily for 5 days than 30mg twice weekly	fever, skin irritation, lung fibrosis

Many cytostatic agents have proved effective in the therapy of advanced malignant lymphomas. The most important of these are listed in Table 1, the dosages given being those used when only one agent is administered. It can be seen that these are generally alkylating agents, metaphase inhibitors (plant alkaloids) or antibiotics. Only CCNU and BCNU seem able to pass the blood-brain barrier because of their lipophilic character.

Today, however, only combination therapy should be administered in general-ised malignant lymphomas. Not only are the results better, but the theoretical aspects also support it; we know that each tumor consists of proliferating cells and the so-called non-proliferating pool, i.e. cells in a resting state. Cytostatic agents have an effect only on proliferating cells. Moreover it is well known that many of these drugs inhibit cell growth only in certain phases of the cell cycle. Because there is only a certain percentage of cells in each phase of the cell cycle in the proliferating pool in any tumour, treat-ment is more effective when several drugs acting on different phases of the cell cycle are administered.

The most useful combination schedule at present seems to be the De Vita-Scheme, which is also called the MOPP-schedule. On day 1 and 8: 1.4 mg/sqm body surface Vincristine plus 6 mg/sqm Nitrogen mustard, day 1 - 14 100mg/sqm Procarbacin plus 60 mg/sqm Prednisolon daily p.o., then 2 weeks pause (2, 3, 10).

It produces remission about 80% of cases even in advanced Hodgkin's disease. Other combinations (Table 2), each with only two drugs, are able to produce nearly the same remission rates (1, 4, 6), but whether the duration of the remission will be the same is not yet known.

After this so-called induction therapy, maintenance therapy must be given. The best maintenance therapy regime seems to be that described by FREI (5); after 6 MOPP courses monthly we continue with another 9 courses at intervals

Table 2

References	Combination		
(7,8)	Day 1 and 8 :	$6mg/m^2$ Nitrogen mustard (or $650mg/m^2$ Cyclophosphamide) $1,4mg/m^2$ Vincristine (or $6mg/m^2$ Vinblastine)	Day 14 - 27 pause
	Day 1 - 13	$100mg/m^2$ Procarbacine $40mg/m^2$ Prednisolone	
(5)	Day 1 and 8 :	$6mg/m^2$ Nitrogen mustard $1,4mg/m^2$ Vincristine $25mg/m^2$ Adriamycin $30mg/m^2$ Bleomycin	Day 14 - 27 pause
	Day 1 - 13	$40mg/m^2$ Prednisolone	
(20)	Bleomycin Cyclophosphamide 6-MP Prednisolon	0,3mg/kg/weekly 1,0mg/kg/day 1,0mg/kg/day 0,6 - 0,8mg/kg/ day	3 month, then consolidation with 0,02mg/ kg/week Vincristine
(10)	Vinblastine	5 - 10mg/weekly + Cyclophosphamide 100-150mg p.o.	
(10,23)	Vinblastine	5 - 10mg/weekly + Procarbacine 100-150mg daily p.o.	
(10,23)	Vinblastine	5 - 10mg/weekly + Chlorambucil 5mg/daily	
(10,23)	Cyclophosphamide 150mg/daily	+ Procarbacine 100-150mg/daily	

of two months. The administration of 6 mg/sqm Vinblastin weekly plus 6 mg/sqm Chlorambuzil daily is also effective as maintenance therapy.

With the development of these forms of chemotherapy the survival time of patients with Hodgkin's disease has been prolonged (11). This has been demonstrated in our patients in stage III and IV. Patients treated with only radiotherapy and cytostatic monotherapy had a median survival time of 3,5 years and a longest survival time of 8 years, while in recent years patients on combined chemotherapy attained a median survival time of 4,5 years, the longest survival time being 16 years. We are sure that the results will be still better in the future.

One must also take note of the new concept of so-called "synchronisation"· therapy. As mentioned above, most cytostatic agents act only in certain phases of the cell cycle. Therapy would therefore be more effective if recruitment of the cells in certain phases could be achieved. The main aim of "synchronisation" therapy is to arrest as many cells as possible in a particular cycle phase without killing them at this stage. "Synchronisation doses" are therefore relative low doses of cytostatic agents. In malignant lymphomas Vincristine as a metaphase inhibitor is most often employed, while in acute leukemias hydroxy-urea or other antimetabolites are used. When partial synchronisation has been obtained a large dose, the so-called "killing-dose", of a cytostatic agent which is effective in the phase in which the cells are synchronized, is administered. This can kill more cells than in a normal asynchronous cell population. An added advantage is that side effects are diminished since the generation time of normal, quickly proliferating tissues such as bone marrow

224   A. Stacher

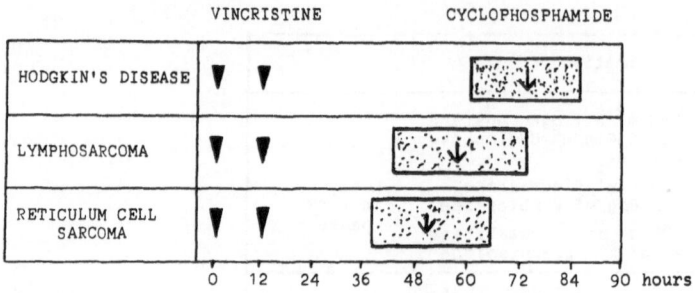

Fig. 1

or intestinal epithelium is shorter than that of tumor cells. If the killing dose is administered after synchronisation, the normal more rapidly proliferating cells have already passed through the phase in which the killing dose is effective, so that they are attacked to a lesser extent than normal. The basic investigations were carried out by KLEIN (7) and his therapy model using Vincristine as a synchronisation drug and cyclophosphamide as a killing drug (Fig. 1) produced really good clinical results.

The only problem is ascertaining the correct interval between the administration of the first and the second agent. In leukemias one can investigate the bone marrow or blood cells by means of the impulse cytophotometer, but this is not possible in lymphomas. Therefore treatment can only be undertaken on the basis of models in controlled trials in an attempt to find the best schedule.

In non-Hodgkin lymphomas the principles of the therapy of lymphomas of high grade malignancy are similar to those of Hodgkin's disease. The so-called lymphosarcomas and reticulosarcomas are generally included in this group. The main aim of treatment must be to eradicate the tumor cells as early as possible. The methods are nearly the same, although some drugs such as Procarbacin are less effective in such cases. Lymphomas of low grade malignancy such as chronic lymphocytic leukemia do not require such an intense chemotherapeutic regime. In such cases, apart from so-called depletion methods such as leukapheresis and extracorporeal irradiation, long lasting cytostatic treatment with lower dosages is necessary.

Finally one may say that in cases of generalised malignant lymphomas where the central nervous system is involved, conventional cytostatic therapy is the best form of treatment, the only preference being for schedules which include CCNU or BCNU. Furthermore the administration of Methotrexate intrathecally usually 0,1 - 0,5 mg/kg, is indicated weekly together with citrovorum factor intramuscularly to neutralize its extracerebral effects. Cytosine-arabinoside, administered intrathecally at a concentration of 1 mg/kg is also effective. The most interesting recently developed substance is, in my opinion, DDMP (Methodichlorophen, 2,4-diamino-5-)3' (4'-dichlorophenyl)-6-methylpyrimidin). It has the long half-life in the plasma of 190 hours and seems to be concentrated in the brain. Up till now it has been given only once weekly in a dose of 1,5 mg/kg, but not more than 75 mg, as higher doses produce convulsions. If its effectiveness in malignant lymphomas is confirmed, we shall have a new and perhaps better cytostatic regime to combat CNS lymphoma.

Acknowledgement: We are indebted to the former Federal President of Austria Dr. h.c. Franz JONAS for supporting our work by means of his "Leukämie-forschungsspende".

REFERENCES

1. DE LENA, M., MONFARDINI, S., BONADONNA, G.: Intensive combination chemotherapy in malignant lymphomas. In A. STACHER (ed.): Leukämien und maligne
   Lymphome. München, Berlin, Wien: Urban & Schwarzenberg 1973
2. DE VITA, V.T., CARBONE, P.T.: Chemotherapeutic implications of staging in
   Hodgkin's disease. Cancer Res. *31*, 1838 (1971)
3. DE VITA, V.T., SERPICK, A.A., CARBONE, P.T.: Combination chemotherapy in
   advanced Hodgkin's disease. Am. Int. Med. *73*, 881 (1970)
4. FISCHER, M., MITROU, P.S., SCHUBERT, J.C.F., MARTIN, H., HÜBNER, K.:
   Zur Therapie des Morbus Hodgkin. Gegenüberstellung der Ergebnisse mit dem
   De Vita-Programm und verschiedenen Zweifach-Kombinationen in Abhängigkeit
   vom histologischen Typ. In A. STACHER (ed.): Leukämien und maligne Lymphome. München, Berlin, Wien: Urban & Schwarzenberg 1973
5. FREI, E.: Recent advances in the management of lymphoma. 1st Meeting Europ.
   Div. Internat. Soc. Hemat., Milano, 1971. Abstract nr. 284
6. KIMURA, K., SAKAI, Y., KONDA, C., SHIMOYAMA, M., SAKANO, T., KITAHARA, T.,
   MIKUNI, M.: Chemotherapy of malignant lymphoma with special references to
   the effects of Bleomycin and sequential therapy of Bleomycin and Vincaalka-
   loids. In A. STACHER (ed.): Leukämien and maligne Lymphome. München,
   Berlin, Wien: Urban & Schwarzenberg 1973
7. KLEIN, H.O., LENNARTZ, K.J., GROSS, R.: Partielle Synchronisation der Tumor-
   zellproliferation and zellphasenspezifisches "Timing" der Zytostatikagabe.
   Erste klinische Ergebnisse bei lymphoretikulären Tumoren, akuter Leukosen
   sowie Bronchialkarzinomen. In A. STACHER (ed.): Leukämien und maligne
   Lymphome. München, Berlin, Wien: Urban & Schwarzenberg 1973
8. LENNERT, K.: Morphology and classification of lymphomas and so-called reticuloses. Acta Neuropath. Suppl. VI, 1 - 16 (1975)
9. LUKES, R.J., CRAVER, L.F., HALL, T.C., RAPPAPORT, H., RUBIN, P.: Report
   of the nomenclature committee. Cancer Res. *26*, 1311, (1966)
10. STACHER, A.: Grundsätze der Therapie des Morbus Hodgkin und der übrigen
    malignen Lymphome. In A. STACHER (ed.): Leukämien und maligne Lymphome.
    München, Berlin, Wien: Urban & Schwarzenberg 1973
11. TREPEL, F.: Zellproliferation in malignen Lymphomen. In A. STACHER (ed.):
    Leukämien und maligne Lymphome. München, Berlin, Wien: Urban & Schwarzen-
    berg 1973
12. Medical News (Leading article): DMP- once discarted for toxicity - combats
    meningeal leukemia. J. amer. Med. Ass. *224*, 1079 (1973)

Prof. Dr. A. STACHER
Ludwig Boltzmann-Institute for Leukemia Research
and Hematology
Heinrich Collinstraße 30
A - 1140, Vienna, Austria

Acta Neuropath. (Berlin), Suppl. VI, 227 - 233 (1975)
© by Springer-Verlag 1975

Immunotherapy of Malignant Disease in Man

J. A. RUSSEL

Chester Beatty Research Institute,
and Royal Marsden Hospital
Sutton, Surrey, U.K.

Summary: At present active specific immunotherapy should only be attempted
where a tumour is shown to be antigenic and immunogenic, patients are immunocompetent, large numbers of tumour cells can be stored and minimal residual
disease can be achieved without heavy immunosuppression. Acute myeloblastic
leukaemia (AML) satisfies such criteria reasonably well and evidence is presented that treatment with BCG and irradiated allogeneic AML cells is of value
in this disease. It is suggested that there is insufficient evidence at present to justify embarking on similar regimes in most of the malignant lymphomas.

Key words: Immunotherapy - Myeloblastic Leukaemia - BCG Treatment - Irradiated
Allogeneic Cells

INTRODUCTION

Although attempts to treat malignant disease by immunological maneouvres have
been made since the turn of the century (1), it is only comparatively recently
that there has been sufficient experimental evidence to put such attempts on ·
a rational basis. With the development of syngeneic animal systems and *in vitro*
methods of studying tumour immunology in man came increasing evidence that many
tumours are capable of provoking an immunological response in the host and that
advantage might be taken of this response in controlling tumour growth (2).

Once it was shown that recurrence of primary tumours in animals following
limited radiotherapy could be delayed or prevented by injection of irradiated
autologous tumour tissue (3), the possibility of using similar maneouvres in
man could be entertained. Later experiments suggested that the use of B.C.C.
which was known to have some non-specific immunological stimulating effect (4)
could enhance the anti-tumour effect of immunisation with autologous tumour
cells (5). It therefore seemed that the best form of immunotherapy might include both specific and non-specific agents, i.e. B.C.G. and tumour cells.

Before any malignant disease in man could be considered suitable for a
clinical trial of this form of immunotherapy, it was apparent that certain
basic conditions had to be satisfied.Acute myeloblastic leukaemia (AML) in
adults was selected as a model for such a trial.

PRE-REQUISITES FOR ACTIVE SPECIFIC IMMUNOTHERAPY

1. Antigenicity and Immunogenicity of Tumour

It is essential that the tumour selected is known to be capable of eliciting
a humoral or cellular immune response in the host. The blastogenic effect of
autologous AML cells on remission lymphocytes has demonstrated that these lym-

phocytes are capable of recognising the leukaemia cells as foreign (6). Moreover, this effect can be enhanced by injecting patients with irradiated autologous tumour cells (6, 7).

2. *Immunocompetent patients*

Depressed cellular immunity has been reported in a large number of malignant diseases. The possible causes may include the disease process itself, treatment with immunosuppressive agents, or inherent immune deficiency which may have pre-disposed to the disease. It is often difficult or impossible to differentiate these causes in a given case.

Remissions can be achieved in AML without using radiotherapy or other excessively immunosuppressive drug regimes and such immune suppression as does occur appears to recover fairly rapidly.

3. *Achievement of Minimal Residual Disease*

The animal experiments referred to above (3) demonstrated that immunotherapy was only of value when the bulk of the tumour had been removed. Other experiments had shown that cytotoxic lymphocytes may only be detectable after removal of the tumour (9). It therefore seemed advisable to choose a situation in which conventional therapy could reduce the tumour burden to a minimum without the excessive immunosuppression referred to above. The state of complete heamatological and clinical remission which can be achieved in some patients with AML is probably a good approximation to this state.

4. *Availability of large numbers of tumour cells*

Experiments with lymphocyte stimulation (6) antibody production (10) and production of cytotoxic lymphocytes (11) have shown that increased immune responses are only demonstrable after injection of between 10^8 and 10^9 tumour cells. Moreover, these responses tend to be transient and in order to be reproduced the injections need to be repeated at intervals of less than two weeks. This means that a large number of tumour cells must be available. The introduction of the IBM cell separator meant that it was possible to obtain up to 10^{12} tumour cells from a single patient with AML (12). It is possible to store these in a viable state without loss of antigenicity (13).

5. *Antigenic identity within tumour type*

In vitro experiments in man have indicated that tumours of similar histological type tend to share tumour associated antigens (14). Skin testing and serological data suggest that this may also be the case in AML. It is important this should be so, first because it has been shown that allogeneic cells may be more immunogenic than autologous cells (15, 16) and second because restriction of immunotherapy to patients from whom autologous tumour cells are available would severely limit the number of patients whom one could treat. This is because only a proportion of those from whom cells are available in fact achieve remission with chemotherapy, and collection of material from those presenting with smaller numbers of tumor cells is more difficult.

6. *Short survival with best conventional treatment*

An advantage of choosing AML as a model for a trial of immunotherapy was that normally remission and survival length in this disease are so poor that any therapeutic effect might become apparent within a few years. There would be less justification for embarking upon such an expensive and time-consuming enterprise in a disease where conventional treatment gives good results, until there is more experimental evidence in favour of doing so.

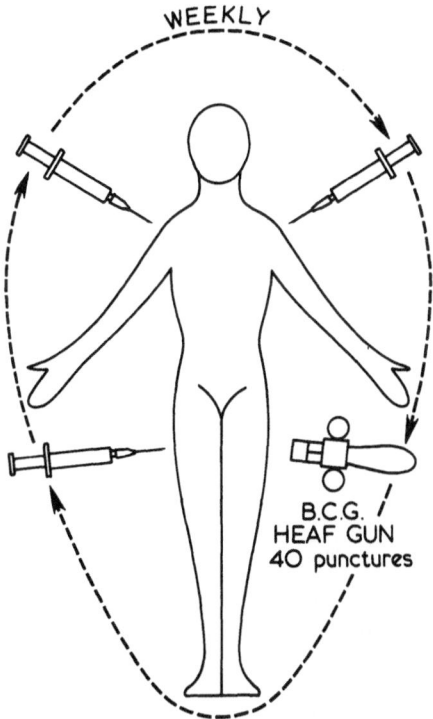

Fig. 1. *Immunisation Schedule.* The syrings represent injection in 3 sites (s.c. and i.d.) of a total of 1 x 10^9 allogeneic AML cells irradiated to 10,000 r. The cells are obtained from AML patients using the IBM cell separator and stored over liquid nitrogen in 10% DMSO.

BCG is given with a Heaf Gun by i.d. injection. About 1 x 10^6 organisms are given each week in one limb so that each limb is injected once every 4 weeks

The effect of treating AML in remission with immunotherapy will now be briefly described. Earlier results have been presented in more detail else-where (8, 17).

PATIENTS AND METHODS

The aim of the first trial was to determine whether immunotherapy could im-prove the results of treating patients in remission with chemotherapy. It in-volved 138 patients presenting to St. Bartholomew's Hospital with a diagnosis of AML (referred to as Barts 2, 3 and 4). The 52 of these patients who achieved complete remission with Daunorubicin (DR) and Cytosine Arasinoside (CA) (18) were then given 12 further courses of chemotherapy consisting of 5 day courses of DR and CA alternating with 6-thioguanine and CA at monthly intervals. 30 of these patients had been allocated at presentation to receive immunotherapy in addition to chemotherapy during remission. The immunotherapy consisted of weekly injections of allogeneic irradiated AML cells and BCG as indicated in Fig. 1. Chemotherapy was stopped in all patients a year after remission and was only restarted if relapse occurred.

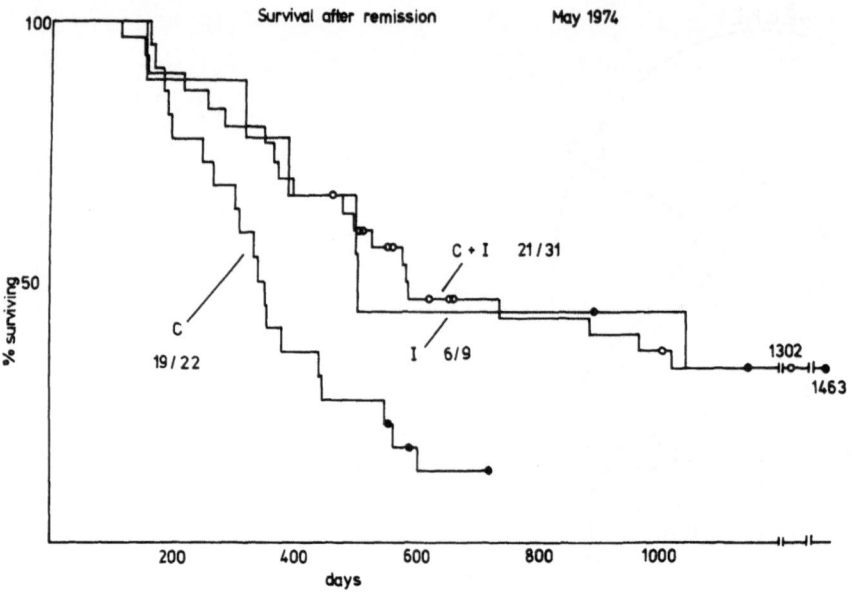

Fig. 2. Raw data analysis of survival after remission induction.

Chemotherapy alone	22 patients)	
	3 alive)	
Chemotherapy plus immunotherapy	30 patients)	– Barts
	10 alive)	2, 3 + 4
Immunotherapy alone	9 patients)	– Marsden I
	3 alive)	

A second smaller study (Marsden I) was designed to investigate the effect of maintenance with immunotherapy given alone in remission. 9 patients in complete remission recieved immunotherapy identical to that described above but without maintenance chemotherapy.

RESULTS

The survival data for all 3 groups of patients are presented schematically in Fig. 2. Of the 30 patients receiving immunotherapy in addition to chemotherapy 10 (33%) remained alive by May 1974 compared with 3 (14%) of the 22 receiving chemotherapy alone. Median survival from remission of the two groups are 586 and 348 days respectively. To obtain overall survival times approximately 60 days has to be added to these figures to account for the time taken to achieve remission.

Statistical analysis of the survival data shows a significant difference between the two groups ($p < 0.01$).

The 9 patients receiving immunotherapy alone were not part of the same controlled trial but as a group are comparable to the others and it is probably legitimate to compare their performance with the above results. Although the median survival (506 days) is less than for the group receiving chemotherapy and immunotherapy it will be seen that the same percentage (3 of 9 or 33%)

remained alive by May 1974 and these patients have survival times ≥ 889 days whereas only 2 patients receiving the combination had reached this point at that time.

DISCUSSION

Our results indicate that immunotherapy as performed in our department is of value in the maintenance treatment of AML in remission and that immunotherapy alone may be as good as immunotherapy and chemotherapy combined. If this is so there are considerable advantages in avoiding maintenance chemotherapy because of the possible immunosuppressive effects of the drugs, production of resistant disease and toxicity to the patients. We have no doubt that the quality of life of patients maintained on immunotherapy alone is much better than on regimes involving intensive chemotherapy. If no evidence exists, therefore, that intensive chemotherapeutic regimes produce significantly longer survivals we feel that immunotherapy alone should be used.

However, the fact that only 10% of the patients who achieve remission then survive for 1000 days shows that long term control or cure of their disease still remains a possibility for only very few patients.

Application to Malignant Lymphomas

It seems appropriate to consider briefly whether the principles outlined above can be applied to the malignant lymphomas. There is some evidence that BCG vaccination may prolong remission in the lymphomas (19). The difficulty in isolating the malignant cell in Hodgkin's disease hinders the study of immunity *in vitro* and we do not know whether the tumour tissue available would be sufficiently immunogenic. There is more *in vivo* and *in vitro* evidence of tumour antigenicity and antigenic cross reactivity in other lymphomas (20). Some of these patients might yield sufficient material for immunotherapy at laparotomy or post-mortem, or by leukapheresis if there were circulating tumour cells.

The debate concerning impairment of cellular immunity in patients with lymphomas has by no means been settled (21, 22, 23). However, it is probably fair to say that those patients with early Hodgkin's disease who tend to have more intact immune responses are a group who do so well with conventional treatment that immunotherapy would be superfluous. The heavily immunosuppressive treatment required to produce remissions in patients with more advanced or rapidly progressive forms of lymphoma would substantially prejudice their chances of responding to immunotherapy. There is, moreover, a possibility that some patients may develop lymphomas because of a pre-existing defect in their immune system. Thus patients with congenital immune deficiency syndromes and those undergoing immunosuppressive treatment for organ transplantation have a greatly increased susceptability to lymphomas particularly those involving the nervous system (24). It is therefore possible that patients with lymphomas of the nervous system have a more marked immunological defect than those without. On the other hand there is not a great deal of evidence to suggest that the nervous system provides a site where tumours may be inaccessible to the immune system. Some primary neurological tumours show lymphoid infiltration (25), it is known that vascular endothelium is permeable to immunocompetent cells, and cells cytotoxic to central nervous system tumours can be demonstrated in the peripheral blood (26). Failure of the trial of immunotherapy in glioblastoma multiforme reported by BLOOM *et al.* (27), could be attributed to other mechanisms in particular the small numbers of cells injected.

It could well be argued that some lymphomas in experimental animals are controllable by immunotherapy, but until more information is available in the human situation it is probably not justifiable to assume that human lymphomas will behave similarly.

The future of immunotherapy

The future of active specific immunotherapy will depend upon increasing sophistication of immunological techniques which will perhaps produce some form of antigenic classification and the production of more effective immunogens.

Such improved understanding might alter the criteria we need to satisfy before considering a disease suitable for immunotherapy. For the present, however, we intend to apply the results of technical advances to AML before embarking on the therapy of other diseases which would seem less likely to respond.

REFERENCES

1. CURRIE, G.A.: Eighty Years of Immunotherapy: A review of Immunological Methods Used for the Treatment of Human Cancer. Br. J. Cancer, *26*, 141 - 153 (1972)
2. FAIRLY, G.H.: Immunity to Malignant Disease in Man. Br. Med. J. *2*, 467 - 473 (1969)
3. HADDOW, A., ALEXANDER, P.: An Immunological Method of Increasing the Sensitivity of Primary Sarcomas to Local Irradiation with X-rays. Lancet, I. 452 - 457 (1964)
4. HALPERN, B.N., BIOZZI, G., STIFFEL, G., MOUTON, D.: Effect de la stimulation du systeme reticuloendothelial par l'inoculation du bacille de Calmette-Guerin sur le developpement d'epithelioma atypique t-8 de Guerin chez le rat. C. R. Soc. Biol. *153*, 919 - 923 (1959)
5. MATHE, G., POILLART, P., LAPEYRAQUE, F.: Active Immunotherapy of L1210 Leukaemia Applied after the Graft of Tumour Cells. Br. J. Cancer *23*, 814 - 824 (1969)
6. POWLES, R.L., BALCHIN, L.A., HAMILTON FAIRLEY, G., ALEXANDER, P.: Recognition of Leukaemic Cells as Foreign Before and After Autoimmunisation. Br. med. J. I. 486 - 489 (1971)
7. GUTTERMAN, J.U., MAVLIGIT, G., McCREDIE, K.B., FREIREICH, E.J., HERSH, E.M.: Auto-immunisation with Acute leukaemia Cells: Demonstration of Increased Lymphocyte Responsiveness. Int. J. Cancer *11*, 3, 521 - 526 (1973)
8. POWLES, R.L., CROWTHER, D., BATEMAN, C.J.T., BEARD, M.E.J., McELWAIN, T.J., RUSSEL, J., LISTER, T.A., WHITEHOUSE, J.M.A., WRIGLEY, P.F.M., PIKE, M., ALEXANDER, P., HAMILTON FAIRLEY, G.: Immunotherapy for Acute Myelogenous Leukaemia. Br. J. Cancer *28*, 365 - 376 (1973)
9. MILCULSKA, Z.B., SMITH, C., ALEXANDER, P.: Evidence for an Immunological Reaction of the Host Directed Against its own actively growing primary Tumour. J. Nat. Cancer Inst. *36*, 29 - 35 (1966)
10. IKONOPISOV, R.L., LEWIS, M.G., HUNTER-CRAIG, I.D., BODENHAM, D.C., PHILLIPS, T.M., COOLING, C.I., PROCTOR, J., HAMILTON FAIRLEY, G., ALEXANDER, P.: Auto-Immunisation with Irradiated Tumour Cells in Human Malignant Melanoma, Br. med. J. II. 752 - 754 (1970)
11. CURRIE, G.A., LEJEUNE, F., FAIRLEY, G.H.: Immunisation with Irradiated Tumour Cells and Specific Lymphocyte Cytotoxicity in Malignant Melanoma. Br. med. J. II. 305 - 310 (1971)
12. POWLES, R.L., LISTER, T.A., OLIVER, R.T.D., RUSSEL, J.A., SMITH, C., KAY, H.E.M., McELWAIN, T.J., HAMILTON FAIRLEY, G.: A safe method of Collecting Leukaemia cells from patients with Acute Leukaemia for use as immunotherapy. Brit. Med. J. In Press
13. POWLES, R.L., GRANT, C.: Some Properties of Cryopreserved Acute Leukaemia Cells. Cryobiology *10*, 290 - 294 (1973)
14. HELLSTROM, I., HELLSTROM, K.E., SJOGREN, H.D., WARNER, G.A.: Demonstration of Cell mediated Immunity to Human Neoplasms of Various Histological Types. Int. J. Cancer *7*, 1 - 16 (1971)

15. GORER, P.A., AMOS, D.B.: Passive Immunity in Mice Against C57Bl Leukosis E.L.4 by Means of Isoimmune Serum. Cancer Res. *16*, 338 - 343 (1956)
16. ALEXANDER, P., HALL, J.G.: The Role of Immunoblasts in Host Resistance and Immunotherapy of Primary Sarcomata. Adv. Cancer Res. *13*, 1 - 37 (1970)
17. POWLES, R.L.: Immunotherapy for Acute Myelogenous Leukaemia. Br. J. Cancer *28*, Suppl. I. 262 - 263 (1973)
18. CROWTHER, D., POWLES, R., BATEMAN, C.J.T., BEARD, M.E.J., GAUCI, C.L., WRIGLEY, P.F.M., MALPAS, J.S., HAMILTON FAIRLEY, G., BRODLEY SCOTT, R.: Management of Adult Acute Myelogenous Leukaemia. Br. med. J. I. 131 - 137 (1973)
19. SOKAL, J.E., AUNGST, C.W., SNYDERMAN, M.: Prolongation and remission in Stage I and II Lymphoma by BCG vaccination. Proc. Amer. Assoc. Cancer Res. *15*, 13 (1974)
20. BRAUN, M., SEN, L., BACHMANN, A.E., PARLORSKY, A.: Cell Migration Inhibition in Human Lymphomas Using Lymph Node and Cell line Antigens. Blood *39*, 3, 268 - 376 (1972)
21. SOKAL, J.E., AUNGST, C.W.: Cellular Immune Responses and Prognosis in Malignant Lymphomas. Nat. Cancer, Inst. Monog. *34*, 109 - 116 (1971)
22. YOUNG, R.C., CORDER, M.P., HAYNES, H.A., DE VITA, V.T.: Delayed Hypersensitivity in Hodgkin's Disease. Amer. J. Med. *52*, 63 - 72 (1972)
23. LAING, J.M., TONGIO, M.M., OBERLING, F., MAYER, S., WAITZ, R.: Mixed lymphocyte reaction as assay for immunological competence of lymphocytes from patients with Hodgkin's Disease. Lancet *1*, 1261 - 1263 (1972)
24. PENN, I., STARZL, T.E.: A Summary of the Status of De Novo Cancer in Transplant Recipients. Trans. Proc. *1V.4*, 719 - 731 (1972)
25. RIDLEY, A., CAVANAGH, J.B.: Lymphocytic Infiltration in Gliomas: Evidence of Possible Host Resistance, Brain *94*, 117 - 124 (1971)
26. LEVY, N.L., MAHALEY, M.S. Jr., DAY, E.D.: In Vitro Demonstration of Cell Mediated Immunity to Human Brain Tumours. Cancer Res. *32*, 477 - 482 (1972)
27. BLOOM, H.J.G., PECKHAM, M.J., RICHARDSON, A.E., ALEXANDER, P., PAYNE, P.M.: Glioblastoma Multiforme : A controlled Trial to Assess the Value of Specific Immunotherapy in Patients Treated by Radical Surgery and Radiotherapy. Br. J. Cancer *27*, 253 - 267 (1973)

J.A. RUSSELL, M.D.
Chester Beatty Research Institute
I.B.M. Blood Cell Separator Unit
Downs Road
Sutton, Surrey, England

Acta Neuropath. (Berlin), Suppl. VI, 235 - 239 (1975)
© by Springer-Verlag 1975

Meningeal Localisation of Acute Leukaemias

G. MATHÉ, P. POUILLART, L. SCHWARZENBERG

Institut de Cancérologie et d'Immunogénétique (INSERM et
Association Claude-Bernard), Hôpital Paul-Brousse, Villejuif, France

Summary: A preventive chemoradiotherapeutic treatment of the central nervous
system has to be started as soon as a complete remission is obtained in acute
lymphoid leukemia. Any meningeal localisation is barely sensitive to treatment
and reduces the long term chances of survival.

The best treatment, according to our study, consists in the intrathecal
administration of methotrexate and cytosine arabinoside followed by an irradiation of the central nervous system at a dose of 1,500 rads. The present
trials have attempted to reduce the number of intrathecal injections, to increase the irradiation dose to 2,400 rads, and to restrict it to the skull.

Key words: Acute lymphoid leukemia - preventive therapy - meningitis - irradiation - central nervous system - relapse

INTRODUCTION

The occurrence of meningeal localisations during the course of treatment of
acute lymphoid leukemia (ALL) indicates a bad prognosis (1). It implies a
double risk: the risk of a severe and recurrent local evolution and the risk
of cellular dissemination originating from this protected tumor site which
acts as a source of systemic recurrences.

Since progress in systemic chemotherapy and immunotherapy has improved the
duration of systemic remissions, the frequency of meningeal localisation is
one of the critical prognosis factors (2). The frequency of meningeal localisations has led to a preventive treatment (3, 4, 5).

In this work are given the results of preventive meningeal treatment applied
to a population of 193 patients treated from 1964 to 1971.

PATIENTS AND METHODS

Between 1964 and 1971, 193 ALL patients were submitted to a treatment protocol
comprising four successive phases: 1) a phase of complete remission-induction-
chemotherapy (RIC) (duration 1 month); 2) a phase of systemic cyto-reductive
combination chemotherapy (CRCC) combining the actions of at least two drugs
(duration 6 to 8 months); 3) a phase of preventive treatment of the central
nervous system (CNS): chemoradiotherapy or chemotherapy alone (during 4 to 8
weeks in conjunction with systemic CRCC); 4) finally, a phase of specific and
non-specific active immunotherapy (AI) (6).

The preventive tretment of meningeal blastic infiltration evolved from 1964
to 1971 : a) 37 patients received 6 to 12 intrathecal injections of methotrexate (MTX) at a rate of 2 injections per week; b) 26 patients received 6
to 12 intrathecal injections of MTX followed by irradiation to the CNS, including the skull and spinal column up to L5, at a mean dose of 1,500 rads
(the dose was always between 1,200 and 1,800 rads); c) 32 patients received

Table 1. *Frequency of Meningeal Leukaemia According to the Prophylactic Treatment*

Treatment	no meningitis	meningitis
0	50	26
Methotrexate alone	28	9
Methotrexate + irradiation	23	3
Irradiation alone	0	3
Methotrexate + cytosine arabinoside	2	0
Methotrexate + cytosine arabinoside + Irradiation	30	2
TOTAL	133	43

12 to 18 injections of MTX + cytosine-arabinoside (CAR) at a rate of 3 injections per week, followed by an irradiation dose of 1,500 rads to the skull; d) 17 patients received 12 intrathecal injections of MTX at a rate of 2 injections per week, followed by irradiation of the skull up to C2 at a dose of 2,400 rads; e) 76 patients received no preventive treatment : they were considered as the reference population in our study as they were submitted to the same type of systemic chemotherapy treatment; f) 3 patients refused all intrathecal injections and were submitted to only one irradiation of the CNS, and 2 patients received only intrathecal injections and refused irradiation.

MTX given at a dose of $5mg/m2$ two to three times a week and CAR at a dose of $10mg/m2$ were administered alternately. When MTX and CAR were combined the patients received 2 MTX injections weekly on the 1st and 6th day of the week, and one injection of CAR on the third day. The drugs were injected after dissolving them in 2ml of saline. In all cases the field of irradiation was extended up to the retroocular zone of the skull, and when limited to the skull the inferior limit was C2.

RESULTS

The results are shown in Table 1. Out of 76 patients receiving no preventive treatment 26 cases of meningeal blastic infiltration were observed (i.e. 34% of cases). Out of 37 patients receiving MTX alone as a preventive treatment, 9 cases of leukemic meningitis were observed during the perceptible phase (24%). Out of 26 patients treated with MTX and complementary irradiation, 3 cases of leukemic meningitis were observed (12%). Out of 32 patients submitted to a combination of MTX and CAR followed by irradiation of the skull, 2 patients later developed leukemic meningitis (6.6%). Out of 17 patients submitted to a combination of irradiation plus MTX, 2 patients had a meningeal blastic infiltration (11.7%). In 2 patients who only received 16 intrathecal injections of MTX and CAR, no meningeal blastic infiltration was observed, whereas 3 patients submitted to a single CNS irradiation at a dose of 1,500 rads developed a meningeal localisation.

The importance of a systemic treatment of the CNS is shown in Fig. 1. It compares the mean survival duration of 2 populations of patients : 1) 45 patients with a meningeal localisation (curve 1); 2) 148 patients in whom this

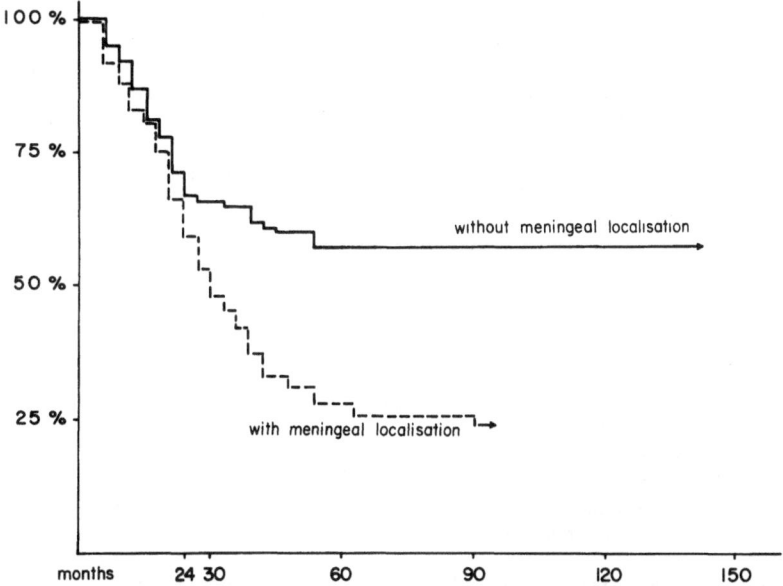

Fig. 1. Actuarial curves of survival of 190 acute lymphoid leukemias with
(------) or without (———) meningeal localisations. Please note that the
time scale is geometrical

complication never appeared (curve 2). A significant difference between the
two groups exists from the first months of evolution. This difference is due
both to a recurrent local, often severe, evolution which is not easily acces-
sible to the therapeutic means used up to now, and to an increased frequency
of systemic relapses. In fact, out of the 45 patients with meningeal localisation, 15 patients had a meningeal relapse and 16 patients relapsed in the
next three months.

TOLERANCE

Irradiation of the skull at 1,500 or 2,400 rads is sometimes accompanied by
slight headaches, easily treated. Alopecia is always present. No severe manifestation of intolerance was observed in any of the patients during this
trial.
    Total CNS irradiation is generally followed by a rarely severe medullary
hypoplasia: only 6 cases with leucopenia below 1,000 per cmm. This irradiation
increases the subsequent hematological sensitivity to systemic chemotherapies
during several weeks, even months, thus constituting an obstacle to the continuation of the general treatment which is essential in this phase of the
disease.
    Intolerance provoked by the intrathecal injections is directly related to
the number of injections. Headache, nausea, anorexia, even a discrete stiffness
of the neck are more frequent after the 12th injection. Sometimes there is an
increase in the albumin level of the spinal fluid up to 1g %, leading to the
interruption of local chemotherapy.
    Out of a population of 7 patients who received more than 35 intrathecal in-
jections of MTX and CAR because of two successive perceptible phases, 4 patients

developed paraplegia without premonitory symptoms. A slight increase in the spinal fluid albumin level was noted. Patients did not show any tendency to recover, and no signs of meningeal blastic infiltration were noticed immediately or even later in the evolution. The additive products used for the storage of MTX and CAR were thought to be the cause, but in the case of MTX its own toxicity on the CNS is well known.

The young patients submitted to the meningeal preventive treatment and who remained in complete remission without any complication had no mental, sensory, motor or schooling problems, and there was no sign of any slowing down in the development of the cranium or in the growth of the spinal column.

DISCUSSION

The frequency of meningeal blastic infiltrations in ALL patients submitted to an efficient systemic treatment without meningeal treatment is usually between 35% and 65% (7, 8).

The results show that MTX alone reduces the percentage of meningeal localisations. Irradiation of the CNS at 1,500 rads, combined with MTX, reduces by 12% the frequency of meningeal localisation. The spinal column represents an important volume of the active bone marrow, and its irradiation temporarily reduces the possibility of systemic chemotherapy for a period which varies according to the patient, often several months, frequently causing the failure of the treatment.

A trial using MTX and CAR followed by irradiation of the skull at 1,500 rads reduces meningeal localisations to 6.6%. In our trial with 17 patients the frequency of meningeal localisations (11.7%) is not statistically different from the results observed when MTX and CAR were combined with total CNS irradiation.

Studies by PINKEL et al. have defined the optimal irradiation dose. His trial showed that doses of 500 and 1,200 rads are insufficient. 2,400 rads to the total CNS do not have a greater preventive effect. But the greater hematological tolerance of the latter makes it the best choice for the moment.

The results in our trial using 1,500 rads irradiation after 18 intrathecal injections of MTX and CAR are comparable to those of AUR (9). Our protocol consists of 8 intrathecal injections (minimal number) and a simultaneous irradiation of the skull at 2,400 rads.

This preventive treatment of meningeal blastic infiltrations defines an efficient therapeutic strategy. Its essential elements are the combined intrathecal injections of MTX and/or CAR to obtain an apparent sterilisation of the cerebrospinal fluid, followed by another irradiation (2,400 rads) limited to the skull; this irradiation is extended to the spinal column if neurological signs indicate that lower regions of the spinal cord or the roots are affected. The immediate and subsequent tolerance to the second irradiation at the same dose is good. The new high energy irradiation techniques which partially protect active bone marrow should be used.

In summary, 1) in ALL patients, it is necessary to start a preventive meningeal treatment immediately after a complete remission is obtained; 2) this treatment should combine intrathecal chemotherapy and irradiation of the skull at 2,400 rads; 3) the occurrence of meningeal blastic infiltrations makes it necessary to restart this treatment according to the same schedule in the case of systemic relapse.

REFERENCES

1. EVANS, A.E., GILBERT, E.S., ZANDSTRA, R.: The increased incidence of central nervous system leukemia in children. Cancer 26, 404 (1970)
2. MATHE, G., AMIEL, J.L., POULLART, P., SCHWARZENBERG, L., HAYAT, M., DE VASSAL, F., BELPOMME, D.: LAFLEUR, M.: Cure expectancy in children with acute lymphoid leukemia. Boll. 1st. Sieroter. Milanese. 53, 282 (1974)

3. MATHE, G.: Operational research in cancer chemotherapy. Chemotherapy in the
   strategy of cancer treatment. p. 72. *In:* Scientific basis of cancer chemotherapy. Berlin, Heidelberg, New York: Springer 1969
4. AUR, R.J.A., HUSTU, O., HERNANDEZ, K., WALTERS, T., SIMONE, J., BORELLA, L.,
   PINKEL, D.: Total therapy of acute lymphocytic leukemia. Proc. Amer. Ass.
   Cancer Res. *10*, 4 (1969)
5. MELHORN, D.K., GROSS, S., FISHER, B.J., NEWMAN, A.J.: Studies on the use of
   "prophylactic" intrathecal amethopterin in childhood leukaemia. Blood *36*,
   55 (1970)
6. MATHE, G., AMIEL, J.L., SCHWARZENBERG, L., SCHNEIDER, M., CATTAN, A., SCHLUM-
   BERGER, J.R., HAYAT, M., DE VASSAL, F.: Démonstration de l'efficacité de
   l'immunothérapie active de la leucémie aiguë lymphoblastique humaine. Rev.
   Fr. Et. Clin. Biol. *13*, 454 (1968)
7. HARDISTY, R.M., NORMAN, P.M.: Meningeal leukaemia. Arch. Dis. Childh. *42*,
   441 (1967)
8. WELLS, C.E., SILVER, R.T.: The neurologic manifestations of the acute leukaemias. Ann. Intern. Med. *46*, 439 (1957)
9. AUR, R.J.A., SIMONE, J., HUSTU, O., WALTERS, T., BORELLA, L., PRATT, C.,
   PINKEL, D.: Central nervous system therapy and combination chemotherapy of
   childhood leukaemia. Blood. *37*, 272 (1971)

Prof. G. MATHE
Institut de Cancérologie et d'immunogénétique
Hôpital Paul-Brousse
14-16, Avenue Paul-Vaillant-Couturier
F - 94800 - Villejuif, France

Acta Neuropath. (Berlin), Suppl. VI, 241 - 245 (1975)

Prevention of Meningeal Leukaemia and Relapses by Cranial Irradiation and Intrathecal MTX in Acute Lymphatic Leukaemia

P. KREPLER, M. KUMMER, J. PAWLOWSKY
St. Anna-Children's Hospital, Vienna, Austria

K. JENTZSCH
Department of Radiotherapy, University of Vienna, Austria

Summary: Experience with CNS prophylaxis in 35 children with acute lymphatic leukaemia is reported.

Before prophylactic irradiation of the skull was given the average survival time in 36 children was 2,8 (2,7) years. Meningeal leukaemia preceeded bone marrow relapse in 9 cases and followed relapse in a further 5 cases (39%).

Between 1971 and 1973 Pinkel's treatment scheme VII was given to 35 children. This included prophylactic skull irradiation and intraspinal MTX injections. 29 children are still in their first remissions which range from 10 - 35 months in length. Meningeal leukaemia has not so far been observed, in this latter group.

Key words: Acute lymphatic leukaemia - meningeal leukaemia - prophylactic irradiation of the brain

The use of Vincristine to induce remission and intensive chemotherapy during remission have significantly extended survival times in acute lymphatic leukaemia (ALL). This has been associated with a marked increase in the frequency of meningeal leukaemia. For this formerly rare complication an occurrence rate as high as 56% has been reported (1) a similar incidence has been found in our patients.

PERSONAL CASE SERIES

From 1967 - 1972 we observed meningeal and CNS leukaemic infiltration in 14 out of 36 children with ALL, (39%), in two collaborating children's hospitals in Vienna. The average survival times in these two groups were 2 years 8 months and 2 years 7 months respectively. In one hospital preventive intrathecal Methotrexate was given at intervals of 1 - 3 months. This reduced the frequency of meningeal relapses to 35% as compared to 46% when no Methotrexate prophylaxis was given. The meningeal leukaemia preceeded bone marrow relapse in 9 cases and followed bone marrow relapse in a further 5 cases. Fig. 1 relates the occurrence of meningeal leukaemia to survival time. It is seen, even from this small series, that meningeal leukaemia may be delayed for several years after the onset of the disease.

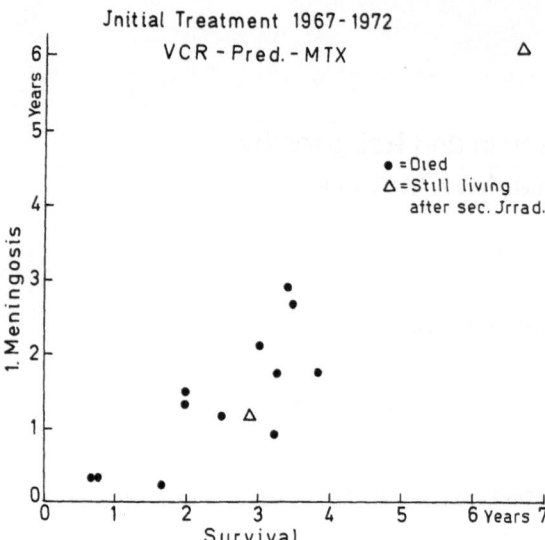

Fig. 1. Relationship of meningeal leukaemia to survival time

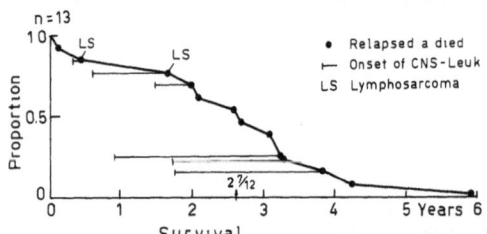

Fig. 2. Survival curve (30. 6. 74) for children with ALL from St. Anna Hospital, where incomplete CNS-prophylaxis was applied. The children received a few injections of MTX intrathecally, and 5 of them underwent CNS irradiation later while in remission

RESULTS

The survival curve (Fig. 2) confirms the high frequency of this complication, with 8 out of 23 patients being affected. The time interval to relapse or death may be as long as 2 years.

The favourable response of leukaemic meningeal infiltration to methotrexate treatment masked the importance of this complication in relation to curative treatment. The importance of the research by PINKEL and his co-workers is that they have established the value of prophylactic treatment of the central nervous system (CNS) in prolonging remission and increasing the chance of cure (2, 3, 4).

In addition to intensive chemotherapy, irradiation of the craniospinal axis has been introduced, as a substitute for chemotherapeutic agents which are un-

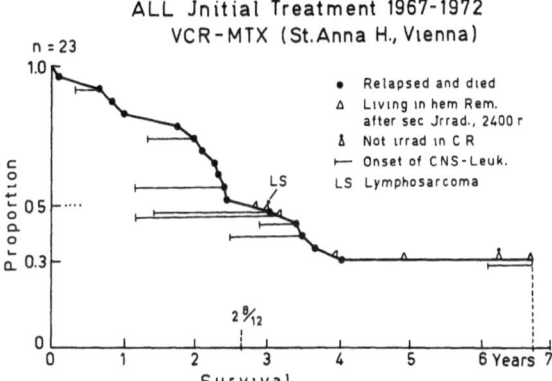

Fig. 3. Survival curve for children with ALL who did not receive any CNS prophylaxis

able to cross the blood CSF barrier in sufficient concentrations. Clinical trials have shown that a dose of 2400 rads to the craniospinal axis is more effective than one of 500 - 1000 rads. Irradiation of the spinal cord can be reinforced by intrathecal Methotrexate injections (5) during the radiotherapy course. This treatment considerably reduces the frequency of bone marrow relapse, so that one can hope, if one excludes prognostically unfavourable cases, that an average remission time of 4 - 5 years can be achieved. If maintenance therapy is discontinued after 2 1/2 - 3 years of full remission, the relapse rate is, so far, only 10%.

In children who have been initially differently treated CNS irradiation seems to have favourable effects, even if applied some months or years after remission has been induced. Five out of seven survivors (Fig. 2) during their first remission, had secondary cranial irradiation. Two had already had meningeal involvement before irradiation, one having developed a tumour. The survival curve now shows a levelling off at 30%. Four patients have been almost 4 - 7 years in their first remission. In the survival curve of a collaborating hospital (Fig. 3), where no CNS prophylaxis was given, this levelling off is not present. In the last two curves 3 cases of lymphosarcoma are included, two of them with CNS involvement. Such patients have been treated as were the children with ALL. The frequency of CNS involvement in lymphosarcoma is even higher than in ALL without CNS prophylaxis.

Besides the well known pseudotumour, in cases with meningeal involvement many forms of clinically localized CNS lesions by leukaemic infiltrations are possible and we have seen these. Especially common are paralysis of cranial nerves and infiltration of the optic nerves with consequent total blindness.

During 1971 - 1973 we treated our patients according to the Pinkel scheme VII, with minor variations.

Irradiation of the skull was carried out in 28 cases at the Institute of Radiotherapy, Vienna University, and in 6 cases in a collaborating hospital in Linz. Deviating somewhat from the original plan, the treatment time was prolonged to 26 days with 21 treatments, instead of 21 days with 12 treatments as suggested by PINKEL. The treatment field must include all the meningeal spaces, which includes the heads of the optic nerves, the pituitary gland and the cervical spine as far as C2/3. During localisation and treatment the child lies on its side and under the simulator the field is defined by fluoroscopy.

The head has to be maintained in the same position during the course of treatment. This is achieved by cutting Styropor mould and fitting the child into

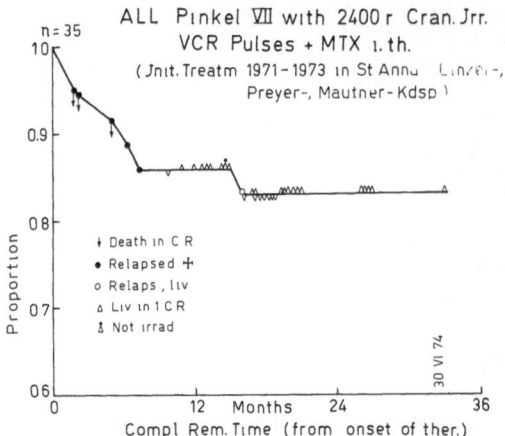

Fig. 4. Duration of remission of 35 children with ALL who were treated according to Pinkel scheme VII, including cranial irradiation

this mould at each treatment. The parts of the face which should be protected from irradiation are shielded with lead. The course of 2400 rads starts with low single dosis, 2 x 50, 2 x 100, 2 x 150 rad to reach daily skin doses of 200 rad, corresponding to a daily dose to the midline of 135 rads.

By the end of 1973, 35 patients (24 from the St. Anna Children's Hospital, the others from collaborating Children Hospitals)[1], underwent this scheme of treatment, with the exception of one child to whom CNS irradiation could not be applied. Fig. 4 demonstrates the preliminary results of treatment and shows the time from diagnosis to first relapse or death. Meningeal relapses have not so far occurred. Unfortunately 3 children died from interstitial pneumonia during the first 5 months of complete remission. Nevertheless the results are favourable. The curve comes to a plateau at 83%. Of 35 children, 29 are still in their first remission, lasting between 10 - 33 months. Only two have died with bone marrow involvement and one is in a second complete remission.

Tolerance of radiotherapy was generally good. Alopecia was always transistory. The somnolence syndrome, described by PINKEL as occurring after irradiation (3, 4), was observed in only a mild form.

Transitory anorexia was common. Brain oedema was never proven. The post irradiation period was complicated in 3 cases by lymphocytic meningitis, encephalitis and convulsions and EEG changes. As chemotherapy was given at the same time these complications could not be ascribed only to radiotherapy. Both drug toxicity and viral infections have also to be considered (5, 6, 7). Loss of immunocompetence is most likely to be caused by the chemotherapy but could be to some extent due to the irradiation (8). The most dangerous complication, sometimes occurring immediately after irradiation, is interstitial pneumonia caused by Pneumocystis Carinii, viral or fungal infection (9).

Since 1974 we together with other pediatricians in an Austrian study group have modified the cytostatic treatment scheme, in order to reduce the number of deaths, of patients in complete remission, due to immune suppression. The scheme of prophylactic radiotherapy remains unchanged.

---

[1] Preyer Kinderspital (Prof. SWOBODA), Mautner Kinderspital (Prof. WOLF), Linzer Kinderspital (Prim. TULZER)

REFERENCES

1. EVANS, A.E., GILBERT, E.S., ZANDSTRA, R.: The increasing incidence of central nervous system leukemia in children. Cancer *26*, 404 - 409 (1970)
2. PINKEL, D.: Five-year follow-up of "total therapy" of childhood lymphocytic leukemia. JAMA *216*, 648 - 652 (1971)
3. PINKEL, D., SIMONE, J., HUSTU, H.O., AUR, R.J.A.: Nine years experience with "total therapy" of childhood acute lymphocytic leukemia. Pediatrics *5o*, 246 - 251 (1972)
4. HUSTU, H.O., AUR, R.J.A., VERZOSA, M.S., SIMONE, J.V., PINKEL, D.: Prevention of central nervous system leukemia by irradiation. Cancer *32*, 585 - 597 (1973)
5. GRÖBE, H., PALM, D.: Vincristininduzierte Encephalopathien unter der Behandlung kindlicher Leukosen. Mschr. Kinderhk. *120*, 23 - 27 (1972)
6. McINTOSCH, S., ASPUES, G.T.: Encephalopathy following CNS prophylaxis in childhood lymphoblastic leukemia. Pediatrics *52*, 612 - 615 (1973)
7. BLEYER, W.A., DRAKE, J.C., CHABNER, B.S., CHABNER, B.A.: Neurotoxicity and elevated cerebrospinal-fluid Methotrexate concentration in meningeal leukemia. New Engl. J. Med. *289*, 770 - 773 (1973)
8. CAMPBELL, A.C., HERSEY, P., MACLENNAN, J.C.M., KAY, H.E.M., PIKE, M.C.: Immunosuppressive consequences of radiotherapy and chemotherapy in patients with acute lymphoblastic leukemia. Brit. med. J. *2*, 385 - 388 (1973)
9. WALZER, P.D., SCHULTZ, M.G., WESTERN, K.A., ROBBINS, J.B.: Pneumocystis carinii pneumonia and primary immune deficiency diseases of infancy and childhood. J. Ped. *82*, 416 - 422 (1973)

Prof. Dr. P. KREPLER
St. Anna Kinderspital
Kinderspitalgasse 6
A - 1090 W i e n

Acta Neuropath. (Berlin), Suppl. VI, 247 - 250 (1975)
© by Springer-Verlag 1975

Atypical Progressive Multifocal Leukoencephalopathy with Plasma-Cell Infiltrates

EDWARD P. RICHARDSON, JR.
Charles S. Kubik Laboratory for Neuropathology
Massachusetts General Hospital, Boston, Mass., USA

PETER C. JOHNSON
Department of Pathology, Letterman General Hospital
San Francisco, Calif., USA

Summary: In rare cases of progressive multifocal leukoencephalopathy (PML) the lesions are atypical in that the characteristic alteration of oligodendrocytic nuclei is infrequent or absent, and the demyelinated foci contain mononuclear inflammatory infiltrates including numerous plasma cells. Otherwise these cases, both as to the topographic features of the lesions, and the background of chronic lymphoproliferative or myeloproliferative disease or immunosuppressive treatment, conform to the usual pattern. In the case here reported, that of a 54-year-old man receiving immunosuppressive drugs for chronic polymyositis, electron microscopy showed papovavirions in astrocytic nuclei and fluorescent antibody studies indicated that these represented JC virus. In this and the 3 previously reported similar cases of atypical PML, the neurologic illness was less devastating than generally occurs in classic PML. Possibly these cases represent instances of unusually strong host-resistance against the disease.

Key words: Progressive multifocal leukoencephalopathy (PML) - Plasma-cell Infiltrates - Papovavirions - JC virus

INTRODUCTION

Although still a rare disease, progressive multifocal leukoencephalopathy (PML) is now well recognized as one of the neurological complications of the overall group of diseases to which this Symposium is devoted - the lymphomas and leukemias. Thanks to the important work that has been done on this disease in recent years, there have been great advances in the understanding of the pathogenesis of this disorder (1). We may now look upon it as an opportunistic infection of the central nervous system by a nearly ubiquitous papovavirus not previously known to be pathogenic for human beings, occurring in patients whose cell-mediated immune responses have been impaired as a result either of the underlying systemic disease or its treatment by immunosuppressive methods. Despite individual variations, its clinicopathologic features have been remarkably uniform from case to case. In a very small group of cases, which from the standpoint of the general medical background and the configuration of the lesions have conformed to the expected pattern, the histopathologic features have been atypical in that the characteristic changes in oligodendrocytic nuclei have been inconspicuous or absent, and the demyelinated foci have been marked by the presence of extensive mononuclear inflammatory infiltrates including numerous plasma cells. One such case was reported in the series from the Massachusetts General Hospital in 1961 (Case 4): that of a 65-year-old man with

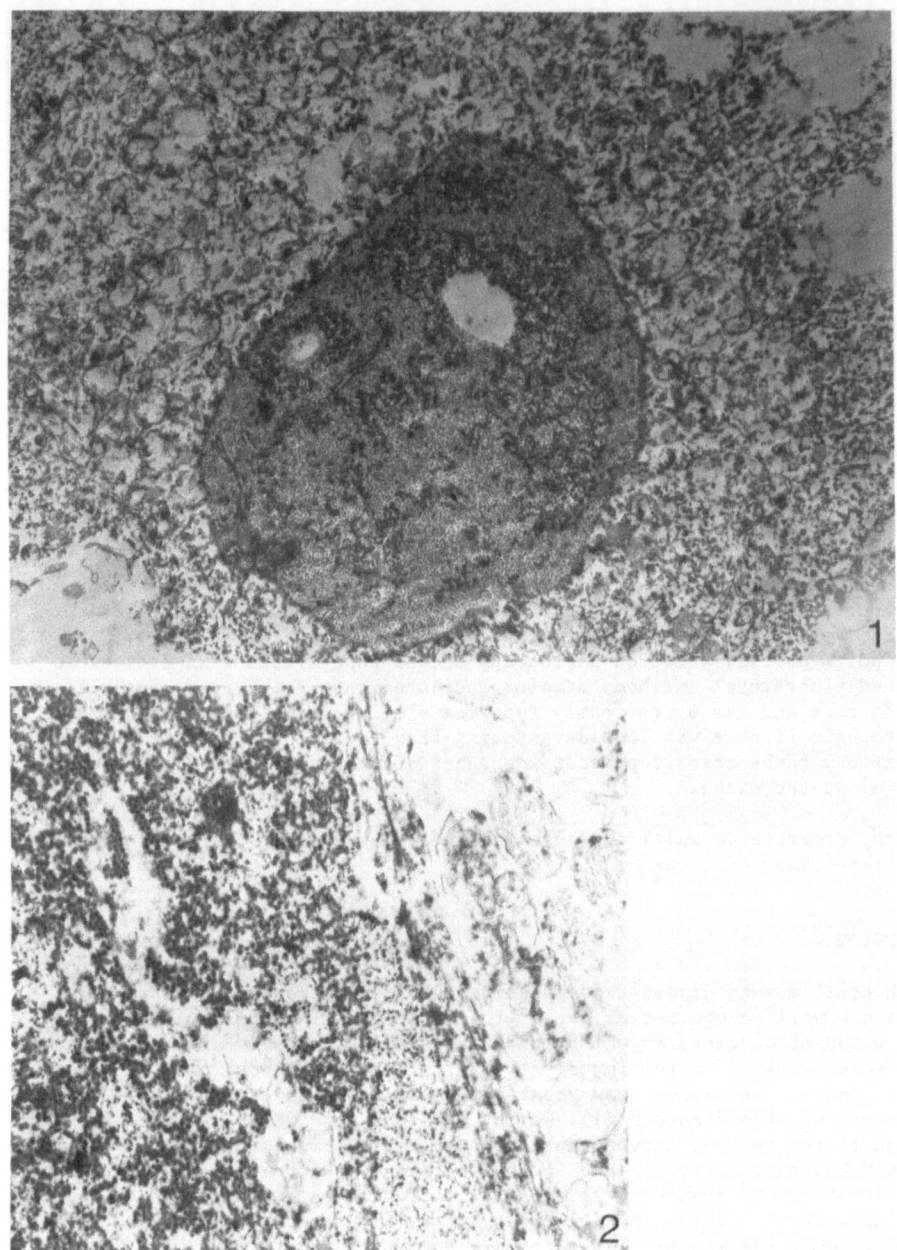

Fig. 1. Low-power EM view of an astrocyte, with abundant intracytoplasmic glial fibrils, containing numerous intranuclear particles typical of papovavirions. (Original magnification 4,000)

Fig. 2. Edge of nucleus with bordering cytoplasmic containing glial fibrils, showing papovavirions in greater detail. (EM photograph; original magnification 15,000)

chronic myelogenous leukemia who in the last 4 months of life had a transitory left hemiparesis and pronounced emotional lability (2). Soon afterward, MANCALL reported a neuropathologically identical case in a 41-year-old man with chronic lymphatic leukemia in whom no neurologic abnormalities were observed except for terminal conculsive seizures (3). More recently, KREMPIEN and his colleagues have described another case with these atypical features (4). This occurred in a 42-year-old woman with sarcoidosis in whom late-developing neurologic deficits showed some improvement before death. Electron-microscopic (EM) studies in this case did not demonstrate papovavirions, whereas they were abundantly present in a typical PML-case studied by these authors.

Since this variant of PML is still relatively unfamiliar, we thought it would be of interest to draw attention to the findings in a case that we have lately been studying.

CASE REPORT

A 54-year-old man had been under treatment with prednisone and chlorambucil because of chronic polymyositis. In the final 5 months of his life, altered behavior, impaired memory, and ataxia were observed. He died of bronchopneumonia. The brain showed multiple cerebral and cerebellar demyelinative lesions which under low magnification were typically those of PML. Histopathologically, the lesions were characterized by conspicuous lymphocytic and plasma-cell infiltrates, with many isolated plasma cells in the parenchyma. There were scattered irregular darkly staining astrocytic nuclei, but no giant astrocytes and no enlarged oligodendroglial nuclei. EM investigation showed that the dark astrocytic nuclei contained typical papovavirions of both filamentous (average thickness: 27 nm) and polyhedral (average diameter: 41 nm) types (Figures 1, 2). Immunofluorescent-antibody studies[1] indicated that the nuclei so affected contained JC virus.

COMMENT

The findings in our case give strong suggestive evidence that the atypical variety of PML with plasma-cell infiltrates may, along with typical PML, be associated with intranuclear papovavirions and may be the result of infection with JC virus. Why the tissue reaction in cases of this kind should deviate to such an extent from what usually occurs is far from clear. A striking feature of all of these cases has been that in comparison with typical PML, the neurologic illness has been less severe, and the course has not been relentless. What we may be seeing, then, is an unusual degree of host-resistance against the cerebral infection. If the nature of this resistance could be discovered, an effective means of combatting the disease might be devised.

The technical assistance of Mr. John BURGESS is gratefully acknowledged.

REFERENCES

1. RICHARDSON, E.P., Jr.: Our Evolving Understanding of Progressive Multifocal Leukoencephalopathy. *In:* Hall, T.C. (ed.): Paraneoplastic Syndromes, p. 358 - 364. New York: Ann. N.Y. Acad. Sci. vol. 230, 1974
2. RICHARDSON, E.P., Jr.: Progressive multifocal leukoencephalopathy. N. Engl. J. Med. *265,* 815 - 823 (1961)

---

[1] These were kindly performed by Dr. O. NARAYAN, Department of Neurology, Johns Hopkins University Medical School, Baltimore, Md.

3. MANCALL, E.L.: Progressive multifocal leukoencephalopathy. Neurology (Minneap.) *15*, 693 - 699 (1965)
4. KREMPIEN, B., KOLKMANN, F.-W., SCHIEMER, H.G., MAYER, P.: Über die progressive multifokale Leukoencephalopathie. Virchows Arch. Abt. A Path. Anat. *355*, 158 - 178 (1972)

RICHARDSON, E.P., Jr., M.D.
C.S. Kubick Lab. of Neuropathology
Massachusetts General Hospital
Boston, Mass. 02114 / U.S.A.

Acta Neuropath. (Berlin), Suppl. VI, 251 - 255 (1975)

Leukoencephalopathy Following Combines Therapy of Central Nervous System Leukemia and Lymphoma

L.J. RUBINSTEIN, M.M. HERMAN, T.F. LONG AND J.R. WILBUR

Stanford University School of Medicine and Children's Hospital, Stanford, California, U.S.A.

Summary: We report a form of disseminated necrotizing leukoencephalopathy observed in five children with acute lymphoblastic leukemia or lymphoma, who received systemic chemotherapy, brain radiation, and intrathecal (IT) methotrexate, cytosine arabinoside and hydrocortisone because of meningeal tumor involvement. Three children developed a progressive neurologic disease at the end of IT therapy or shortly thereafter. The lesions consisted in discrete, apparently coalescent foci of coagulative necrosis in the white matter, with a remarkable absence of inflammatory cells, little or no tissue breakdown, and striking axonal swellings. The adjacent tissue showed status spongiosus and moderate astrocytic hypertrophy. Vascular lesions were few and inconstant.

Key words: Leukoencephalopathy - CNS leukemia - Intrathecal methotrexate and cytosine arabinoside - Brain radiation

INTRODUCTION

Central nervous system (CNS) involvement in childhood leukemia has been reported to be demonstrable in 50 to 75% of the cases (1). The CNS is also the most frequent site of initial relapse in acute leukemia treated with systemic chemotherapy. As a result, therapy to the CNS, including prophylactic treatment, has been increasingly vigorous in recent years (2, 3). The modes of treatment consist of craniospinal radiation (3), or a combination of whole brain radiation and courses of intrathecal (IT) methotrexate (MT) (2) with or without IT cytosine arabinoside (CA) and hydrocortisone (HC) (4).

Complications following IT chemotherapy in childhood leukemia have included chemical meningitis (5), motor and sensory losses, usually but not invariably (6) transient; and a type of encephalopathy characterized by confusion, somnolence, ataxia, spasticity and major seizures, which may progress to dementia, coma and death (7). Pathologic descriptions of this form of encephalopathy have so far been few (4, 7).

We report the neuropathologic findings of a disseminated type of necrotizing leukoencephalopathy (DNL) whose features are highly distinctive. The patients in our series include four children with acute lymphoblastic leukemia and one child with Burkitt's lymphoma and terminal lymphoblastic leukemia. All were treated with systemic chemotherapy, and with IT MT, CA and HC because of meningeal tumor involvement. Whole brain radiation (in the range of 3,500 R) was given before or during IT therapy. Three children developed, immediately or shortly after completing IT treatment, a neurologic illness characterized by irritability, agitation, confusion, ataxia and slurred speech, progressing to increasing lethargy, decerebrate posture and repeated seizures. Death occurred approximately 2 months after the onset of the encephalopathy.

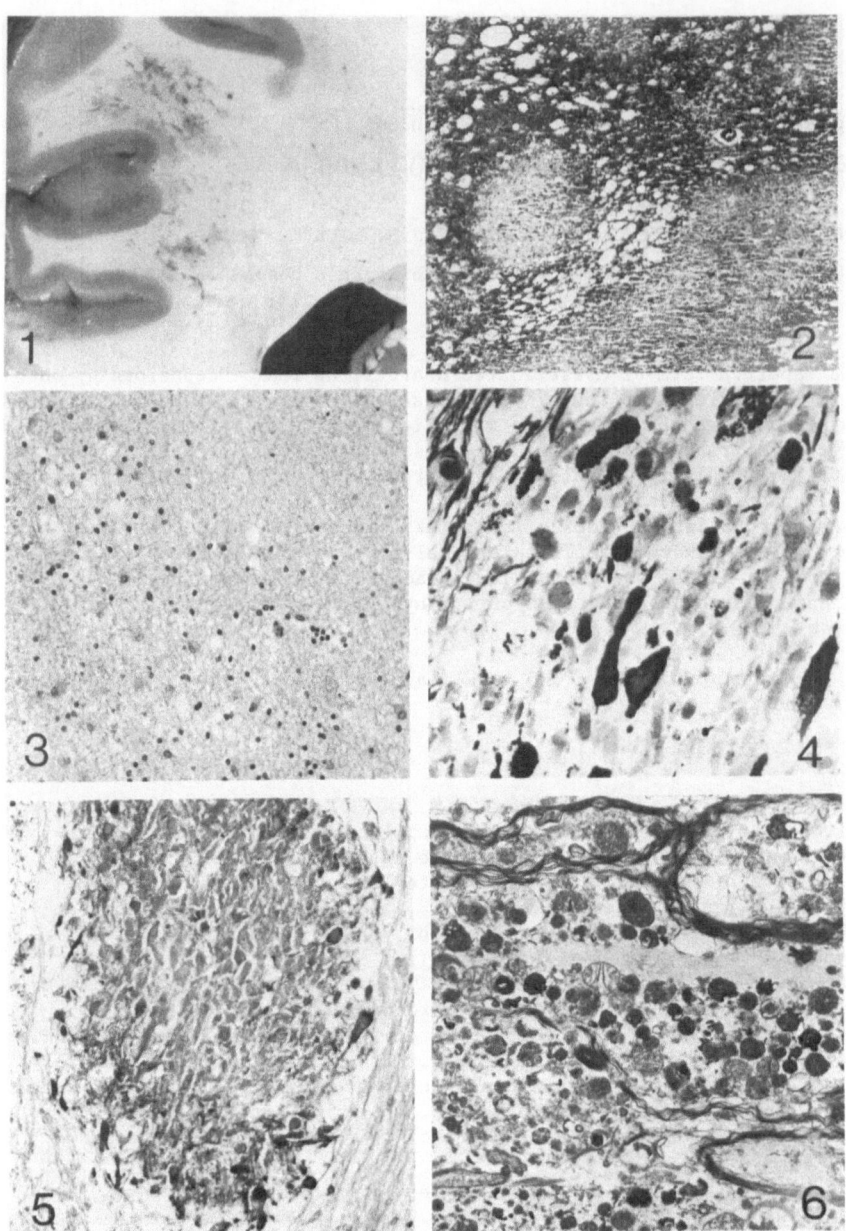

Fig. 1. Multiple discrete grey foci of softening in cerebral white matter

Fig. 2. Irregular foci of demyelination, with adjacent status spongiosus. Myelin stain, x 30

Fig. 3. Acellular coagulative necrosis (upper right). Reactive astrocytes in adjacent brain. H.-E., x 120

The clinical and pathologic data of these patients will be detailed elsewhere. We here summarize the apparent sequential evolution of the lesions in
an attempt to characterize the pathologic process and briefly discuss its
possible relationship to the modalities of treatment to which these patients
were subjected.

NEUROPATHOLOGIC FINDINGS

The early gross lesions, best seen in the freshly cut brain, consist of discrete foci of gray-pink to brown softening randomly distributed in the digitate
cerebral white matter (Fig. 1). They are often accompanied by petechial or
ring-shaped hemorrhages. The cerebellar white matter, midbrain, pons and medulla
may also be involved. In one case, the brain showed extensive symmetrical necroses in the centra ovalia, associated with masses of petechial hemorrhages
in the frontal lobes.
   Microscopically, the early lesions consist in disseminated foci of coagulative
necrosis in the white matter, unrelated to the blood vessels (Figs. 2 and 3).
Loss of myelin, and severe to complete loss of oligodendroglia are evident.
Little or no tissue breakdown usually accompanies the necrosis (Fig. 3). Macrophages are few. Compared to the extent of the necrosis, only sparse neutral
fat is demonstrable, and then usually only at the edges of the foci. There is
a remarkable paucity of inflammatory cells. In more severely affected areas,
there is coalescence of the lesions. A characteristic irregular map-like pattern
of necrosis is then apparent. The adjacent tissue often shows marked status
spongiosus (Fig. 2) and a moderate hypertrophic astrocytic response (Fig. 3).
   Axonal damage is constant and characteristic, both at the edges of the necrotic foci and within them. It ranges from scattered focal axonal enlargement
and fragmentation (Fig. 4) to massive collections of closely packed swellings
that may progress to calcification (Fig. 5). Electron microscopy in one case
confirmed the presence of striking changes in both myelinated and non-myelinated
axons (Fig. 6). These were distended by mitochondria, smooth vesicles, dense
bodies containing membrane fragments, autophagic vacuoles, and microfilaments.
some were packed almost entirely with mitochondria.
   The necrotic foci may or may not be associated with viable tumour cells or
with the ghosts of dead tumour cells. Perivascular distribution of the lesions
is exceptional. Fibrinoid necrosis of the vessel walls and parenchymatous fibrin
extravasation may be present, but are as a rule neither severe nor frequent. In
the one case where bilateral lesions were unusually massive, the necrosis consisted in a mixture of the lesions described above with extensive areas of
parenchymatous fibrin extravasation and fibrinoid necrosis of the vessel walls.
In the less affected areas, small discrete lesions typical of DNL were found.

DISCUSSION

The salient neuropathologic features of DNL are highly distinctive. Although
all the patients received brain radiation before or during IT therapy, the

Fig. 4. Axonal swellings in necrotic focus. Bielschowsky silver, x 300

Fig. 5. Closely packed, occasionally calcified axonal swellings in pons.
H.-E., x 135

Fig. 6. Axonal swellings involving myelinated and non myelinated axons.
x 6,600

lesions differ from those of cerebral radionecrosis in that, with the exception of the one case with massive bilateral lesions, they lacked the conspicuous vascular fibrinoid necroses and extensive parenchymatous fibrin extravasations diagnostic of radiation damage (8).

The mechanism of the lesions is obscure. Stains and cultures for bacteria, fungi or parasites were consistently negative. Neither inclusions nor viral particles were seen by light or electron microscopy. The evidence that links the necroses to IT therapy is circumstantial only. If a relation exists, the selective involvement of the white matter is puzzling. No correlation has been obtained between the extent and severity of the structural changes, and the dosage and duration of IT and systemic chemotherapy or the amount of brain radiation. Unlike the cases which received intraventricular MT for the treatment of posterior fossa tumors (9, 10), the juxtaventricular zones of the cerebral white matter were not preferentially involved. The spinal cord has not so far shown any such lesions. The lack of relationship between the necrotizing lesions and the vascular architecture, and the rarity of changes involving the blood vessel walls speak against a toxicity mechanism that would be primarily related to a breakdown of the blood-brain barrier. They also argue against brain radiation being the primary pathogenetic factor. However, it is conceivable that radiation may play a part in increasing the vulnerability of the white matter to the neurotoxic effects of IT and systemically administered chemotherapeutic drugs. Whether meningeal tumor infiltration could play a role in the pathogenesis of DNL through the production of obstructive hydrocephalus should also be considered in view of the suggestion that encephalopathy resulting from intraventricular instillation of MT may be enhanced by the presence of ventricular obstruction (10, 11). However, such a hypothesis would be difficult to reconcile with the neuroanatomic distribution of the lesions in our cases.

Attention is drawn to the presence of numerous axonal swellings, a constant and early feature in DNL. These common axonal changes are of course known to occur in a wide range of clinical and experimental conditions, and are believed to reflect a non-specific reaction of the axon to various toxic, biochemical, genetic or traumatic agents. The metabolism or function of the axoplasm is presumed to be implicated in this process, perhaps as a catabolic event due to changes in neuronal metabolism (12). The pathogenesis of axonal swelling is, however, still poorly understood. Its constancy and severity in DNL merit further investigation. The antimetabolic properties of MT and CA are based on their inhibiting action on DNA synthesis. Whether these drugs might also conceivably exert specific neurotoxicity by interfering with the structural integrity of the axoplasm needs to be elucidated.

REFERENCES

1. PRICE, R.A., JOHNSON, W.W.: The central nervous system in childhood leukemia: I. The arachnoid. Cancer *31*, 520 - 533 (1973)
2. BRODER, L.E., CARTER, S.K.: Meningeal leukemia. pp. 109 - 122. New York: Plenum Press 1972
3. HUSTU, H.O., AUR, R.J.A., VERZOSA, M.S., SIMONE, J.V., PINKEL, D.: Prevention of central nervous system leukemia by irradiation. Cancer *32*, 585 - 597 (1973)
4. HENDIN, B., DEVIVO, D.C., TORACK, R., LELL, M-E, RAGAB, A.H., VIETTI, T.J.: Parenchymatous degeneration of the central nervous system in childhood leukemia. Cancer *33*, 468 - 482 (1974)
5. DUTTERA, M.J., BLEYER, W.A., POMEROY, T.C., LEVENTHAL, C.M., LEVENTHAL, B.G.: Irradiation, methotrexate toxicity, and the treatment of meningeal leukaemia. Lancet *2*, 703 - 707 (1973)

6. SAIKI, J.H., THOMPSON, S., SMITH, F., ATKINSON, R.: Paraplegia following
   intrathecal chemotherapy. Cancer *29*, 370 - 374 (1972)
7. KAY, H.E.M., KNAPTON, P.J., O'SULLIVAN, J.P., WELLS, D.G., HARRIS, R.F.,
   INNES, E.M., STUART, J., SCHWARTZ, F.C.M., THOMPSON, E.N.: Encephalopathy
   in acute leukemia associated with methotrexate therapy. Arch. Dis. Childh.
   47, 344 - 354 (1972)
8. RUBINSTEIN, L.J.: Tumors of the central nervous system. Atlas of tumor
   pathology, second series, fasc. 6 pp. 352 - 360, Washington: Armed Forces
   Institute of Pathology 1972
9. BRESNAN, M.J., GILLES, F.H., LORENZO, A.V., WATTERS, G.V., BARLOW, C.F.:
   Leukoencephalopathy following combined irradiation and intraventricular
   methotrexate therapy of brain tumors in childhood. Trans. Amer. Neurol.
   Assoc. *97*, 204 - 206 (1972)
10. SHAPIRO, W.R., CHERNIK, N.L., POSNER, J.B.: Necrotizing encephalopathy
    following intraventricular instillation of methotrexate. Arch. Neurol.
    28, 96 - 102 (1973)
11. NORRELL, H., WILSON, C.B., SLAGEL, D.E., CLARK, D.B.: Leukoencephalopathy
    following the administration of methotrexate into the cerebrospinal fluid
    in the treatment of primary brain tumors. Cancer *33*, 923 - 932 (1974)
12. JELLINGER, K.: Neuroaxonal dystrophy: its natural history and related
    disorders. In: Progress in Neuropathology, vol. 2, pp. 129 - 180, H.M.
    Zimmerman (ed.) New York: Grune & Stratton 1973

L.J. RUBINSTEIN, M.D.
Department of Pathology (Neuropathology)
Stanford University School of Medicine
Stanford, California, 94305, U.S.A.

Acta Neuropath. (Berlin), Suppl. VI, 257 - 260 (1975)

Diffuse Reticulosis with Leukomalacia

L. LISS AND S.A. GOGATE

Neuropathology Division, Department of Pathology
Ohio State University, College of Medicine
Columbus, Ohio

Summary: A malignant lymphoproliferative disease with acute clinical course and selective clinical CNS involvement is described. The metastatic lesions in the brain are compared with a primary microglioma of the brain.

Key words: Reticulosis - Leukomalacia - Microglioma - Lymphoproliferative disease

The neoplastic lymphoproliferative disease problem is illustrated on two clinico-pathological studies. The clinical course in both patients indicated primary involvement of the central nervous system.

CASE REPORTS

Case I. Clinical History: A 56 year old Negro woman was a known alcoholic with a past history of documented nutritional cirrhosis and portal hypertension. She entered the hospital because of progressive neurologic deterioration consisting primarily of increasing lethargy, speech difficulty, and a right hemiparesis. On admission the neurological examination revealed a disoriented, lethargic patient with inability to adduct the left eye, droop of the right labial fold, increased flexor tone of the right elbow and knee with right-sided weakness, and a positive Babinski on the right, negative on the left. The blood ammonia was slightly elevated. Spinal fluid contained 175 red cells and 6 white cells and the protein was elevated (95 mg %). No evidence of AFB or fungi. C.S.F. sugar was 100 mg %, simultaneous blood sugar 124 mg %.
    Hematologic Data: Admission hemoglobin was 11.7, Hct. 35.0, RBC 3.28. Reticulocytes 4.6% (range from 2.0-4.6% during hospitalization). The smear showed numerous macrocytes, toxic granulation of lymphocytes, and markedly reduced platelets. Admission platelet count was 22,000 (reaching a maximum of 55,000 during hospitalization, then dropping to a minimum of 3,000 just prior to death). WBC: 11,700 on admission (73% PMN's, 8% lymphs, 19% monocytes, no immature forms). This ranged between 8,000 to 15,000 during hospitalization. Bone marrow biopsy was interpreted as hypercellular, somewhat megaloblastic, with numerous megakaryocytes. Coagulation work-up showed, in addition to thrombocytopenia, a prolonged prothrombin time, increased fibrinogen split products, and numerous "helmet cells" on the smear consistent with a consumptive coagulopathy.
    The patient was put on a hepatic coma regime and arterial ammonia fell to normal range. In spite of this, her neurologic status continued to deteriorate, casting doubt on a metabolic etiology for her neurologic disorder. She was not oriented and showed very little response to painful stimuli over her legs, arms, and trunk. She had nuchal rigidity. She continued to have right hemiparesis, greater in the arm than in the leg, and hyperreflexia greater on the right

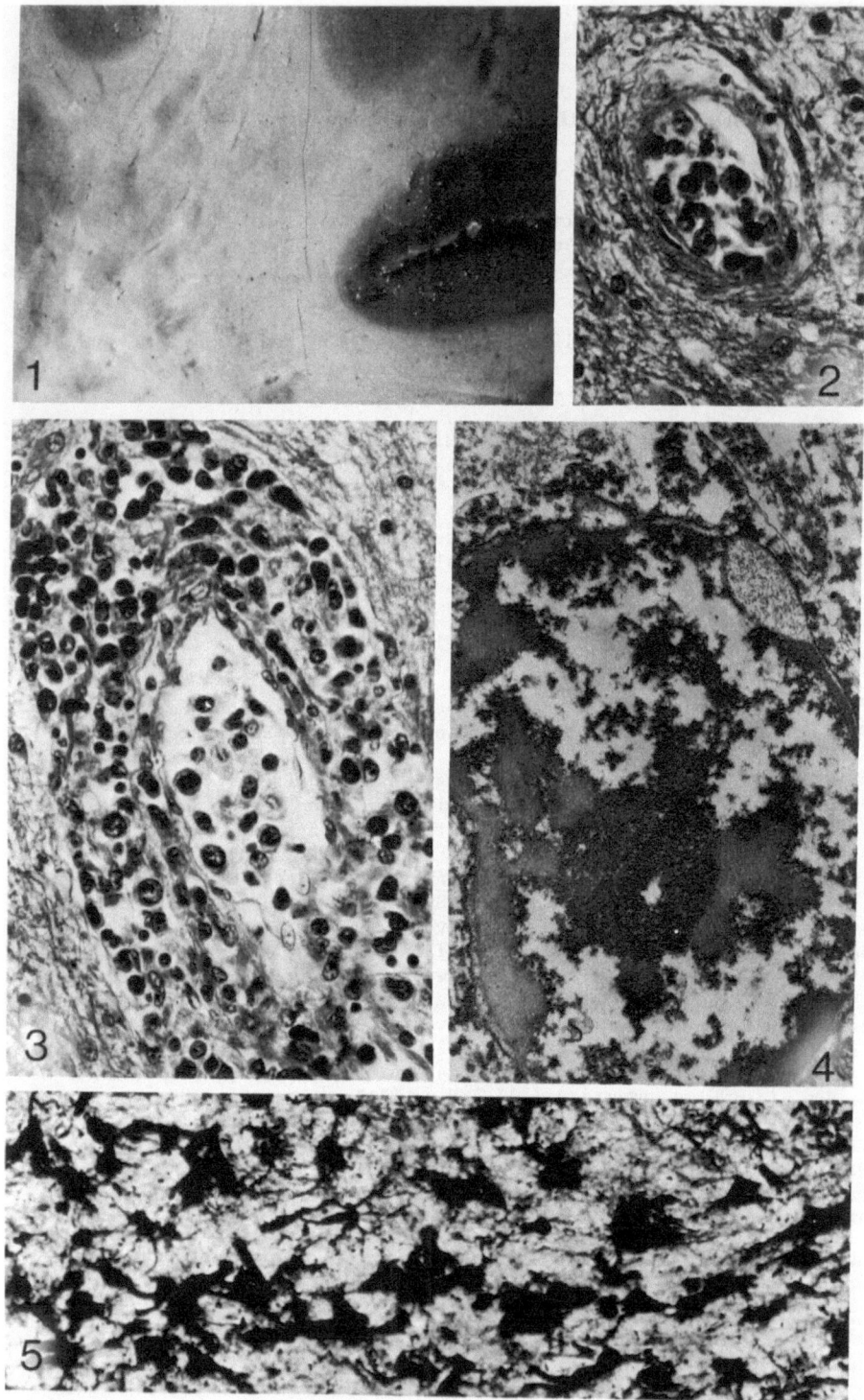

than on the left. The brain scan was interpreted as normal. A left carotid
angiogram was also performed and showed no evidence of a space-occupying
intracranial lesion. Hepatic dysfunction was never pronounced; bilirubin
never exceeded 2.5 total, enzymes were not elevated, and ascites was minimal
or absent. She had periodic evidence of GI bleeding and received several trans-
fusions. Her thrombocytopenia persisted, but she was not heparinized for presumed intravascular coagulopathy. As her coma deepened, she developed acidosis
and expired, in spite of vigorous efforts. The exact nature of both her neurologic and hematologic disorders remained unresolved at the time of death.

On *post mortem examination* the abdominal cavity contained 1000 cc. of clear
yellow fluid. The liver cirrhosis of nutritional type was confirmed. The sinu-
soids, central veins and portal areas were infiltrated with cells which were
large, with hyperchromatic nuclei and with multinucleated cells. The spleen
and lymph nodes showed loss of normal architecture and infiltration with malignant cells, nucleated red blood cells and multinucleated giant cells. The large
cells had hyperchromatic nuclei and many had bizarre appearance. Infiltration
by the undifferentiated malignant cells was documented in the submucosa of the
gall bladder, the subepicardial fat and in myocardium, esophagus submucosa, in
the mucosa and submucosa of the stomach, pancreas, thyroid, adrenals, in the
glomeruli and capillaries of the kidneys, and in the ovaries. The capillaries
in all the affected organs were filled with neoplastic cells. The perivascular
tissue was infiltrated to a varying degree and the multiple hemorrhages were
accompanying the tumor cells.

The brain weight was 1100 grams - the meninges were thickened and cloudy with
areas of subarachnoid hemorrhages. On coronal sections multiple hemorrhagic infarcts were scattered throughout the cortex and white matter and involving
basal ganglia and cerebellum. In addition to these hemorrhagic infarcts areas
of gray discolored white matter indicating demyelinization were identified
(Fig. 1). On microscopic examination the blood vessels contained neoplastic cells.
The perivascular reaction was most pronounced in areas where the infiltration
by tumor cells was minimal. The astrocytic proliferation was accompanied by
edema (Fig. 2). There was also evidence of perivascular cuffing and extensive
infiltration of brain tissue by the neoplastic cells (Fig. 3). The tumor cells
were large in size, the nuclei varying in density, but mainly hyperchromatic.
Frequent mitotic figures were encountered and abnormal divisions were present.
The myelin was intact around some of the vessels which showed presence of neoplastic cells in their lumina and extensive perivascular infiltration by neoplastic cells. The demyelinated foci were frequently no related to either the
severity or even presence of the neoplastic cells. In contrast the extravasation of the red blood cells was found both in areas of most pronounced infiltration and in the region around the third ventricle, where they represented
agonal changes.

The neoplastic process which infiltrated all organs originated apparently
in the lymph nodes and in the spleen, where no residual of normal architecture
was found. The cerebral changes were mainly secondary to direct invasion of
neoplasm, vascular occlusions, and hemorrhagic diathesis. Some difficulty

---

Fig. 1. (Case I). Necrotic lesions in the white matter and in the cortex

Fig. 2. (Case I). A blood vessel filled with neoplastic cells. Astrocytic
proliferation in the surrounding tissue (300 x)

Fig. 3. (Case I). Intra- and perivascular neoplastic cells. (300 x)

Fig. 4. (Case I). Fine electron dense intranuclear material. (17,200 x)

Fig. 5. (Case II). Characteristic cells of microglioma impregnated with
Hortega's triple silver carbonate technique. Unlike other glial elements,
the bodies of the microglia cells are frequently elongated and their processes fern-like. (350 x)

presented correlation between areas of malacia in regions relatively spared by the tumor cells. The electron microscopy suggested presence of aggregation of dense, fine granular particles, but no definite identification was possible in the post mortem material (Fig. 4).

Case II. An eleven year old boy was admitted to the hospital with history of headaches and "difficulties at school" of about six weeks duration and recent left-sided weakness. The arterial contrast studies and ventriculogram indicated a space-occupying lesion in the right fronto-parietal region which resulted in brain shift. Subsequently a craniotomy was performed and a neoplasm was subtotally removed. The patient had first radiation treatment following the surgery and a second eleven months later when there was indication of the tumor recurring in the same area. Death occurred 14 months after surgery with no clinical indication of involvement of other organs.

A post mortem examination was not obtained, therefore only clinical indication was present of a solitary intracerebral lesion. The histological examination of the craniotomy specimen indicated a cellular neoplasm with slight pleomorphism. The cells were predominantly oval and in silver carbonate impregnation displayed fine fern-like processes characteristic for microglia (Fig. 5).

It is most likely that the microglioma (1, 2, 3) was a primary intracranial solitary lesion which responded poorly to treatment, and eventually caused demise of the patient by infiltration or recurrence and increased pressure.

DISCUSSION

These two examples illustrate that in a case of generalized lymphoproliferative neoplasm which we labeled as reticulosis (4) the conventional histological techniques applicable to post mortem material leave a number of questions unanswered. The site of origin of the tumor can be assumed to be lymphatic tissue and spleen. The diffuse origin from the vessel wall elements, although suggestive in some slides seems unlikely (5). The involvement of the brain is most likely of metastatic type. The correlation between the polio- and leukomalacia and the neoplastic process presents little difficulty with the former, but leaves considerable doubt as to the origin of many white matter lesions. Possibility of an additional etiological factor such as a viral agent cannot be excluded.

The microglioma represent, in contrast to the above, a neoplasm originating from intracerebral elements and can therefore be a solitary lesion, mimicking gliomas and not associated with a systemic disease (6).

REFERENCES

1. RUSSEL, D.S., MARSHALL, A.H.E., SMITH, F.B.: Microgliomatosis: A form of reticulosis affecting brain. Brain *71*, 1 - 15 (1948)
2. HSU, Y.K.: Primary intracranial sarcomas. Arch. Neurol. *43*, 901 - 924 (1940)
3. FISHER, E.R., DAVIS, E.R., LEMMEN, L.J.: Reticulum cell sarcoma of brain (microglioma). Arch. Neurol. *81*, 591 - 598 (1959)
4. BERTELSEN, K.: Primary cerebral reticulosarcoma. Path. Microbiol. *78*, 209 - 214 (1970)
5. DICKINSON, E.S.: Sarcoid meningoencephalitis. Dis. Nerv. Syst. *32*, 118 - 124 (1971)
6. NEAULT, R.W., SCOV, R.E., VAN OKAZAKI, H., McCARTY, C.S.: Uveitis associated with isolated reticulum cell sarcoma of the brain. Amer. J. Ophthal. *73*, 431 - 436 (1972)

L. LISS, M.D.
Neuropathology Division
Upham Hall
Ohio State University
Columbus, Ohio 43210

Acta Neuropath. (Berlin), Supp. VI, 261 - 265 (1975)

Unusual Infections of the Nervous System in Malignant Lymphomas

NITYA R. GHATAK

Department of Pathology (Neuropathology)
Bowman Gray School of Medicine of the
Wake Forest University
Winston-Salem, N.C. 27103. U.S.A.

Summary: Infection of the nervous system by toxoplasma, cytomegalovirus and varicella-zoster virus is described in three adult patients with malignant lymphoma. Morphologic identification of these organisms in otherwise non-specific lesions is emphasized. Since such intercurrent infections are not usually diagnosed clinically in debiliated patients, their recognition at autopsy is important, particularly in view of the wide spread distribution of these organisms in normal population.

Key words: Toxoplasma - Cytomegalovirus - Varicella-zoster - Lymphoma

INTRODUCTION

This report describes three examples of intercurrent infection of the nervous system by toxoplasma, cytomegalovirus (CMV) and varicella-zoster (V-Z) virus respectively in patients with malignant lymphoma. In addition, certain aspects of these infections in immunologically compromised patients are briefly discussed.

MATERIALS AND METHODS

Complete autopsy examination was done on the following patients:

Case 1. An 83-year old woman died about one year after a diagnosis of chronic lymphocytic leukemia. No neurologic symptoms were noted during her illness.

Case 2. A 78-year old woman was diagnosed to have generalized lymphosarcoma about one year prior to death. Her terminal illness was characterized by fever and semi-stuporous state.

Case 3. A 50-year old woman with known Hodgkin's disease for two years developed herpetic rash in the distribution of left 11th and 12th thoracic dermatomes. One week later the rash became generalized and she died 3 weeks after the onset of the localized rash. The V-Z complement fixation titer, 3 days prior to death was 1:16.

All three patients were treated with various cytotoxic agents and prednisone. Two patients (Cases 2 and 3) received irradiation.

In addition to the routine light microscopy, selected areas of the brain in Cases 1 and 2, lung in Case 2, and spinal ganglia in Case 3 were examined by the electron microscope (EM).

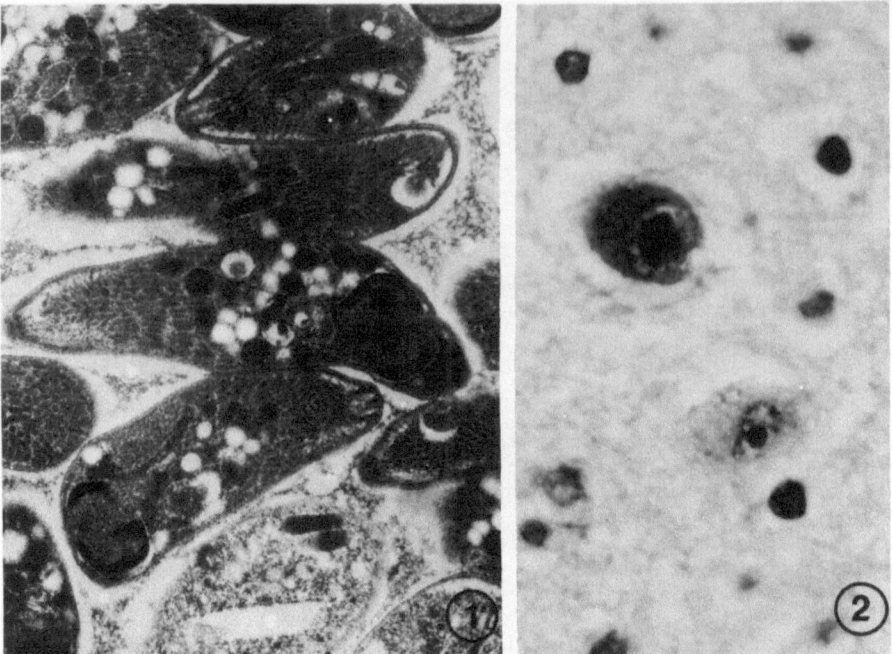

Fig. 1. Electron micrograph of toxoplasma in cyst sectioned at various planes
(x 18,000)

Fig. 2. Cytomegalic inclusions in two neurons surrounded by apparently normal
neuropil. Hematoxylin and eosin (x 500)

RESULTS

Case 1. The brain appeared normal on macroscopic examination with the exception
of an ill-defined grayish area in the right globus pallidus. Microscopically,
this area revealed a necrotizing subacute inflammatory lesion containing both
encysted and free toxoplasma organisms. In addition, scattered glial nodules
were present in otherwise normally appearing areas. Electron microscopic study
not only defined the characteristic morphology of toxoplasma (Fig. 1) in the
lesions, but revealed isolated organisms in the glial nodules which were not
appreciated at the time of initial examination. Furthermore, various stages of
multiplication and encystment of the organisms in the human brain in this study
were found similar to those observed experimentally (1). Toxoplasma infection
in this case was limited to the brain.

Case 2: The brain appeared normal on gross examination. Random sections from
various parts showed scattered aggregates of microglia and astrocytes resulting
in the formation of glial nodules mostly in the cortex. Only on rare occasions,
neurons were seen containing slightly basophilic type A intranuclear inclusions
(Fig. 2). Such neurons were considerably larger than normal and occasionally
contained coarse cytoplasmic granules in addition to the Nissl substance. Most
of the inclusion-bearing neurons were unrelated to the glial nodules and
occurred in apparently normal neuropil. There was no inflammatory cellular
reaction. Inclusion-bearing large cells were also seen in the lungs in abun-

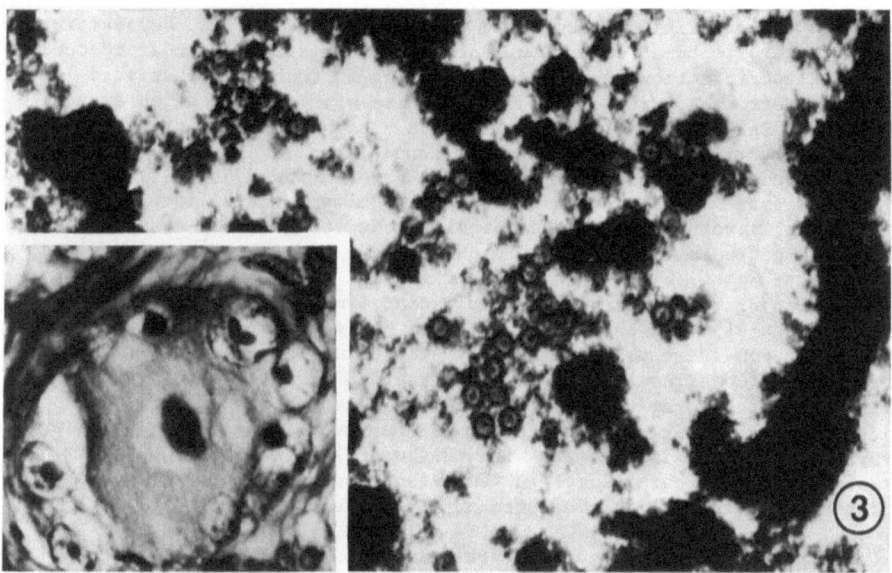

Fig. 3. Electron micrograph showing herpesvirus in a satellite cell nucleus
in spinal ganglion (x 30,000); inset shows light microscopic appearance of
a neuron with its satellite cells containing intranuclear inclusions (x 500)

dance and to a variable extent in the kidneys, adrenals and adenohypophysis.
Although attempted demonstration of virus particles in the relatively rare
inclusion-bearing neurons was unsuccessful, clusters of herpesvirus virions
(HV) were seen in the nucleus and cytoplasm of similar cells in the pulmonary
alveolar linings.

Case 3: The changes in the nervous system were essentially confined to the
left 11th and 12th thoracic ganglia and the related nerve fibers. In addition
to hemorrhagic necrosis, the remaining neurons and satellite cells contained
eosinophilic intranuclear inclusions (Fig. 3). Rarely, a neuron appeared to
contain more than one nuclei and more interestingly, an occasional neuron
appeared to be in mitosis. The skin lesions were typical of herpetic vesicles
and showed nuclear inclusions and multinucleation of the epidermal cells.
Occasional inclusions were also seen in the pancreas and neurons of myenteric
plexus. EM study of the affected spinal ganglia and skin showed HV (Fig. 3).
Isolation of V-Z virus from skin lesions and lungs was successful at autopsy.

DISCUSSION

A similar spectrum of unusual infection of the nervous system in patients with
malignant lymphoma and following organ transplantation strongly suggests an
immunologic impairment as the major predisposing factor (2-6). Toxoplasma, CMV
and V-Z viruses appear to be of particular interest in this regard since
severe infections by these organisms in such patients are now considered to
be the result of activation of a latent infection (4, 7-10). This would indicate the obvious difficulty in the prevention of such infections in susceptible
individuals.
     Toxoplasma is currently recognized as an intestinal coccidian parasite in
cats with wide distribution in a variety of animals (11). Interestingly, toxo-

plasma bears certain striking resemblance to CMV, a member of the herpesvirus family, with regard to human infection. Both organisms are well known to cause severe generalized infection in neonates resulting in such characteristic lesions as chorioretinitis, periventricular necrosis with calcification among others (10, 12). Epidemiologic studies indicate a high incidence of subclinical infection by both organisms in normal adult population (7, 10). In immunologically impaired patients, the infection is usually severe, frequently affecting the central nervous system (CNS) (4-6, 12-16) and resemble neonatal infection in some respects. Indeed, several instances of simultaneous infection by toxoplasma and CMV in such patients as well as in neonates have been described (13, 17 - 19).

The association of V-Z infection with malignant lymphoma is now well established (3, 20-21). Not only the incidence, but severity of the infection under this condition seems to be remarkably altered as indicated by frequent dissemination with occasional involvement of the CNS (22). Although V-Z virus has long been considered as the etiologic agent of herpes zoster (HZ), its identification in the affected sensory ganglia has been achieved very recently and suprisingly, only in patients with malignant lymphoma (23 - 25). The presence of unusual nuclear changes in the affected neurons as described here might further suggest a possible altered pathologic expression of HZ in abnormal hosts.

An increasing number of viruses are currently known to affect the CNS in immunologically impaired patients. Recognition of such cases is mostly based on autopsy studies (26 - 28). In clinically unsuspected patients, a positive identification of the infectious agent in the CNS lesions is often difficult at autopsy. Therefore, only an increased awareness of pathologists and clinicians alike might shed some light regarding the true incidence of such potentially serious intercurrent infection.

Acknowledgement: The author gratefully acknowledges the help and suggestions of H.M. ZIMMERMAN, M.D.

REFERENCES

1. GHATAK, N.R., ZIMMERMAN, H.M.: Fine structure of Toxoplasma in the human brain. Arch. Path. *95*, 276 - 283 (1973)
2. CASAZZA, A.R., DUVALL, C.P., CARBONE, P.P.: Infection in lymphoma. J. Am. Med. Assoc. *197*, 710 - 716 (1966)
3. HARRIS, J.E., SINKOVICS, J.G.: The Immunology of Malignant Disease. St. Louis: C.V. Mosby Co. 1970
4. GHATAK, N.R., POON, T.P., ZIMMERMAN, H.M.: Toxoplasmosis of the central nervous system in the adult. Arch. Path. *89*, 337 - 348 (1970)
5. SCHNECK, S.A.: Neuropathological features of human organ transplantation: 1. Probable cytomegalovirus infection. J. Neuropath. Exp. Neurol. *24*, 415 - 429 (1965)
6. SCHOBER, R., HERMAN, M.M.: Neuropathology of cardiac transplantation. Survey of 31 cases. Lancet *1*, 962 - 967 (1973)
7. FELDMAN, H.A.: Toxoplasmosis. New Engl. J. Med. *279*, 1370 - 1375, 1431 - 1437 (1968)
8. COHEN, S.N.: Toxoplasmosis in patients receiving immunosuppressive therapy. J. Amer. Med. Assoc. *211*, 657 - 660 (1970)
9. BLANK, H., EAGLSTEIN, W.H., GOLDFADEN, G.L.: Zoster, a recrudescence of VZ virus infection. Postgrad. Med. *46*, 653 - 658 (1970)
10. WELLER, T.H.: The cytomegaloviruses: Ubiquitous agents with protean clinical manifestations. New Engl. J. Med. *285*, 203 - 214 (1971)

11. HUTCHISON, W.M., DUNACHIE, J.F.: The life cycle of the coccidian parasite, Toxoplasma gondii, in domestic cat. Trans. R. Soc. Trop. Med. Hyg. *65*, 380 - 399 (1971)
12. FRENKEL, J.K.: Toxoplasmosis. *In:* MINCKLER, J. (ed.): Pathology of the Nervous System. Vol. 3, 2521 - 2538. New York: McGraw-Hill Book Co. 1972
13. VIETZKE, W.M., GELDERMAN, A.H., GRIMLEY, P.M., VALSAMIS, M.P.: Toxoplasmosis complicating malignancy: Experience at the National Cancer Institute. Cancer *21*, 816 - 827 (1968)
14. REMINGTON, J.S.: Toxoplasmosis in the adult. Bull. N. Y. Acad. Med. *50*, 211 - 227 (1974)
15. TOWNSEND, J.J., WOLINSKY, J.S., BARINGER, R., JOHNSON, P.: Toxoplasmosis: A neglected cause of treatable nervous system disease. Neurology (Minn.) *24*, 381 (1974)
16. DORFMAN, L.J.: Cytomegalovirus encephalitis in adults. Neurology (Minn.) *23*, 136 - 144 (1973)
17. GELDERMAN, A.H., GRIMLEY, P.M., LUNDE, M.N., RABSON, A.S.: Toxoplasma gondii and cytomegalovirus: Mixed infection by a parasite and a virus. Science *160*, 1130 - 1132 (1968)
18. LUNA, M.L., LICHTIGER, B.: Disseminated Toxoplasmosis and cytomegalovirus infection complicating Hodgkin's disease. Amer. J. Clin. Path. *55*, 499 - 505 (1971)
19. DEMIAN, S.D.E., DONNELLY, W.H., Jr., MONIF, G.R.G.: Coexistent congenital cytomegalovirus and toxoplasmosis in a stillborn. Amer. J. Dis. Child. *125*, 420 - 421 (1973)
20. WILSON, J.R., MARSA, G.W., JOHNSON, R.E.: Herpes zoster in Hodgkin's disease: Clinical, histologic and immunologic correlations. Cancer *29*, 461 - 465 (1972)
21. FELDMAN, S., HUGHES, W.T., KIM, H.Y.: Herpes zoster in children with cancer. Amer. J. Dis. Child. *216*, 178 - 184 (1973)
22. McCORMICK, W.F., RODNITZKY, R.L., SCHOCHET, S.S., McKEE, A.P.: Varicella-zoster encephalomyelitis: A morphologic and virologic study. Arch. Neurol. *21*, 559 - 570 (1969)
23. ESIRI, M.M., TOMLINSON, A.H.: Herpes zoster: Demonstration of virus in trigeminal nerve and ganglion by immunofluorescence and electron microscopy. J. Neurol. Sci. *15*, 35 - 48 (1972)
24. GHATAK, N.R., ZIMMERMAN, H.M.: Spinal ganglion in Herpes zoster. Arch. Path. *95*, 411 - 415 (1973)
25. BASTIAN, F.O., RABSON, A.S., YEE, C.L., TRALKA, T.S.: Herpesvirus varicellae. Isolated from human dorsal root ganglia. Arch. Path. *97*, 331 - 333 (1974)
26. CHOU, S.M., ROOS, R., BURRELL, R., GUTMANN, L.: Subacute focal adenovirus encephalitis. J. Neuropath. Exp. Neurol. *32*, 34 - 50 (1973)
27. BREITFELD, V., HASHIDA, Y., SHERMAN, F.E., ODAGIRI, K., YUNIS, E.J.: Fatal measles infection in children with leukemia. Lab. Invest. *28*, 279 - 291 (1973)
28. WEINER, L.P., NARAYAN, O., PENNY, J.B., HERNDON, R.M., FERINGA, E.R., TOURTELLOTTE, W.W., JOHNSON, R.T.: Papovavirus of JC type in progressive multifocal leukoencephalopathy. Arch. Neurol. *29*, 1 - 3 (1973)

NITYA R. GHATAK, M.D.
Department of Pathology
Bowman Gray School of Medicine
Winston-Salem, North Carolina 27103, U.S.A.

Acta Neuropath. (Berlin), Suppl. VI, 267 - 272 (1975)

SSPE-Like Inclusion Body Disorder in Treated Childhood Leukemia

E. SLUGA, H. BUDKA, K. JELLINGER and E. PICHLER

Neurological Institute and Pediatric Clinic
University of Vienna, Austria

Summary: Clinico-pathological report on a boy with cytostatically treated
leukemia, dying with cerebral symptoms after passing clinical measles 10
weeks before death. At autopsy, numerous nuclear inclusion bodies in glial
and nerve cells were found. By electron microscopy, nuclear inclusions
appeared as loosely arranged smooth tubules, corresponding to paramyxovirus
nucleocapsids. Frequently, cytoplasmic changes appeared too, consisting of
incomplete tubular structures and an abundant dense "fuzzy" material. No
regular tubuli of the coated granular type were present, as in common measles
virus infection, nor any mature viral structures or differentiation of the
surface membrane. The lack of maturation in cytoplasm together with a predominance of nuclear changes suggested a slow type of measles virus infection,
while the particular cytoplasmic changes suggested a defect in synthesis of
granular nucleocapsids, possibly a basic factor for the slow type of the
viral infection. Possible pathogenetic factors are discussed.

Key words: SSPE - Slow Virus Infection - Measles Virus Encephalitis - Leukemia -
Cytostatic Drugs

INTRODUCTION

The occurrence of unusual viral infections in the course of lymphoproliferative
diseases is known, e.g. progressive multifocal leukoencephalopathy in CNS. Subacute sclerosing panencephalitis (SSPE), now considered as a slow measles virus
infection, has been recently observed as a secondary disease in leukemia. In
1973, BREITFELD *et al.* (1) first described SSPE-like syndromes in two infantile
cases of leukemia. Our report is concerned with a similar observation.

CASE REPORT

Acute lymphoblastic leukemia was diagnosed in a boy of 2 years and 2 months.
Initial remission was induced by treatment with prednisone, vincristine and
1-asparaginase; the ensuing complete hematological remission was sustained
till death by administration of 6-mercapto-purine, methotrexate and cyclophosphamide. Intermittent re-induction therapy was done in intervals of 10
weeks with prednisone, vincristine, occasional adriamycine and intrathecal
methotrexate. Gammatron irradiation of the skull (2416 r) was performed once
(1 year before death).
  10 weeks before death, measles virus infection, running an inconspicuous
course, was diagnosed clinically.
  15 days before death, there was a sudden onset of neurological symptoms with
hemiparesis, focal epileptic seizures and progressive somnolence; focal leukemic

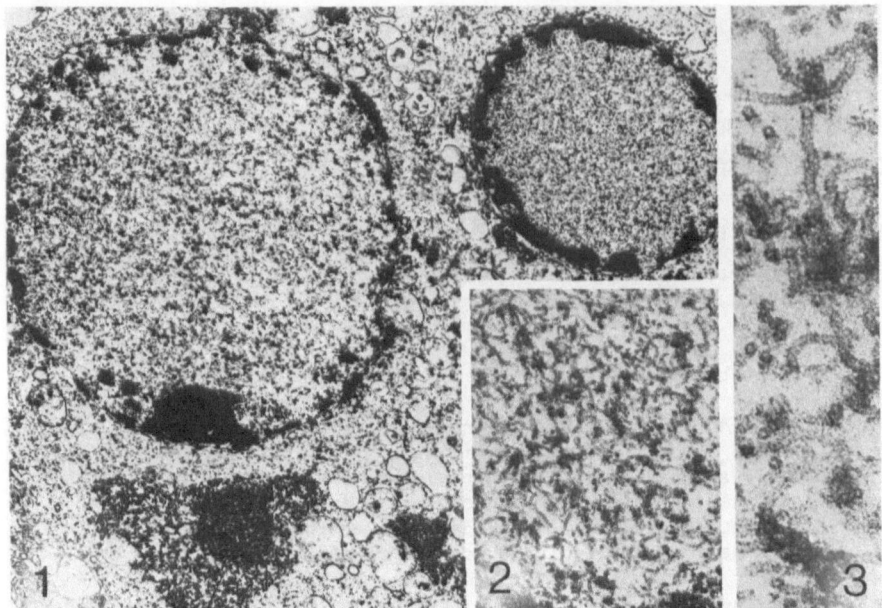

Figs. 1-3. Nuclear inclusions. Fig. 1. Randomly arranged fine tubular structures
in the nuclei of two glial cells; a large and a small cluster of electron-dense
material in the cytoplasm. x 6000. Fig. 2. Higher magnification: The tubular
character of the included structures becomes visible. x 24900. Fig. 3. High
magnification: The fine cross striation becomes visible and the diameter measur-
able. x 87000

infiltration of the brain was clinically suspected, and focal cobalt irradiation (900 r) to the right cerebrum was tried. No serological nor virologi-
cal investigations were performed. Generalised epileptic seizures, electrolyte
disturbances and hyperpyrexia preceded death at the age of 3 years and 3 months.
    At *autopsy*, complete remission from leukemia was confirmed; multifocal inter-
stitial pneumonia with occasional multinucleated giant cells, lacking any inclusion bodies, was present in both lungs. In the brain, there were multifocal
spongy tissue changes with gliosis and nerve cell degeneration, but without
any significant perivascular inflammatory response. However, the most impressive findings were numerous eosino- and pyroninophilic intranuclear inclusions
(type Cowdry A) in many glial cells and some neurones; giant cells (without
inclusions) were very rare.
    The impressive nuclear inclusions and the associated cellular changes were
subjected to a detailed *electron microscopic (EM) study*. Autopsy material
had to be used and was taken from the predominantly affected left frontal
region. Many cells, especially glial ones, were affected and contained nuclear
inclusions (Figs. 1 - 3). These consisted of clearly defined tubular structures
with a diameter of 160 Å and a fine cross striation of approximately 60 Å
periodicity (Figs. 2, 3) - structures identical to the well-described nucleocapsids of paramyxoviruses, especially of measles strains. The nuclear tubuli
had sharp limits and no coating material around (Fig. 3), representing the
"smooth" tubular type. The arrangement of the tubules in the nuclei was most
frequently at random (Figs. 1, 2), but sometimes a paracrystalline array was
present. In most of these cells with intranuclear viral structures, cytoplasmic

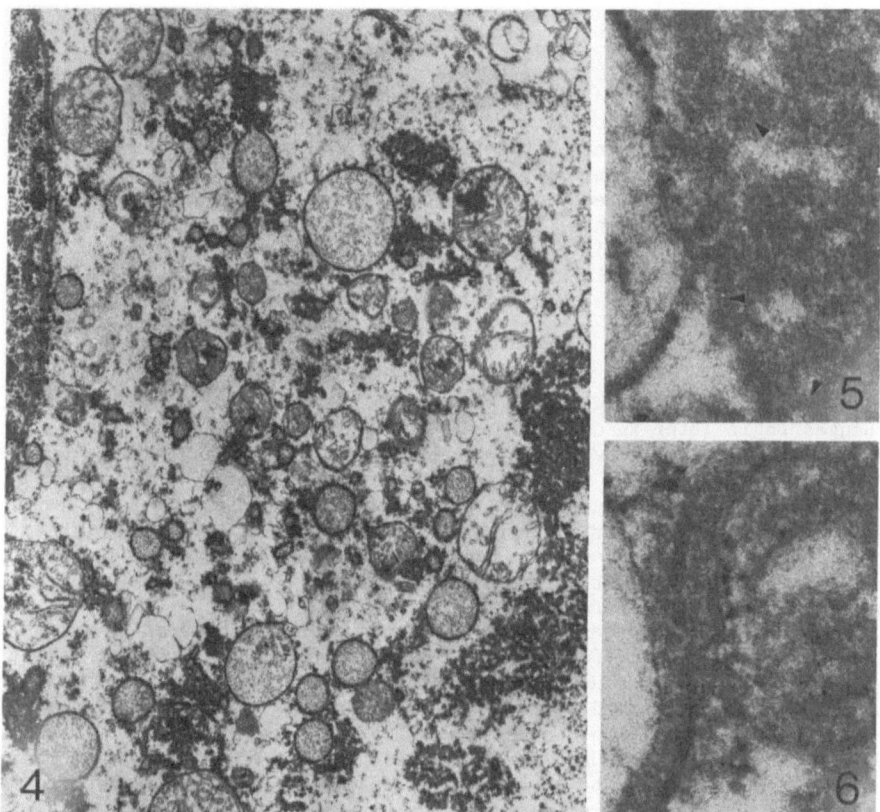

Figs. 4-6. Cytoplasmic inclusions. Fig. 4. Highly activated cytoplasm with
ribosome-occupied endoplasmic reticulum (ER) and many clusters of an electron-
dense "fuzzy" material. x 15000. Fig. 5. Intimate contact of the dense "fuzzy"
material with membranes of the ER; the dense material remains nearly unresolv-
able, only borderlines of tubular structures appear (arrowheads). x 87000.
Fig. 6. Long unusual tubular structures with cross striation and central filamentous structure in intimate contact with the membranes of the ER. x 87000

changes appeared too (Figs. 1, 4), but they were much more difficult to eluci-
date. The cytoplasm was highly activated, exhibiting a strongly ribosome-
occupied endoplasmic reticulum (ER) (Fig. 4) and clusters of an unusual electron-
dense "fuzzy" material (Figs. 1, 4, 5). This material often had intimate contact with the activated ER (Fig. 5) and was not readily resolvable. Its strongly electron-dense matrix appeared homogenous rather than finely granular; in
some areas, borderlines of short tubular structures seemed to appear, but only
indistinctly (Fig. 5). This suggested that in the cytoplasm, besides an abundant
production of "fuzzy" material, formation of tubular structures took place, but
only in an incomplete, unusual manner. This suggestion was supported by frequently found long, distinct tubules in close contact with membranes of the ER
(Fig. 6); they had a fine cross striation and sometimes a central filamentous
structure. No alignment of tubules beneath the outer cell membrane nor budding
of mature paramyxovirus particles could be seen.

DISCUSSION

CNS changes of our case, most impressive in EM, gave evidence of viral structures identifiable as replicated paramyxovirus nucleocapsids, suggesting a measles virus infection in retrospect of clinical measles 10 weeks before death. The pattern of changes in the virus-attacked cells was quite unusual for a common measles virus encephalitis.

Measles virus infections, especially in the CNS, have already been investigated in human (2) and experimental (3, 4) encephalitis, also in virus-infected tissue cultures (5, 6, 7, 8); therefore, structures of viral replication as well as changes in the host cells are well elucidated for the common strains; tubular nucleocapsids are produced early and predominantly in the cytoplasm, with alignment beneath the cell membrane, and show maturation by membrane envelopping; mature virions are finally released by budding. Nucleocapsids in the cytoplasm are "granular" (8, 9), coated by a non-structured electron-dense "fuzzy" material, also present at the cell membrane in areas of budding. Nuclear changes begin later in common measles virus infection and are much less prominent (6, 7, 8, 9). The tubular-structured nucleocapsids in the nucleus are everywhere without coating, representing the type of "smooth" tubules. It is therefore evident that replication of measles virus occurs with formation of two distinct types of tubular nucleocapsids. The longer an infection lasted, the more prominent nuclear inclusions became, while the cytoplasmic replication went on constantly unchanged. The prevalence of nuclear changes is then considered as a sign of chronic infection (9).

In our case, the striking prominence of nuclear nucleocapsids combined with unusual cytoplasmic changes differs markedly from the typical pattern of common measles virus infection. The abundance of nuclear inclusions, associated with absence of mature structures and surface-cell-membrane differentiation, is much more like the pattern of a chronic or slow measles virus infection. Such a slow measles virus infection of the CNS is represented by human SSPE. Here a multitude of nuclear inclusions is the most prominent and most often described feature (see 10, 11); data which are in good accordance with our observation. The cytoplasmic changes appear less prominent in SSPE; their ultrastructural analysis has been limited to few papers, and the delineated structural data are not uniform. Some of the authors stressed ill-defined tubular structures in an amorphous cytoplasmic material (12, 13), while others described clearly defined tubules especially in axonal cytoplasm (11, 14). In SSPE, there is uniform description and general agreement about the absence of mature viral structures, about lack of cell membrane differentiation and lack of membrane relationship of cytoplasmic inclusions; this again is in accord with our observations on the cytoplasmic changes.

Without doubt, the pattern of our findings is in good agreement with a slow virus infection; it is even identical with SSPE, if we except the abnormal, rich cytoplasmic material and its indistinct structures, the special changes of our case. This material seems to correspond to the "fuzzy" coating material of cytoplasmic measles virus nucleocapsids; its abundant production suggests in our case a disturbance in the proportion of coating material to proper tubular structures, resulting in a malformation of the cytoplasmic viral elements, while intranuclear "smooth" viral structures remain unchanged. The lack of further maturation in cytoplasm, the characteristic sign of slow measles virus processes like SSPE, seems to be a necessary consequence.

The abnormal behaviour of measles virus replication in SSPE has been subject of many investigations. In tissue cultures infected with SSPE-measles virus isolated by cocultivation (8, 10), replication occurred in a manner similar to the pattern of SSPE and to those changes in our case comparable with it. But while the signs of maturation were lacking obligatorily, coated nucleocapsids were produced in quantity in the cytoplasm. Recently, more searching investigations were done with productive and latent SSPE-virus infected cell cultures (15); with the latent strains, not only the hitherto well-known absence of virion maturation and surface-membrane differentiation was found, but also a lack of coating of cytoplasmic nucleocapsids; only "smooth" tubules appeared, and they gave no labelling with immunoperoxydase, a feature which means that they are not antigenic for the host; a defect in synthesis or in interaction of one of the virus proteins with the nucleocapsids was suggested; the protein involved in latent conditions might represent the "fuzzy" coating material of the cytoplasmic tubules.

Such an alteration in production or interaction of the amorphous coating material with tubular structures of the "granular" nucleocapsid type is also very likely to be the basic defect of the special changes in our observation, leading finally to a slow type of the measles virus infection.

Factors causing such an altered virus protein reproduction are still looked for, as well as the conditions for a slow type of infection. In human SSPE, on the one hand abnormal immunological host response is considered, especially impairment of the T-cell-system (16; extensively reviewed by 17); on the other hand, virus changes like short subgenomic RNA (18), changed ratio of low to high weight RNA (19), and changes in the nucleotide sequence (20) have been reported. In our case, there are some possibilities of starting factors for the slow type of infection or the altered viral nucleocapsid synthesis in cytoplasm: first, leukemia itself might alter the immunological state; and second, the administered cytotoxical drugs might impair host immune response (as experimentally proved with cyclophosphamide - 21) or interfere with RNA, DNA or protein metabolism (22). Although in our case definite potentially causative factors are present, exact evaluation of their significance remains obscure.

It seemed important to demonstrate the observation that in children with leukemia and/or cytostatic treatment, simple measles virus infection may lead to the fatal process of a CNS slow virus disease. And the described disturbance of cytoplasmic nucleocapsid formation, as an interesting and possible mechanism for the slow type of viral infection, should be stressed.

REFERENCES

1. BREITFELD, V., HASHIDA, Y., SHERMAN, F.E., ODAGIRI, K., YUNIS, E.J.: Fatal measles infection in children with leukemia. Lab. Invest. 28, 279 - 291 (1973)
2. ADAMS, J.M., BAIRD, C., FILLOY, L.: Inclusion bodies in measles encephalitis. JAMA 195, 290 - 298 (1966)
3. WEAR, D.J., RABIN, E.R., RICHARDSON, L.S., RAPP, F.: Virus replication and ultrastructural changes after induction of encephalitis in mice by measles virus. Exp. Mol. Path. 9, 405 - 417 (1968)
4. BARINGER, J.R., GRIFFITH, J.F.: Experimental measles virus encephalitis. A light, phase, fluorescence, and electron microscopic study. Lab. Invest. 23, 335 - 346 (1970)
5. MANNWEILER, K.: Ultrastructural examination of tissue cultures after infection with measles virus. Arch. ges. Virusforsch. 16, 89 - 96 (1965)
6. NAKAI, M., IMAGAWA, D.T.: Electron microscopy of measles virus replication. J. Virol. 3, 187 - 197 (1969)
7. RAINE, C.S., FELDMAN, L.A., SHEPPARD, R.D., BORNSTEIN, M.B.: Ultrastructure of measles virus in cultures of hamster cerebellum. J. Virol. 4, 169 - 181 (1969)
8. OYANAGI, S., MEULEN, V. ter, KATZ, M., KOPROWSKI, H.: Comparison of subacute sclerosing panencephalitis and measles viruses: an electron microscope study. J. Virol. 7, 176 - 187 (1971)

9. RAINE, C.S., FELDMAN, L.A., SHEPPARD, R.D., BORNSTEIN, M.B.: Ultrastructural study of long-term measles infection in cultures of hamster dorsal-
   root ganglion. J. Virol. *8*, 318 - 329 (1971)
10. MEULEN, V. ter, KATZ, M., MÜLLER, D.: Subacute sclerosing panencephalitis:
    a review. Curr. Top. Microbiol. Immunol. (Berl.) *57*, 1 - 38 (1972)
11. MARTINEZ, A.J., OHYA, T., JABBOUR, J.T., DUENAS, D.: Subacute sclerosing
    panencephalitis (SSPE). Reappraisal of nuclear, cytoplasmic and axonal
    inclusions. Ultrastructural study of eight cases. Acta neuropath. (Berl.)
    28, 1 - 13 (1974)
12. TELLEZ-NAGEL, I., HARTER, D.H.: Subacute sclerosing leukoencephalitis:
    Ultrastructure of intranuclear and intracytoplasmic inclusions. Science
    154, 899 - 901 (1966)
13. HERNDON, R.M., RUBINSTEIN, L.J.: Light and electron microscopy observations
    on the development of viral particles in the inclusions of Dawson's ence-
    phalitis (subacute sclerosing panencephalitis). Neurology (Minn.) *18*,
    Part 2, 8 - 18 (1968)
14. TOGA, M., DUBOIS, D., BERARD, M., TRIPIER, M.F., CESARINI, J.P., CHOUX, R.:
    Étude ultrastructurale de quatre cas de leuco-encéphalite sclérosante
    subaiguë. Acta neuropath. (Berl.) *14*, 1 - 13 (1969)
15. DUBOIS-DALCQ, M., BARBOSA, L.H., HAMILTON, R., SEVER, J.L.: Comparison bet-
    ween productive and latent subacute sclerosing panencephalitis viral in-
    fection in vitro. Lab. Invest. *30*, 241 - 250 (1974)
16. BURNET, F.M.: Measles as an index of immunological function. Lancet *1968*
    II, 610 - 613
17. DU PASQUIER, P., VITAL, CL., HENRY, P., LOISEAU, P., LATINVILLE, D.,
    PATY, J.: Étude d'un cas de panencéphalite sclérosante subaiguë. Recherches
    virologiques et immunologiques. Rev. neurol. (Paris) *128*, 401 - 418 (1973)
18. KILEY, M.P., GRAY, R.H., PAYNE, F.E.: Replication of measles virus:
    distinct species of short nucleocapsids in cytoplasmic extracts of in-
    fected cells. J. Virol. *13*, 721 - 728 (1974)
19. WINSTON, S.H., RUSTIGIAN, R., BRATT, M.S.: Persistent infection of cells
    in culture of measles virus. III. Comparison of virus specific RNA syn-
    thesized in primary and persistent infection in HeLa-cells. J. Virol.
    11, 926 - 932 (1973)
20. YEH, J.: Characterization of virus-specific RNAs from subacute sclerosing
    panencephalitis virus-infected CV-1 cells. J. Virol. *12*, 962 - 968 (1973)
21. WEAR, D.J., RAPP, F.: Latent measles virus infection of the hamster central
    nervous system. J. Immunol. *107*, 1593 - 1598 (1971)
22. PÜTTER, J.: Über die biochemische Wirkung von Cytostatica auf Tumorzellen.
    In: Therapie maligner Tumoren, Bd. 1: Pathologie und Chemotherapie.
    Meythaler, F. (ed.). Stuttgart: F. Enke 1966

Dr. ELFRIEDE SLUGA
Neurologisches Institut der
Universität Wien
Schwarzspanierstr. 17
A - 1090 Wien, Austria

Acta Neuropath. (Berlin), Suppl. VI, 273 - 278 (1975)
© by Springer-Verlag 1975

The Ultrastructure of Normal and Reactive Microglia

W.F. BLAKEMORE

Wellcome Laboratory for Comparative Neurology,
School of Veterinary Medicine
Madingley Road, Cambridge

Summary: Normal microglia have a distinct morphology. In rapidly, but not
in slowly evolving pathological states the features used to identify the
resting cell are often lost. When there is invasion by haematogenous monocytes, phagocytes develop whose origin - cerebral or haematogenous - cannot
be ascertained on morphological features alone. These observations stress
that microglia are part of the reticulo-endothelial system.

Key words: Glia - microglia - ultrastructure - reticulo-endothelial system

INTRODUCTION

Microglial cells are components of the reticulo-endothelium system (RE), as
such they have a communal as well as an individual identity. Some of the confusion concerning their ultrastructural identification has arisen because their
close relationship to extraneural cells has been ignored (1, 2, 3). In the past
microglia have been confused with oligodendrocytes (4) and dark shrunken neurones (5). In addition cells with similar ultrastructural appearance and
showing behaviour in pathological situations typical of classical microglia
have been termed 'third neuroglial type' (6), M cells (7), phagocytic oligodendrocytes (8), and microglia (9). As the term microglia has established roots
in neuropathology it is preferable that this term be retained and the ultrastructural appearance of this cell type defined. In order to attain this goal
a number of different approaches have been followed; MORI and LEBLOND (10)
made ultrastructural observations on specific metallic impregnations, BLAKEMORE
obviated confusion between oligodendrocytes and microglia by examining areas
where oligodendrocytes are absent such as the periependymal zones (11) and
the retina (unpublished observations), others have examined pathological
situations (9), or looked for cells in normal brain which resemble other components of the RE system. All these workers have identified a morphologically
similar cell and equated it with the classical microglia cell of RIO-HORTEGA
(12).

MATERIAL

Brain and spinal cord, both normal and pathological, has been examined from the
following species: rat, mouse, rabbit, cat, dog, horse, pig, sheep and ox,
liver of rats and mice and peripheral blood of rats. Inflammatory lesions from
other sites have also been examined.

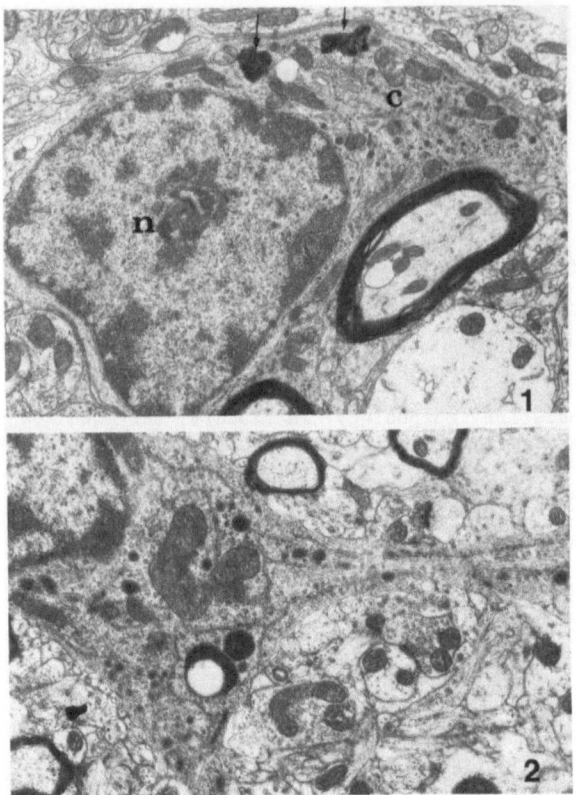

Fig. 1. Microglial cell in normal rat cerebellum. n = nucleolus, c = centriole surrounded by primary lysosomes, arrow = secondary lysosomes. x 11,500

Fig. 2. Microglial cell in normal mouse cerebral cortex. Endoplasmic reticulum and microtubules extend into the processes. x 13,500

RESULTS

Normal.

A cell with the following features can be separated from the other glia in normal animals. It has a small irregularly shaped nucleus with coarsely clumped chromatin and a small nucleolus (Fig. 1). The cytoplasm is of medium electron density and contains long single strands of endoplasmic reticulum (Fig. 1, 2), the lumen of which contains material of similar density to the surrounding cytoplasm (Fig. 3) and on which are attached short chains of ribosomes. Poly-ribosomes occur in small numbers throughout the cytoplasm. A centriole may sometimes be detected but all cells contain numbers of primary lysosomes and variable numbers of secondary lysosomes (Fig. 1, 2). Processes extend from the perinuclear cytoplasm, these contain microtubules and endoplasmic reticulum and often have an irregular outline which contrasts with the smooth regular contoured processes of oligodendrocytes (Fig. 2). Cells with these features have been found at different sites in the CNS of all the species so far examined. This cell type is equated with the classical microglial cell. Any variations in morphology which are present can be related either to the presence or absence of processes, age, activity of the cell, or sub-optimal fixation.

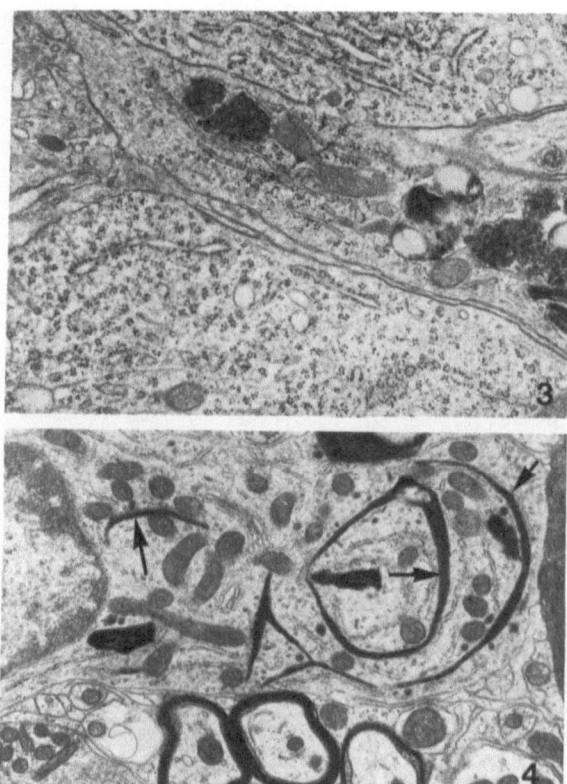

Fig. 3. A process of a microglial cell interposed between the cytoplasm of two oligodendrocytes. The lumen of the endoplasmic reticulum in the microglial cell contains material of similar density to the surrounding cytoplasm whereas that in the oligodendrocytes is electron lucent. x 25,000

Fig. 4. Microglial cell from the cerebellum of a rat which had a long term porto-caval anastomosis. The appearance of the cell is very similar to those found in normal brain, but the cytoplasm contains several 'lyre' shaped bodies (arrow), a form of inclusion commonly found in microglial cells in areas of chronic degeneration. x 15,300

Pathological states.

In slowly evolving conditions where there is no massive influx of haematogenous cells, microglia retain many of the features used to identify them in the normal tissue. They may increase in number and the area of perinuclear cytoplasm and the number and complexity of secondary lysosomes may be greater (Fig. 4), but the rapid and marked alterations in cell morphology seen in cerebral oedema and primary demyelination (13, 14) do not occur, so identification presents few problems. Whereas, in rapidly evolving situations identification of cells becomes difficult, not only do cerebral cells lose their resting morphology, as a result of reactive changes, but other cells invade the area and undergo reactive changes which obscure their identity as well.

In oedematous areas surrounding necrotic lesions microglia lose many of their resting features as a result of rapid increase in size and activity; these changes have been described in detail elsewhere (13). Monocytes which enter such lesions have many morphological features in common with microglial cells

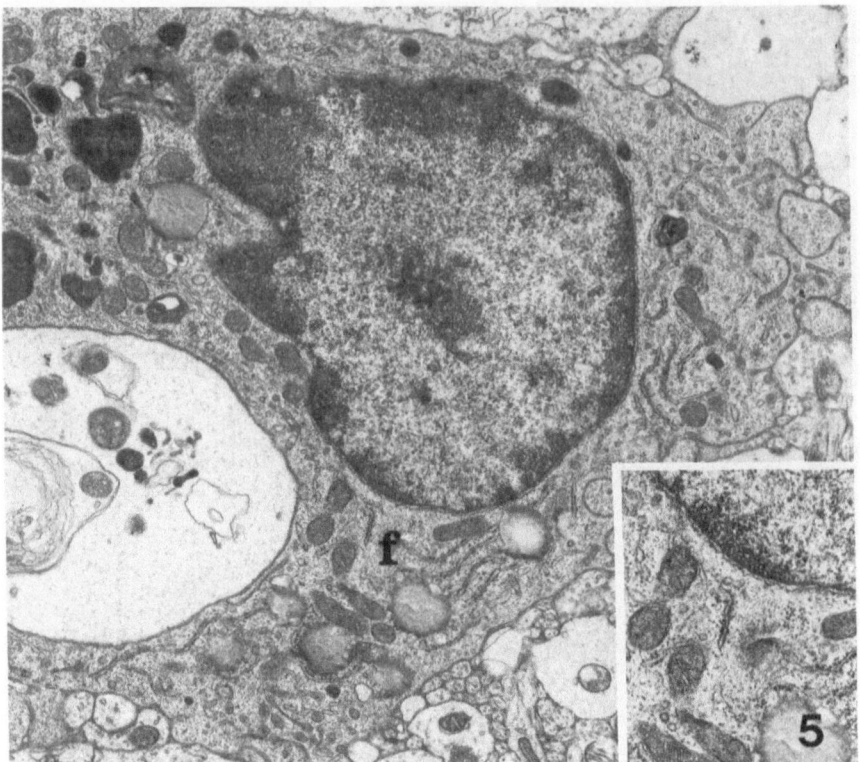

Fig. 5. A phagocytic cell in oedematous area of 3 days duration. Although many of its features are similar to those of the microglial cell, i.e. appearance of the nucleus and endoplasmic reticulum, the presence of primary and secondary lysosomes, the periphery of the cell is ruffled and a few indistinct fibrils (F) are present. These structures are found in monocytes but not microglial cells. x 12,000, inset x 20, 000

but contain bundles of 7 nm fibrils and no microtubules. Following their entry the fibrils are lost and a population of phagocytic cells develop which possess neither fibrils or microtubules. In the late stages of the reaction (7 days onwards) all the cells showing evidence of past phagocytic activity resemble microglia as they contain microtubules rather than the fibrils found in monocytes and their derivative phagocytes elsewhere in the body.

In situations where there is little or no entry of monocytes, such as tract degeneration (15), the transformation of microglia into phagocytes is accompanied by loss of microtubules, decrease in cytoplasmic density and ruffling of the cell surface in the early stages. In the later stages apart from containing large numbers of secondary lysosomes and fat droplets the phagocytic cells closely resemble resting microglia.

In areas of primary demyelination many cells similar to normal microglia are present. In the later stages they contain large numbers of fat droplets and have features common to resting microglia and microglia seen in slowly evolving or late pathologies. But at the time myelin breakdown commences, when they are closely associated with the degenerating myelin sheath they differ as their cytoplasm contains glycogen granules (Fig. 7). That these are microglia although they contain glycogen granules (structures not present in resting microglia) can be confirmed by the absence of fibrils (a feature of astrocytes) and by a

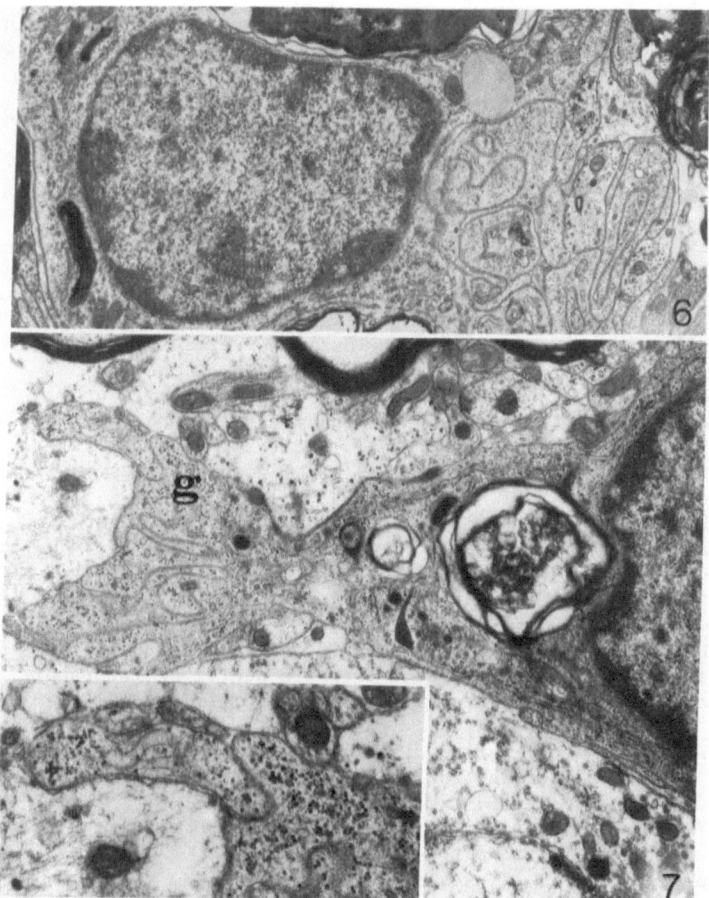

Fig. 6. A phagocytic cell in a degenerating tract in rat spinal cord. The cell surface is ruffled and the cytoplasm contains neither fibrils or microtubules. x 12,000

Fig. 7. A phagocytic cell with many features of a microglial cell in an area of primary demyelination. Glycogen granules (g) are present in the cytoplasm which contains neither fibrils or microtubules. x 11,000, inset x 21,500

process of exclusion similar to that used to identify microglia in the oedematous situation (13).

CONCLUSION

In the resting state microglia have certain unique features which enable them to be differentiated not only from the other types of glial cells in the brain, but also from the circulating elements of the RE system. In slowly evolving pathological states they retain many of their resting features, but in rapidly evolving pathological states they may lose some of them. When there is frank invasion by monocytes, macrophages develop whose origin - cerebral or haematogenous - cannot be determined on morphological criteria alone. This merging of identity of cells of different origin supports the view that microglia are part of the RE system and suggests that any unique morphological features which microglia may possess result from their cerebral sojourn rather than indicating that they are an unrelated cell type.

Acknowledgements: This work was supported by grants from the Wellcome Trust and the National Fund for Research into Crippling Diseases.

REFERENCES

1. ROESSMANN, U., FRIEDE, R.L.: Entry of labelled monocytic cells into the central nervous system. Acta neuropath. (Berl.) *10*, 359 - 362 (1968)
2. ADRIAN, E.K., SMOTHERMAN, R.D.: Leucocytic infiltration into the hypoglossal nucleus following injury to the hypoglossal nerve. Anat. Rec. *166*, 99 - 115 (1970)
3. OEHMICHEN, M., GRÜNINGER, H., SAEBISCH, R., NARITA, Y.: Mikroglia und Pericyten als Transformationsformen des Blut-Monocyten mit erhaltener Proliferationsfähigkeit. Acta neuropath. (Berl.) *23*, 200 - 218 (1973)
4. KRUGER, L., MAXWELL, D.S.: Electron microscopy of oligodendrocytes in normal rat cerebrum. Amer. J. Anat. *118*, 411 - 436 (1966)
5. MUGNAINI, K., WALBERG, F.: Ultrastructure of neuroglia. Ergebn. Anat. Entwickl.-Gesch. *37*, 194 - 236 (1964)
6. VAUGHN, J.E., HINDS, P.L., SKOFF, R.P.: Electron microscopic studies of Wallerian degeneration in rat optic nerves. I. The multipotential glial. J. comp. Neurol. *140*, 175 - 205 (1970)
7. MATHEWS, M.A., KRUGER, L.: Electron microscopy of non-neuronal cellular changes accompanying neural degeneration in thalamic nuclei of the rabbit. II. Reactive elements within the neuropil. J. comp. Neurol. *148*, 313 - 346 (1973)
8. MAXWELL, D.S., KRUGER, L.: The reactive oligodendrocyte. An electron microscopic study of cerebral cortex following alpha particle irradiation. Amer. J. Anat. *118*, 437 - 460 (1966)
9. TORVIK, A., SKJÖRTEN, F.: Electron microscopic observations on nerve cell regeneration and degeneration after axon lesions. II. Changes in glial cells. Acta neuropath. (Berl.) *17*, 265 - 282 (1971)
10. MORI, S., LEBLOND, C.P.: Identification of microglia in light and electron microscopy. J. Comp. Neurol. *135*, 57 - 80 (1969)
11. BLAKEMORE, W.F.: The ultrastructure of the subependymal plate in the rat. J. Anat. (Lond.) *104*, 423 - 433 (1969)
12. RIO-HORTEGA, P. del: Microglia. *In:* Penfield, W. (ed.): Cytology and Cellular Pathology of the Nervous System, vol. 2, p. 481 - 534. New York: Paul B. Hoeber, Inc. 1932
13. BLAKEMORE, W.F.: Microglia reactions following thermal necrosis of the rat cortex: An electron microscopic study. Acta neuropath. (Berl). *21*, 11 - 22 (1972)
14. BLAKEMORE, W.F.: Demyelination of the superior cerebellar peduncle in the mouse induced by cuprizone. J. neurol. Sci. *20*, 63 - 72 (1973)
15. STENWIG, A.E.: The origin of brain macrophages in traumatic lesions, Wallerian degeneration, and retrograde degeneration. J. Neuropath. exp. Neurol. *31*, 696 - 704 (1972)

W.F. BLAKEMORE, M.D.
Department of Veterinary Clinical Studies
University of Cambridge
Madingley Road
Cambridge, CB3 OES
England

Acta Neuropath. (Berlin), Suppl. VI, 279 - 283 (1975)
© by Springer-Verlag 1975

EM Findings on the Source of Reactive Microglia on the Mammalian Brain

H. HAGER

Department of Neuropathology
Justus-Liebig University
Giessen, F.R.G.

Summary: In traumatic brain lesions microglia cells are often plastered on the
outer surface of capillaries. Basement membranes delimit these juxtacapillary
cells from pericytes and endothelial cells. In altered nervous tissue many
stages in the activation of pericytes may be seen at the same time. It is clearly demonstrable that these pericytes attack the basement membrane vigorously
from inside. After penetration of the basement membrane these cells propel
themselves between the perivascular feet processes of astrocytes and squeeze
between the intracellular gaps, becoming surrounded by the cell processes of
the neuropil. The observations suggest that in reactive stages the microglia
cells may, at least in part, originate from the perivascular mesenchymal tissue.

Key words: Neuroglia - Electron microscopy - Reactive Microglia - Brain Injury

Knowledge of the microglia in the mammalian C.N.S. dates from the years 1919 -
1921 when del RIO-HORTEGA studied the histogenesis of microglia, its morphological evolution to form rod cells and phagocytising elements (9). The functional
assimilation of the microglia with the reticuloendothelial system postulated by
HORTEGA has been accepted by many investigators.

Little attention was directed to the source of reactive microglia cells under
pathological conditions. HORTEGA, who has emphasized the migratory activity of
microglia cells, claimed that the reactive elements originate mainly from
resting microglia cells, which are able to invade from the vicinity in the
altered neuropil.

RIO-HORTEGA and PENFIELD (8) observed that after traumatisation of the brain
of kittens, the cerebral cortex which is still almost completely deprived of
microglia is soon filled in the neighbourhood of the wound with cells which
according to the authors, are derived from the white matter. These authors were
not able to observe migration and extravasation of leucocytes under such conditions.

In recent years autoradiographic experiments have indicated that brain macrophages may originate from haematogenous elements (6, 7).

Further studies with labeled blood monocytes (10) suggested an exclusively
endogenous origin of macrophages in Wallerian and retrograde degeneration.

In view of these conflicting observations the source of cells forming reactive
microglia and macrophages in the C.N.S. is still of acute concern.

The electron microscopical studies to be illustrated here were made during the
last 12 years on experimental mammalian brains (1 - 5).

HORTEGA has shown that the microglia cells are sometimes closely adjoining
the walls of the vessels, resting on the outer surface of the adventitia. In

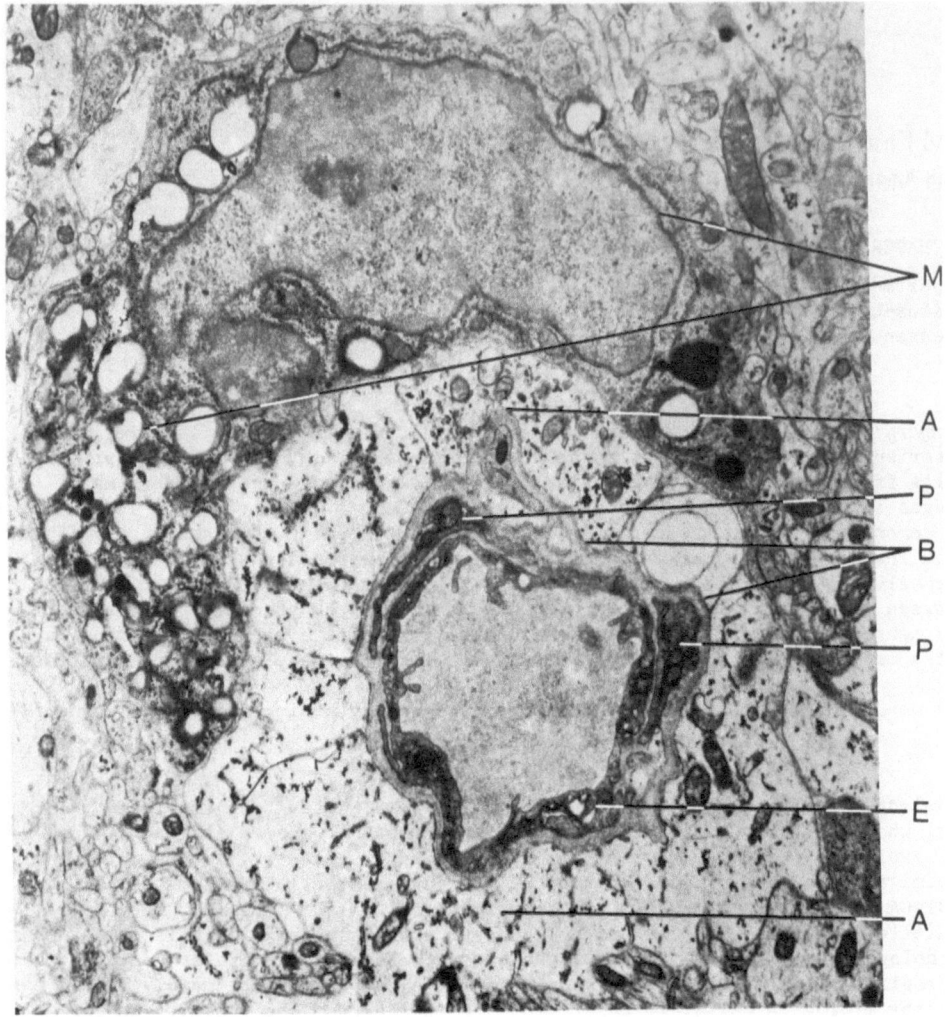

Fig. 1. A reactive microglia cell in juxtacapillary position.
M = Microglia cell. Many phagosomes are to be seen in the cytoplasm.
A = Swollen astrocytic feet.
B = Basement membrane.
P = Processes of pericytes.
E = Endothelium.
From the region of a traumatic lesion (puncture wound) in the cerebral
cortex of a syrian hamster, five days after injury. 9000 : 1

other cases these cells are connected with the capillaries only by lamellar
cytoplasmic prolongations.

   According to our observations in experimental traumatic brain lesions, reactive microglia cells are often plastered on the outer surface of capillaries.

   Astrocytic perivascular sheets and basement membranes delimit these juxtacapillary cells from pericytes and endothelial cells. The microglia cells

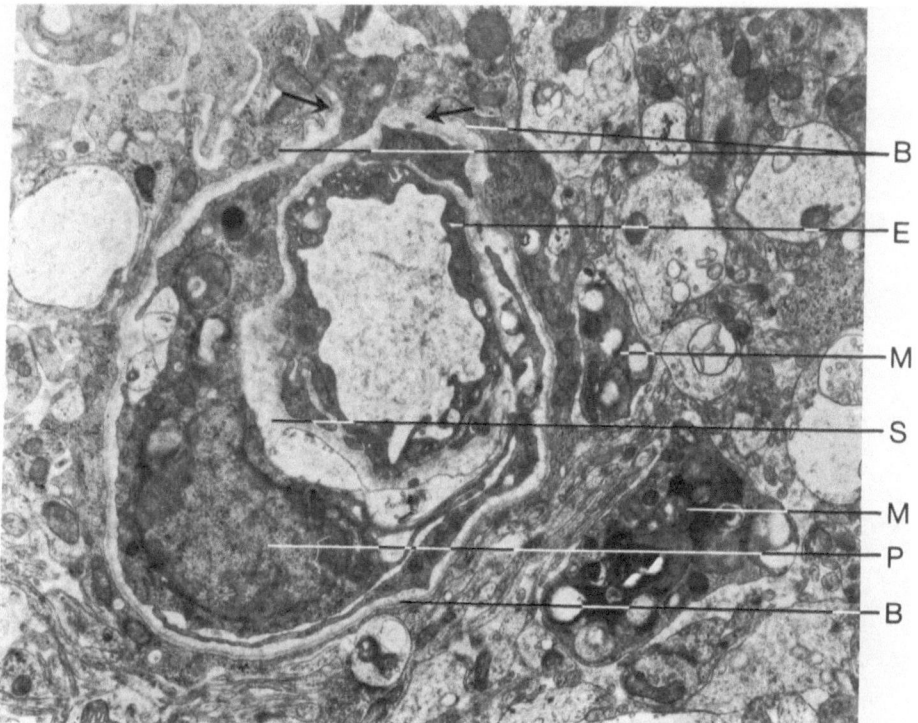

Fig. 2. Further stage of mobilisation of capillary pericyte.
P = Pericyte; between arrows: a process which penetrates through the basement
    membrane (B)
E = Endothelium.
S = Dilatated pericapillary space.
M = Processes of microglia cells, which are embedded in neuropil.
From the region of a traumatic lesion (puncture wound) in cortex of a syrian
hamster, five days after injury. 9000 : 1

which are closely embedded in the neuropil, show phagosomes as an indication
of intracytoplasmatic ingestive and digestive activities (Fig. 1).

Besides these juxtacapillary cells many stages of the activation of pericytes
may be seen at any given time (Fig. 2).

The basement membrane, which envelopes the pericytes, is extended. Occasionally inclusions are seen in the cytoplasm.

Further stages of mobilisation of capillary pericytes show a broader pericapillary space (Fig. 2).

The figure shows the mobilized pericyte still in the pericapillary space, but
a process extends through the basement membrane and the gaps in the surrounding
neuropil. In more progressive stages the mobilized cells which have an elongated shape, leave the pericapillary space (Fig. 3).

A cell process penetrates the basement membrane and propels itself between
the components of the surrounding neuropil. These mobile cells squeeze between
the intercellular gaps and become entirely surrounded by the cell processes of
the neuropil.

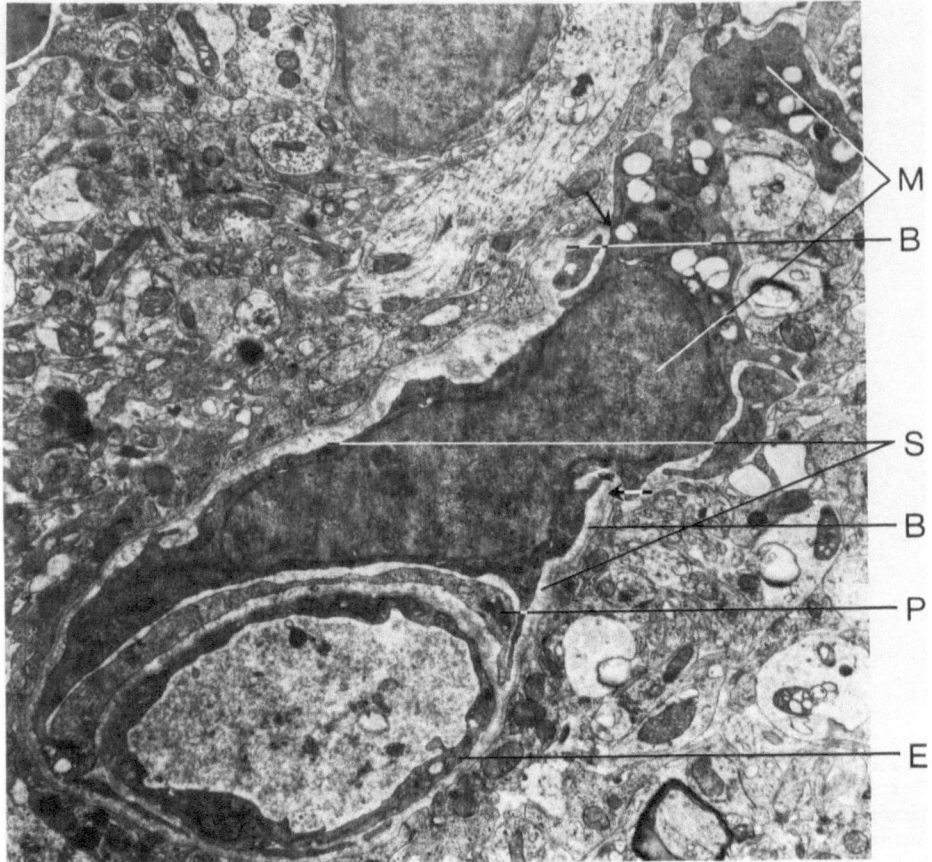

Fig. 3. A mobilized cell (M) leaves the pericapillary space.
Arrows: The cell extends through the basement membrane.
B = Basement membrane.
S = Pericapillary space.
P = Process of a pericyte.
E = Endothelium.
From the region of a traumatic lesion (puncture wound) in cortex of a syrian
hamster, five days after injury. 9000 : 1

These observations suggest that in reactive stages the microglia cells may,
at least in part, originate from the perivascular mesenchymal tissue.

REFERENCES

1. BLINZINGER, K., HAGER, H.: Elektronenmikroskopische Untersuchungen über die
   Feinstruktur ruhender und progressiver Mikrogliazellen im Säugetiergehirn.
   Beitr. path. Anat. *127*, 173 - 192 (1962)
2. BLINZINGER, K., HAGER, H.: Elektronenmikroskopische Untersuchungen zur Fein-
   struktur ruhender und progressiver Mikrogliazellen im ZNS des Goldhamsters.
   Progr. Brain Res. *6*, 99 - 111 (1964)

3. HAGER, H.: Die feinere Cytologie und Cytopathologie des Nervensystems.
   Stuttgart: Fischer 1964
4. HAGER, H.: Ultrastruktur der Makro- und Mikroglia im elektronenmikrosko-
   pischen Bild. Acta neuropath. (Berl.) Suppl. *4*, 86 - 97 (1968)
5. HAGER, H.: Allgemeine morphologische Pathologie des Nervengewebes. Handbuch
   der allgemeinen Pathologie Band III, Teil 3, 1 - 385. Berlin-Heidelberg-
   New York: Springer 1968
6. HUNTINGTON, H.W., TERRY, R.D.: The origin of the reactive cells in cerebral
   stab wounds. J. Neuropath. exp. Neurol. *25*, 646 (1966)
7. KÖNIGSMARK, B.W., SIDMAN, R.L.: Origin of brain macrophages in the mouse.
   J. Neuropath. exp. Neurol. *22*, 643 - 676 (1963)
8. RIO-HORTEGA, P. DEL, PENFIELD, W.: Cerebral cicatrix. The reaction of
   neuroglia and microglia to brain wounds. Bull. Johns Hopkins Hosp. *41*,
   278 (1927)
9. RIO-HORTEGA, P. DEL: Microglia. *In:* Cytology and cellular pathology of the
   nervous system. PENFIELD, W. (ed.), Vol. 2, 481 - 534. New York: Hafner 1932
10. STENWIG, A.E.: The origin of brain macrophages in traumatic lesions,
    Wallerian degeneration and retrograde degeneration. J. Neuropath. exp.
    Neurol. *31*, 696 - 704 (1972)

Prof. Dr. Dr. H. HAGER
Institut für Neuropathologie
im Zentrum Neurologie
Justus-Liebig Universität
Arndtstraße 16
D-63 Giessen/BRD

Acta Neuropath. (Berlin), Suppl. VI, 285 - 290 (1975)
© by Springer-Verlag 1975

Experimental Studies on Kinetics and Functions of Monuclear Phagozytes of the Central Nervous System

M. OEHMICHEN,
with the technical assistance of H. GRÜNINGER and

M. GENČIĆ

Institut für Hirnforschung der Universität Tübingen, G.F.R.

Summary: The described experimental studies on rabbits gave evidence of the hematogenous - obviously monocytic - origin, the lymphatic drainage, and the IgG- and complement-receptor sites of monocytoid CSF-cells, epiplexus cells, perivascular cells of the intracerebral vessels, and of some cells within damaged brain tissue - so-called progressive microglia. - Because of their identical kinetics and functions these types of mononuclear cells of the CNS were placed in a system known as 'Mononuclear Phagocyte System'.

Key words: Monocytoid CSF-cell - perivascular cell - progressive microglia - kinetics - receptor sites

INTRODUCTION

The purpose of this investigation is to find some answers to three different problems relating to the so-called mononuclear phagocytes (MP) of the CNS on the basis of experimental studies on rabbits. This report deals with their hematogenous origin, their lymphatic drainage, and their IgG- and complement-receptor sites. Finally, the term 'MP of the CNS' should be defined on the ground of similar kinetic behaviour and of comparable receptor sites.

I. The hematogenous origin of MP of the CNS

In the literature evidence is given of the hematogenous origin of some intra-cerebral, perivascular (1, 2), epiplexus (3), and CSF-cells (4) using experimental procedures which achieved a labelling of peripheral mononuclear blood cells. As labelling agents there were used ^{3}H-thymidine (2), and carbon (5). These studies could not totally exclude the possibility that activated local cells incorporate or phagocytize the tritiated substances or the carbon released at the degeneration of labelled blood cells. In contrast to these studies we now used tritiated diisopropyl-fluorophosphate (^{3}H-DFP) as a tracer which irreversibly binds on esterase. This agent has several advantages (see 6): The ^{3}H-DFP binds rapidly and irreversibly to leukocytes, lymphocytes bind little or no ^{3}H-DFP, and the label is not reutilized.

Experimental procedure: About 70 to 100 ml blood was withdrawn by cardiac puncture of 2 or 3 rabbits and collected in a bottle containing 20 ml ACD. Subsequently 2 µCi/ml ^{3}H-DFP [2], dissolved in propylene glycol, was injected into the bottle, mixed, and incubated at room temperature for 1 hr.

---

[1] These studies have been supported by a grant from the Deutsche Forschungs-gemeinschaft.

[2] Radiochemical Center, Amersham (England); spec. act. about 10 Ci/mM.

Then the blood was returned to another rabbit which had received an intracerebral injection of herpes viruses (see 1) 4 days earlier. 24 hrs. later the acceptor animal was sacrificed and fixed by cardiac perfusion with formalin. Sections of the paraffin-embedded material were processed autoradiographically using the dipping technique and an exposure time of 28 days.

Results: Autoradiographs of smears of the transfused blood showed that 95-100% of monocytes and neutrophils were labelled whereas the majority of lymphocytes were not labelled significantly. On the autoradiographically processed sections we could observe clearly labelled mononuclear cells (Fig. 1) within the subarachnoid space, within the neuropil, and within the immediate vicinity of intracerebral vessels. We assumed that at least under pathological conditions mononuclear cells - obviously monocytes - may leave the vessels and - based on their localisation - may be called monocytoid CSF-cells, progressive microglia, and intracerebral perivascular cells. Though we could not find labelled epiplexus cells we cannot deny their hematogenous origin.

II. The lymphatic drainage of MP of the CNS

The fate of MP of the CNS is still unknown. Three different possibilities are to be discussed: A local degeneration, an absorption or migration directly into the blood stream, and a lymphatic drainage. Whereas there is nearly no indication of a local degeneration under normal conditions, some experimental evidence is given of the appearance of intracerebrally injected red blood cells in the peripheral blood (7) and in the deep cervical lymph nodes (8). Using similar experimental procedures we tried to find an indication of a lymphatic drainage of intracerebrally injected peritoneal macrophages.

Experimental procedure: To get some information of lymphatic drainage under timebound conditions at first 0.1 ml sterilized ferritin[3] or colloidal carbon[4] were injected intracerebrally. In a 2nd series an increase of peritoneal macrophages in rabbits was obtained by intraperitoneal injections of sterile paraffin oil. The macrophages in vitro were labelled by three different agents: Ferritin, colloidal carbon, and ^{3}H-DFP. About 10^5 to 10^6 peritoneal cells were injected intracerebrally.

Results: In cervical lymph nodes ferritin and carbon were primarily observed one hour after the intracerebral injection, but not 30 min. after the injection. Within 4 hrs. single labelled peritoneal macrophages could be found in the deep cervical lymph nodes (Fig. 2). In the brain the peritoneal macrophages were localised (Fig. 3) in the immediate vicinity of the needle wound and within the preformed spaces of the leptomeninges, the ventricle, and around the intracerebral vessels. We conclude that intracerebrally injected peritoneal macrophages are localised like monocytoid CSF-cells, intracerebral perivascular cells, progressive microglia, and epiplexus cells and they are - at least partly - drained by the cervical lymph ducts.

III. IgG- and complement-receptor sites on MP of the CNS

The high phagocytic activity of monocytoid CSF-cells, intracerebral perivascular cells, and progressive microglia is well known, but only a few studies are published concerning their activity in immunological processes. Supposing these cells were comparable with macrophages of the body (9, 10) we have tried in collaboration with Dr. H. HUBER to demonstrate IgG- and complement-receptor sites on their surface.

Experimental procedure: Sheep red blood cells (SRBC) were coated with rabbit anti-erythrocyte-antibodies and partly with complement; the inhibitory effect of IgG and complement was proved (Table 1). Washed and pretreated SRBC alone

---

[3] Serva Feinbiochemica, 6900 Heidelberg (GFR); code - 21321
[4] Günther Wagner, 3000 Hannover (GFR); Pelikan C11/1431

Table 1. *Representative experiments demonstrating IgG- and complement-receptor sites on cells within the brain and on brain cells adhering to glass*

used antisera	red cell complexes	inhibitor	phagocytosis by MP of CNS
	homolog. E	-	(-)
	sheep E	-	(-)
7 S anti-Forssman			
1 : 500	E A	-	+++
1 : 2000	E A	-	+
1 : 8000	E A	-	(+)
1 : 500	E A	IgG 1mg/ml	(-)
1 : 500	E A C	IgG 1mg/ml	++
19 S anti-Forssman	E A	-	(-)
	E A C	-	++
	E A C	C 1 : 80	(-)

and in combination with inhibitory agents as well as washed homologous SRBC were injected into the brain of a rabbit after cardiac perfusion with phosphate buffered saline for one hour. After the cell-injection the perfusion was continued for another hour. Subsequently the brain was fixed by formalin. - In a 2nd series of experiments glass-slides were implanted intracerebrally for 7 days and then withdrawn. The cells adhering to the glass surface were incubated with untreated and pretreated SRBC. - The number of erythrocytes-containing cells and of rosette-forming cells was compared in the different experiments. *Results:* IgG- and complement-receptor sites were shown on some types of cells according to Table 1 which summarizes the representative experiments. Receptor sites could be demonstrated by means of phagocytizing and rosette-forming (Fig. 4a, b, d) on monocytoid CSF-cells, on intracerebral perivascular cells and on epiplexus cells. The glass-adherent cells (Fig. 4c) have been considered to be progressive microglia because of the histological examination of the brain-wounds after glass-implantation and because of the mesenchymal feature of this type of cell on glass. Morphologically these cells are to be compared with macrophages in culture (11). These cells showed the same receptor sites as known on macrophages and monocytes and therefore we have to assume a comparable function of these cells in the process of immune response.

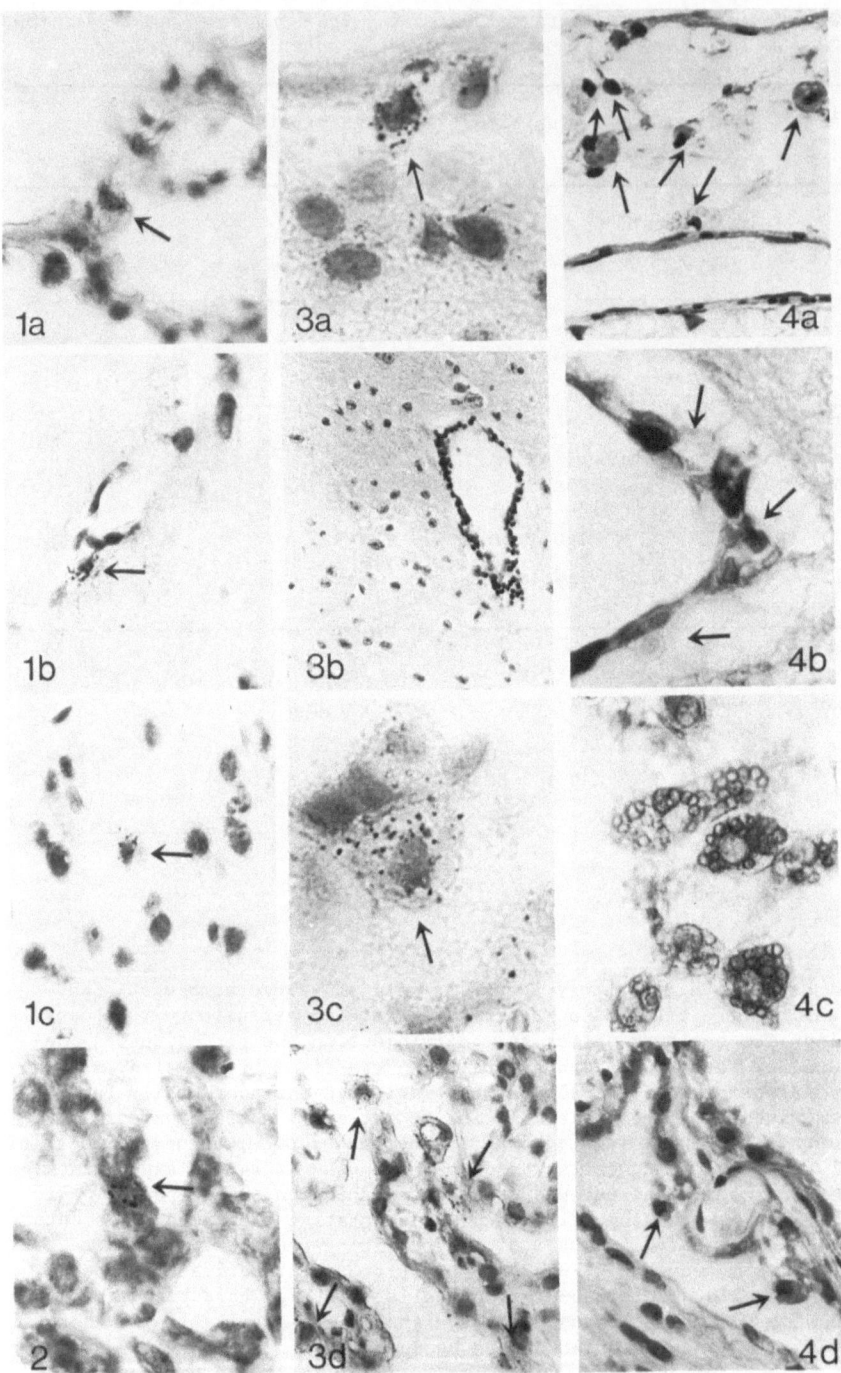

Fig. 1. Demonstration of the hematogenous origin of mononuclear cells of the CNS by transfusion of ³H-DFP-labelled blood-cells into herpes virus-infected rabbits. The labelled cells (arrows) are localized as monocytoid CSF-cells (a), pericytes (b) and progressive microglia (c). (HE-stain; x 500)

CONCLUSION

Summarizing these findings we could observe that monocytoid CSF-cells, perivascular cells of intracerebral vessels, and so-called progressive microglia are derived from mononuclear blood cells and that these cells as well as epiplexus cells have IgG- and complement-receptor sites. Within the CNS peritoneal macrophages injected intracerebrally showed a distribution-pattern comparable with all these cells and additionally they showed a lymphatic drainage. Because of these common features we wanted to put together the different cell-types which are mainly distinguishable by their different localisation.

In 1970 VAN FURTH *et al.* (12) stated that highly phagocytic mononuclear cells of the body and their precursors could be placed in one system, the so-called 'Mononuclear Phagocyte System'. I think our experiments showed that the phagocytic cells of the CNS fulfilled the criteria applicable to known mononuclear phagocytes: The different cell-types are of hematogenous - obviously monocytic-origin (exception: the cytogenesis of epiplexus cells couldn't be proved), they contain comparable receptor sites, and - by means of their localization - they cannot be distinguished from intracerebrally injected peritoneal macrophages.

REFERENCES

1. OEHMICHEN, M., GRÜNINGER, H., SAEBISCH, R., NARITA, Y.: Mikroglia and Pericyten als Transformationsformen der Blut-Monocyten mit erhaltener Proliferationsfähigkeit. Acta neuropath. (Berlin) *23*, 200 - 218 (1973)
2. OEHMICHEN, M.: Monocytic origin of microglia cells. Report on: Second Conference on Mononuclear Phagocytes, Leiden 1973 (in press)
3. KITAMURA, T., HATTORI, T., FUJITA, S.: Autoradiographic studies on histogenesis of brain macrophages in the mouse. J. Neuropath. exp. Neurol. *31*, 502 - 518 (1972)
4. OEHMICHEN, M., GRÜNINGER, H.: Cytokinetic studies on the origin of cells of the cerebrospinal fluid. J. neurol. Sci. *22*, 165 - 176 (1974)
5. STENWIG, A.E.: The origin of brain macrophages in traumatic lesions, wallerian degeneration, and retrograde degeneration. J. Neuropath. exp. Neurol. *31*, 696 - 704 (1972)
6. ATHENS, J.W., MAUER, A.M., ASHENBRUCKER, H., CARTWRIGHT, G.E., WINTROBE, M.M.: A method for labelling leukocytes with radioactive diisopropylfluorophosphate (DFP[32]). Ann. N.Y. Acad. Sci. *77*, 773 - 776 (1959)
7. USUI, K.: The actions and absorption of subarachnoid blood. Nagoya J. med. Sci. *31*, 1 - 23 (1968)

Fig. 2. Demonstration of the lymphatic drainage of intracerebrally injected ^{3}H-DFP-labelled peritoneal macrophages. A labelled cell (arrow) is seen in the deep cervical lymph node (HE-stain; x 1.200)

Fig. 3. Distribution pattern of intracerebrally injected peritoneal macrophages within the brain. The cells (arrows) are localized as monocytoid CSF-cells (a, x 1.200), pericytes (b, x 200), progressive microglia (c, x 1.200), and epiplexus cells (d, x 500). (HE-stain)

Fig. 4. Erythrophagocytosis (arrows) of coated SRBC by different cells of the CNS after intracerebral injection of erythrocytes into sacrificed rabbits (a, b, d,) and on glass-adherent cells 7 days after the intracerebral implantation of the glass (c). The phagocytizing cells were interpreted to be monocytoid CSF-cells (a, x 500), perivascular cells (b, x 1.200), progressive microglia (c, x 1.200), and epiplexus cells (d, x 500). (HE-stain)

8. SIMMONDS, W.J.: The absorption of blood from the cerebrospinal fluid in animals. Austral. J. exp. Biol. Med. Sci. *30*, 261 - 270 (1952)
9. LOBUGLIO, A.F., COTRAN, R.S., JANDL, J.H.: Red cells coated with immunoglobulin G: binding and sphering by mononuclear cells in man. Science *158*, 1582 - 1585 (1967)
10. HUBER, H., MICHLMAYR, G., MÜLLER-EBERHARD, H.J., FUDENBERG, H.H.: Rezeptoren an menschlichen Monozyten für IgG und Komplement. Schweiz. med. Wschr. *100*, 344 - 347 (1970)
11. BENNETT, B.: Isolation and cultivation in vitro of macrophages from various sources in the mouse. Amer. J. Path. *48*, 165 - 181 (1966)
12. VAN FURTH, R.: Mononuclear phagocytes. Oxford - Edinburgh: Blackwell Scientific Publ. 1970

Dr. med. M. OEHMICHEN
Institut für Hirnforschung der
Universität
Belthle Str. 15
7400 Tübingen, GFR

Acta Neuropath. (Berlin), Suppl. VI, 291 - 296 (1975)

Origin of Brain Macrophages and the Nature of the So-Called Microglia

S. FUJITA AND T. KITAMURA

Department of Pathology
Kyoto Prefectural University of Medicine
Kyoto, Japan

Summary: Two aspects of the so-called microglia were studied by silver impregnation and ^{3}H-TdR ARG in light and electron microscopy. (1) So-called microglioblasts are glioblasts differentiated from matrix cells. They are progenitors of the so-called resting microglia as well as of astrocytes and oligodendroglia. (2) Brain macrophages in stab wounds, experimental Japanese encephalitis and retrograde degeneration of the facial nucleus are all found to be of hematogenous origin. Infiltrating hematogenous cells cannot stay permanently in the brain parenchyma unless pathological alterations persist indefinitely.

Key words: Monocytes - Brain macrophages - Microglia - Autoradiography - Electron microscopy

INTRODUCTION

HORTEGA's concept of the so-called microglia (1) was created on the basis of the unification of separate observations on 3 types of cells that are selectively stained by his silver carbonate method: microglioblasts in newborn animals, the so-called resting microglia and macrophages in damaged brains. He regarded these 3 types of cells as 3 aspects of the same kind of mesodermal cells, the microglia. Recently, however, the interrelationship between these 3 groups of cells has been interpreted very differently from the original theory of HORTEGA. The present paper is aimed to discuss the following controversial points concerned with the microglial system;
1. Do the so-called microglioblasts, which are now believed to be the direct progeny of matrix cells and to differentiate into astrocytes and oligodendroglia, now called glioblasts (2, 3), also differentiate into the resting microglia?
2. Are there any possibilities for endogenous cells in the brain to become macrophages?

MATERIALS AND METHODS

Morphological studies with silver carbonate staining

Human and rabbit brains at various fetal and postnatal stages were used. They were fixed in ammonium bromide fixative and stained by HORTEGA's silver carbonate method for microglia or by several modifications thereof.

Autoradiographic studies

1. Adult mice received successive 18 subcutaneous injections of ^{3}H-thymidine (^{3}H-TdR) at 6 hours' interval. These mice were divided into 3 groups. Twelve

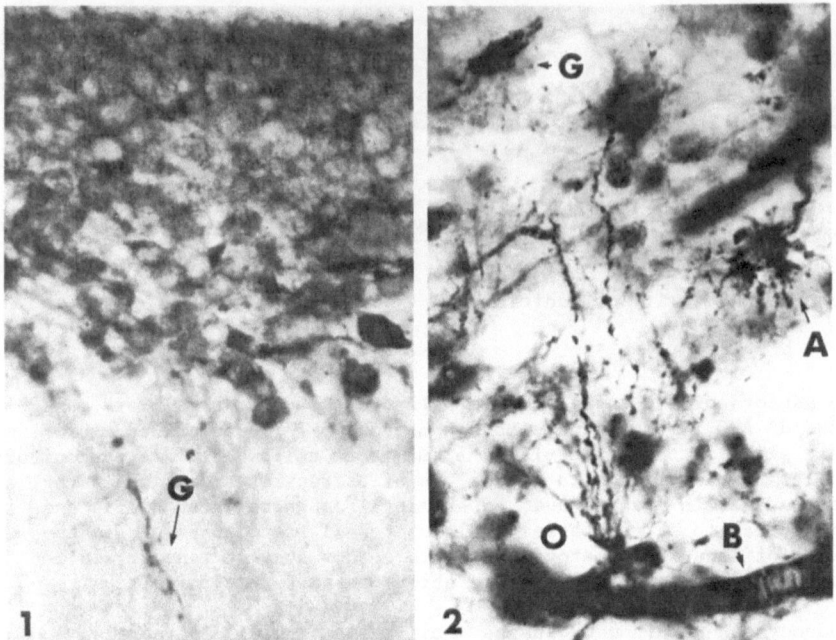

Fig. 1. Periventricular layer of the cerebrum of fetal rabbit on 22nd day of gestation. Silver carbonate staining. All the cells in this layer are stained. Perikarya of the glioblasts in this subependymal layer are lemon-shaped. No glioblasts are found in the deeper layer of the brain parenchyma at this stage. One glioblast (G) now begins to migrate out from the layer. x 400

Fig. 2. Differentiation of neuroglial cells in the white substance of the cerebrum of a human newborn. Silver carbonate staining. Migrating glioblasts (G), immature astrocytes with a vascular foot (A) and oligodendroglia (O) with typical ribbon-shaped processes. B indicates a blood vessel to which the oligo-dendroglia attaches with a sessile foot. x 400

to 14 hours after the last injection, mice of the 1st group received a stab wound in the cerebrum; those of the 2nd group were injected with the Japanese encephalitis virus intracerebrally; and those belonging to the 3rd group were given a left facial nerve transection. Each mouse was sacrificed at a series of postoperative periods ranging from 6 hours to 6 days.
2. Fourty-eight hours after the stab wounding 4 mice received 4 successive injections of ^{3}H-TdR at 6 hours' interval and sacrificed 2 hours and 20 days after the last injection. All the injured cerebra and facial nuclei were processed for light and electron microscopic autoradiography. The procedures for autoradiography were outlined in detail elsewhere (2, 4).

RESULTS

Differentiation of glioblasts into three kinds of neuroglia

In the rabbit cerebral hemisphere, stage III of cytogenesis (2) starts on 22nd day of gestation. At this day cells stained by silver carbonate method were

Table 1. *Labelling indices counted in blood smears and brain sections at various times after stab wounding, inoculation of Japanese encephalitis virus or transection of the left facial nerve. This labelling indices (expressed in %) in the neural tissue were counted on autoradiographs using semithin or ultrathin sections. The mice were cumulatively labelled with ^3H-TdR for 4,3 days and experiments started 12-14 hours after the final injection when extracellular ^3H-TdR was completely cleared away*

Tissue & cell type	Time	after stab-wounding		after JEV inoculation		after nerve transection	
Blood		0 days	3 days	0 days	4 days	0 days	4 days
neutrophils		94	100	97	100	97	100
monocytes		74	87	77	86	77	86
large lymphocytes		45	43	38	48	38	48
small lymphocytes		10	18	4	10	4	10
Brain							
neutrophils		-	100	-	-	-	-
transformed monocytes		-	87	-	81	-	86
macrophages		-	75	-	89	-	-
pericytes		0	0	0.3	0	0	0
endothelium		1.8		0.2		1.1	1.2
neuroglia		1.2		0.6		1.2	1.4

restricted to the periventricular layer (Fig. 1). On the 24th day of gestation, we found many impregnated glioblasts now migrating in the white substance along the nerve fibers. In new born rabbits, numerous glioblasts were found in the white and gray substance. Some of them did not lose their affinity for the silver carbonate during further development and finally differentiated into the so-called resting microglia. In respect of this point we completely agree white and gray substance. Some of them did not lose their affinity for the really precursors of the so-called resting microglia. Besides this line of differentiation, the glioblasts also differentiate into oligodendroglia and astrocytes (2, 3). Differentiation of glioblasts into three kinds of neuroglia could be confirmed in the human brain. From 20 weeks of pregnancy glioblasts appeared in the human cerebrum, and the silver carbonate method stained all their transitional forms up to the so-called microglia, oligodendroglia and astrocytes (Fig. 2).

Origin of macrophages in the stab wound, encephalitis and retrograde degeneration

Three kinds of experimental lesions, mentioned above, were made in the mouse brains in which circulating leukocytes were selectively labelled with ^3H-TdR (Tab. 1). Common to these 3 types of lesion, labelled inflammatory cells appeared in number in response to the brain damage. Their labelling indices were almost comparable with those of the circulating monocytes (Tab. 1). Because the experimental periods were restricted to the early phase of alterations, there had been little, if any, labelled degradation products to be reutilized before the labelled cells began to increase in the brain. Therefore, we conclude that these inflammatory cells are all derived from blood monocytes and that few endogenous cells contribute to the macrophage formation. The morphological characteristics of labelled cells appearing in the

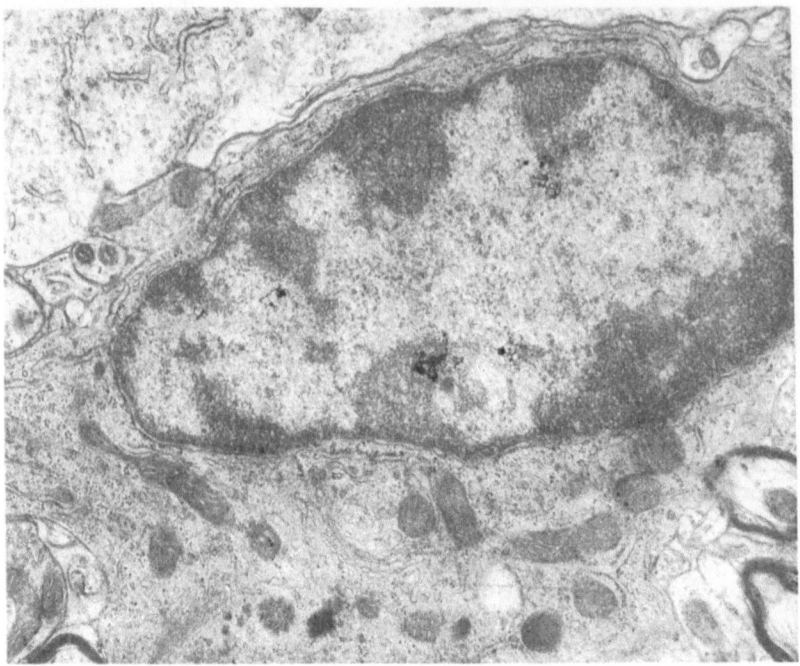

Fig. 3. Electron microscopic autoradiograph of the perineuronal transformed
monocyte appearing in the facial nucleus under retrograde degeneration. This
cell shows well-developed Golgi apparatus. Several lysosomal dense bodies are
seen. The overall density of the cytoplasmic matrix is relatively high.
x 20000

facial nucleus under retrograde degeneration (Fig. 3) completely agree with
those of the cells that have been described by previous investigators as a
type of endogenous cells, the microglia, in the same kind of brain lesions
(5, 6). However, their high labelling index indicates unequivocally that they
originate from blood monocytes and not from any type of endogenous cells.
The fine structural characteristics of these transformed monocytes are the
diffuse density of the cytoplasmic matrix, long, thin and stringy endoplasmic
reticulum, which frequently runs parallel to the surface of the cell, and the
presence of lysosomal dense bodies (Fig. 3). In this context, it is important
to note that TORVIK *et al.* (6) as well as the present authors have not found
this type of cell in the normal facial nuclei of control animals. The fate of
these infiltrating monocytes in the neural tissue was studied by the pulse
labelling method of ^{3}H-TdR applied to the stab wounding in the mouse brain
(Tab. 2). Two days after the stab wound was made, a large number of DNA-syn-
thesizing cells, of which the majority were transformed monocytes, were found
scattered in the cerebrum. In 20 days the labelled blood cells decreased
greatly in number and were virtually eliminated in areas distant from the
wound. This fact indicates that blood monocytes, once infiltrating in the
neural tissue, cannot persist as one of the endogenous elements indefinitely
in the normally recovered neural tissue, even if they may proliferate and
stay temporarily as long as the pathological alterations persist.

Table 2. *Proliferating cells shortly after the stab wounding and their fate.*
Mice received 4 injections of ^{3}H-TdR between 38 to 66 hours after the stab
wounding. Two mice each were sacrificed 2 hours and 20 days after the final
injection and the number of labelled cells were counted on autoradiographs
of one whole coronal sections (5μ in thickness) of one mouse. At the same
time, ratio of various labelled cell type were examined by electron micro-
scopic autoradiography on another mouse (EM-ARG) and the total number of
labelled cells was allotted to each cell type. Note initial active prolifera-
tion and subsequent marked decrease of the infiltrated monocytes

| Time after ^{3}H-TdR | | 0 day | | 20 days | |
Time after injury		2 days		22 days	
Number of labeled cells in a coronal section		1035	→	226	
Type of labeled cells	(EM-ARG)		(EM-ARG)		
transformed monocytes	(37/46)	833	(6/106)	9	
astrocytes	(1/46)	22 }202	(88/106)	188 }217	
oligodendroglia	(8/46)	180	(12/106)	29	

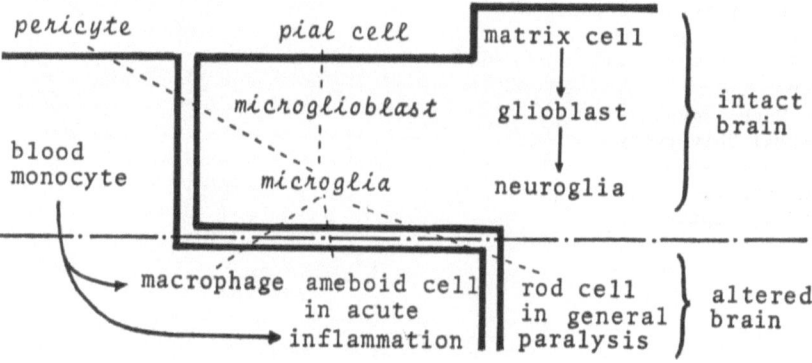

Fig. 4. Origin of macrophages and the nature of the so-called microglia.
Classical concepts of microglia are shown with broken lines (----) and
italics. In this scheme, we propose that macrophages and amoeboid inflammatory cells are exclusively derived from circulating monocytes. Neuroglial
cells in the brain and proper pericytes do not contribute the brain macrophages. The so-called resting "microglia" and the microglioblasts belong to
neuroglia of matrix cell origin. As a consequence, the so-called microglial
system is separated into two groups of cells different in origin and function
as indicated by bold lines; monocyte-macrophage system and system of neuroglial
cells

COMMENTS

The simplest way to interpret these autoradiographic and silver carbonate
findings on the histogenesis of the brain macrophages and the so-called
resting microglia is to accept the conclusions that inflammatory amoeboid
cells and macrophages are exclusively originated from circulating monocytes,
and that their precursors are not present in the normal central nervous
system (Fig. 4).

REFERENCES

1. HORTEGA, P. DEL RIO: Microglia. *In:* PENFIELD, W. (ed.): Cytology and
   Cellular Pathology of the Nervous System, p. 481 - 534. New York: Hafner
   Publish. Co. 1932 (Reprint edition, 1965)
2. FUJITA, S.: Application of light and electron microscopic autoradiography ot the study of cytogenesis of the forebrain. *In:* HASSLER, R.,
   STEPHAN, H. (eds.): Evolution of the Forebrain, p. 180 - 196. Stuttgart:
   Thieme 1966
3. PATERSON, J.A., PRIVAT, A., LING, E.A., LEBLOND, C.P.: Investigation of
   glial cells in semithin sections. III Transformation of subependymal
   cells into glial cells, as shown by radioautography after ^{3}H-thymidine
   injection into the lateral ventricle of the brain of young rats. J.
   comp. Neurol. *149*, 83 - 102 (1973)
4. KITAMURA, T., HATTORI, H., FUJITA, S.: Autoradiographic studies on histogenesis of brain macrophages in the mouse. J. Neuropath. exp. Neurol.
   31, 502 - 518 (1972)
5. KREUTZBERG, G.W.: Über perineuronale Mikrogliazellen (Autoradiographische
   Untersuchungen). Acta neuropath. (Berl.) Suppl. IV, 141 - 145 (1968)
6. TORVIK, A., SKJÖRTEN, F.: Electron microscopic observations on nerve
   cell regeneration and degeneration after axon lesions. I. Changes in the
   nerve cell cytoplasm. II. Changes in the glial cells. Acta neuropath.(Berl.)
   17, 248 - 282 (1971)

S. FUJITA, M.D.
Department of Pathology
Kyoto Prefectural University
of Medicine
Kawaramachi-Hirokoji,
Kamikyoku, Kyoto, Japan

Acta Neuropath. (Berlin), Suppl VI, 297 - 300 (1975)
© by Springer-Verlag 1975

The Relationship between Microglia and Brain Macrophages. Experimental Investigations

ANSGAR TORVIK

Laboratory of Neuropathology
Ulleval Hospital,
Oslo, Norway

Summary: A series of experiments are reported which indicate that the microglia
are endogenous cells which may constitute the only source of phagocytes in certain mild degenerative conditions, such as Wallerian degeneration and retrograde nerve cell disintegration. In more extensive lesions with increased
vascular permeability a substantial number of the phagocytes are derived from
the blood monocytes.

Key words: Microglia - Macrophages - Monocytes

INTRODUCTION

The present paper summarizes a series of investigations from the Laboratory
of neuropathology, Ulleval Hospital, Oslo, concerning the identification,
function and origin of microglia (1 - 8). Three types of experimental models
have been studied, viz. retrograde nerve cell reaction, Wallerian degeneration,
and traumatic lesions. Carbon labelling of blood monocytes has been employed
to examine whether some of the reactive cells are of hematogenous origin.

MATERIAL AND METHODS

Details concerning the materials have been reported elsewhere (1 - 6). Adult
mice and rats and newborn rabbits were used as experimental animals. The
retrograde nerve cell reaction was studied after crush lesion, transection,
or evulsion of the facial nerve. These lesions were performed in adult mice
and rats and newborn rabbits. Wallerian degeneration was studied after lesions of the posterior columns in newborn rabbits. Stab wounds of the spinal
cord in newborn rabbits served as models for traumatic lesions.

   Electron microscopy was performed after vascular perfusion with glutaraldehyde. Silver impregnation for microglia was performed with the Hortega
method on formalin fixed frozen sections. Carbon labelling of the blood
monocytes was obtained by intravenous injection of carbon suspensions in
newborn rabbits and the lesions were made after the blood was cleared of
free carbon. Examination of the various lesions for extravascular labelled
cells was performed on serial sections of formalin fixed and paraffin-
embedded material.

RESULTS

Retrograde Nerve Cell Reaction

All types of lesions of the facial nerve were followed by a proliferation of
small elongated perineuronal cells in all examined species (1 - 4, 7). The

cells had characteristic ultrastructural features with coarse and marginated nuclear chromatin, conspicuously long and narrow strands of endoplasmic reticulum, and many dense bodies. Only minor species variations in the ultrastructure were observed. The reactive perineuronal cells were impregnated as microglia with the Hortega method (3).

In mice and rabbits the microglial reaction was extensive after nerve transection or evulsion, and only slight after crush lesions (1 - 4). Since transection and evulsion of the nerve caused neuronal disintegration whereas crush lesions were followed by complete neuronal recovery, it was first suggested that the microglial reaction was mainly determined by the degree of neuronal degeneration. However, later studies habe shown that in adult rats the microglial reaction is equally severe after crush lesion and evulsion of the facial nerve (7). In certain species the microglia may thus react extensively also in non-destructive conditions.

Phagocytosis. After evulsion of the nerve in newborn rabbits an extensive disintegration of the nerve cells was observed within a few days. Electron microscopy showed that the disintegrating neurons were phagocytized by the perineuronal microglia (3). Phagocytosis was only rarely observed after nerve transection in adult mice (1, 2). This was probably due to the slow disintegration of the neurons in mice, with less probability of encountering necrotic neurons.

Origin of phagocytes. In order to determine whether the phagocytic cells were of hematogenous origin, the blood monocytes of newborn rabbits were labelled by intravenous injections of carbon before the evulsion of the facial nerve (5). No labelled extravascular cells were seen in the facial nucleus 3 days later, although there was an extensive phagocytosis by this time. Since labelled cells were present in traumatic lesions under similar experimental conditions (see below), the most likely explanation for the negative findings is that the phagocytic microglial cells during retrograde degeneration are of endogenous and not of hematogenous origin.

Wallerian Degeneration

Electron microscopy of the posterior columns of newborn rabbits showed phagocytosis of disintegrating material from the first day after the lesion. Hortega preparations demonstrated a brisk proliferation of microglia in the same areas (8). No labelled cells were found in areas with Wallerian degeneration when the blood monocytes were labelled with carbon before the lesions (5). It is likely, therefore, that also in Wallerian degeneration the phagocytosis is performed by endogenous cells only.

Traumatic Lesions

After stab lesions of the spinal cord in newborn rabbits the necrotic area was filled with lipid macrophages within a few days. A substantial number of these phagocytes were labelled after intravenous injection of carbon before the injury (5). Similar findings were made in peripheral nerves in which labelled phagocytes were present in areas with traumatic lesions but absent in areas with pure Wallerian digeneration (6).

DISCUSSION

The small reactive cells observed during retrograde and Wallerian degeneration have been described by many electron microscopists under various names, such as "microglia", "the third neuroglial type", "multipotential glia", "M-cells", and "reactive oligodendrocytes" (for reviews see references 2 and 9 - 14). Since the same cells are impregnated as microglia with the classical silver methods (3, 8, 15), the name microglia probably should be retained. Autoradio-graphic studies concerning their origin are controversial (10, 16, 21). The present investigations indicate that they are endogenous cells but the experi-ments do not give any further information about their histogenesis.

Some investigators apparently doubt that the proliferating microglia after axotomy are phagocytic cells (17). However, the phagocytic potential of the cells is readily observed in models with extensive and rapid neuronal dis-integration after axotomy (3).

There are considerable species variations in the extent of the microglial reaction after axotomy. The reaction also varies with the type of nerve lesion. Thus the microglial reaction was slight after crush lesions and severe after transection or evulsion of the facial nerve in adult mice and newborn rabbits (2, 4). Adult rats, on the other hand, showed equally severe reactions after crush lesion and evulsion (7). The functional significance of the microglial reaction in non-destructive processes is obscure.

There may also be other regional or species variations in the tissue reaction after axotomy. Thus MATTHEWS and KRUGER (18) and BARRON *et al.* (19) reported invasion of polymorphs and mononuclear leucocytes in the thalamus following cortical lesions in rabbits and rats. Such changes have not been observed in any of the models mentioned above.

The present investigations suggest that there are at least two sources of brain phagocytes, viz. endogenous microglia and hematogenous macrophages. Furthermore, it seems that the hematogenous source is activated only in cer-tain types of degenerative conditions, such as traumatic lesions. A similar graded response from different sources of phagocytes has been suggested by VAUGHN and PEASE (20) and VAUGHN and SKOFF (9). It may be significant that the blood-brain barrier for proteins is intact in retrograde (21) and Wallerian (22) degeneration and disturbed in mechanical lesions (23), thus indicating that an increased vascular permeability may be necessary to acti-vate the hematogenous macrophages.

REFERENCES

1. TORVIK, A., SKJÖRTEN, F.: Electron microscopic observations on nerve cell regeneration and degeneration after axon lesions. I. Changes in the nerve cell cytoplasm. Acta neuropath. (Berl.) *17*, 248 - 264 (1971)
2. TORVIK, A., SKJÖRTEN, F.: Electron microscopic observations on nerve cell regeneration and degeneration after axon lesions. II. Changes in the glial cells. Acta neuropath. (Berl.) *17*, 265 - 282 (1971)
3. TORVIK, A.: Phagocytosis of nerve cells during retrograde degeneration. An electron microscopic study. J. Neuropath. exp. Neurol. *31*, 132 - 146 (1972)
4. TORVIK, A., SÖREIDE, A.: Nerve cell regeneration after axon lesions in newborn rabbits. Light and electron microscopic study. J. Neuropath. exp. Neurol. *31*, 683 - 695 (1972)
5. STENWIG, A.E.: The origin of brain macrophages in traumatic lesions, Wallerian degeneration, and retrograde degeneration. J. Neuropath. exp. Neurol. *31*, 696 - 704 (1972)
6. BERNER, AA., TORVIK, A., STENWIG, A.E.: Origin of macrophages in traumatic lesions and Wallerian degeneration in perpheral nerves. Acta neuropath. (Berl.) *25*, 228 - 236 (1973)
7. SÖREIDE, A.: Personal communications
8. STENWIG, A.E.: Personal communications
9. VAUGHN, J.E., SKOFF, R.P.: Neuroglia in experimentally altered central nervous system. *In:* The Structure and Function of Nervous Tissue, p. 39 - 72. New York: Academic Press 1972

10. OEHMICHEN, M., GRÜNINGER, H., SAEBISCH, R., NARITA, Y.: Mikroglia und Pericyten als Transformationsformen der Blut-Monocyten mit erhaltener Proliferationsfähigkeit. Acta neuropath. (Berl.) *23*, 200 - 218 (1973)
11. KERNS, J.M., HINSMAN, E.: Neuroglial response to sciatic neurectomy. II. Electron microscopy. J. comp. Neurol. *151*, 255 - 280 (1973)
12. MATTHEWS, M.A.: Mikroglia and reactive "M" cells of degenerating nervous system: Does similar morphology and function imply a common origin? Cell. Tiss. Res. *148*, 477 - 491 (1974)
13. COOK, R.D., WISNIEWSKI, H.M.: The role of oligodendroglia and astroglia in Wallerian degeneration of the optic nerve. Brain Res. *61*, 191 - 206 (1973)
14. ADRIAN, E.K., WILLIAMS, M.G.: Cell proliferation in the injured spinal cord. An electron microscopic study. J. comp. Neurol. *151*, 1 - 24 (1974)
15. KREUTZBERG, G.W.: Über perineuronale Mikrogliazellen (Autoradiographische Untersuchungen). Acta neuropath. (Berl.) Suppl. IV, 141 - 145 (1968)
16. ADRIAN, E.K., SMOTHERMON, R.D.: Leucocytic infiltration into the hypoglossal nucleus followi g injury to the hypoglossal nerve. Anat. Rec. *166*, 99 - 116 (1970)
17. WATSON, W.E.: Cellular r sponses to axotomy and to related procedures. Brit. med. Bull. *30*, 112 - 115 (1974)
18. MATTHEWS, M.A., KRUGER, ..: Electron microscopy of non-neuronal cellular changes accompanying neu al degeneration in thalamic nuclei of the rabbit. I. Reactive hematogenous and perivascular elements within the basal lamina. J. comp. Neurol. *148*, 28! - 312 (1973)
19. BARRON, K.D., MEANS, E.D., FENG, T., HARRIS, H.: Ultrastructure of retrograde degeneration in the .amus of rat. 2. Changes in vascular elements and transvascular migration c leucocytes. Exp. molec. Path. *20*, 344 - 362 (1974)
20. VAUGHN, J.E., PEASE, D.C. Electron microscopic studies of Wallerian degeneration of optic ner es. II. Astrocytes, oligodendrocytes and adventitial cells. J. comp. Neurol. *140*, 207 - 226 (1970)
21. SJÖSTRAND, J.: Morphologic l changes in glial cells during nerve regeneration. Acta physiol. scar l. Suppl. *270*, 19 - 43 (1966)
22. OSTERBERG, K.A., WATTENBER, L.W.: Inductive factors in gliosis. Proc. Soc. exp. Biol. (N.Y.) *111* 452 - 455 (1962)
23. HIRANO, A., BECKER, N.H., : IMMERMAN, H.M.: Pathological alterations in the cerebral endothelial cell l arrier to peroxidase. Arch. Neurol. (Chic.) *20*, 300 - 317 (1969)

Prof. Dr. A. TORVIK
Laboratory of Neuropathology
Ullevaal Hospital
Oslo / Norway

Acta Neuropath. (Berlin), Suppl. VI, 301 (1975)
© by Springer-Verlag 1975

Conclusions

H.M. ZIMMERMAN AND K. LENNERT

It must be recognized that currently there is no general acceptance of a single classification of malignant lymphomas that involve the nervous system. This is even true for a classification of extracranial lymphomas. Yet progress has been made in this direction, notably by LENNERT, whose proposal for such a classification has been presented in some detail. It is expected that attempts will be made in the future to apply this classification to the tumors of this category that affect the brain and spinal cord. Hopefully some order will result from such efforts in an admittedly very complex subject.

The consensus of the participants in this symposium is that certain avenues of approach are both available and feasible in studying the problems of primary lymphomas of the nervous system. These include the following:

1. Light microscopic studies with a variety of staining techniques, especially applied to imprints of lesions obtained from fresh material.
2. Electron microscopic studies of such lesions with the aim of cell identification.
3. Immunological approaches utilizing surface markers (immunoglobulins, C_3-receptors, Fc-receptors, sheep red blood cell receptors, etc.) studied in cell suspensions (CSF!) or sections. There is some evidence indicating that some tumor cell types can be morphologically correlated with immunological data, while other tumors have yet to be clarified.
4. Determinations of DNA content in neoplastic and normal cells.
5. Chromosome analysis.
6. Cell, tissue, and organ cultures. It may be especially fruitful to establish and characterize continuous cell culture lines of human malignant lymphomas. It is now also possible to study the intracerebral heterotransplantation of lymphoma tissue in the nude athymic mouse.
7. Cerebrospinal fluid analyses for cells and M gradients.
8. Histo- and cytochemical studies of sections and imprints respectively.
9. Search for animal models of lymphomas, especially of Hodgkin's disease.
10. Intensive clinical studies on lymphomas, these to include epidemiological investigations as well as clinical-anatomical correlations.
11. Viral studies of lymphoma lesions.

It is felt by at least some participants of this symposium that the active pursuit of these approaches may yield results that would warrant a second follow-up conference on this subject in the foreseeable future.

Allocortex
Bearbeitet von H. Stephan
Etwa 465 Abbildungen
Etwa 1080 Seiten. 1975
(Handbuch der mikros-
kopischen Anatomie des
Menschen, Band 4:
Nervensystem, Teil 9)
In Vorbereitung
ISBN 3-540-07037-0

S.L. Palay, V. Chan-Palay
Cerebellar Cortex
Cytology and Organiza-
tion
267 figures incl. 203 plates
X, 348 pages. 1974
Cloth DM 156,—,
US $67.10
ISBN 3-540-06228-9
Distribution rights for
Japan: Igaku Shoin Ltd.,
Tokyo

K.J. Zülch
**Atlas of Gross
Neurosurgical Pathology**
379 figures. V, 228 pages
1975. Cloth DM 120,—;
US $51.60
ISBN 3-540-06480-X
Distribution rights for
Japan: Nankodo Co.
Ltd., Tokyo

**Neurosecretion —
The Final
Neuroendocrine Pathway**
6th International Sym-
posium on Neurosecretion,
London 1973
Editors: F. Knowles,
L. Vollrath
92 figures. X, 345 pages
1974. Cloth DM 118,—
US $50.80
ISBN 3-540-06821-X

K.J. Zülch
**Atlas of the Histology
of Brain Tumors**
Title and text in six
languages (English,
German, French, Spanish,
Russian, and Japanese)
100 figures
XVI, 261 pages
Cloth DM 96,—;
US $41.30
ISBN 3-540-05274-7
Distribution rights for
Japan: Nankodo Co. Ltd.,
Tokyo

T. Edinger
**Paleoneurology
1804 – 1966,
an annotated bibliography**
Approx. 275 pages. 1975
(Advances in Anatomy,
Embryology and Cell
Biology, Volume 49)
DM 80,—; US $34.40
ISBN 3-540-07060-5

Intracranial Pressure
Experimental
and Clinical Aspects
Editors: M. Brock,
H. Dietz
142 figures
XVI, 383 pages. 1972
Cloth DM 86,—;
US $37.00
ISBN 3-540-06039-1
Distribution rights for
Japan: Igaku Shoin Ltd.,
Tokyo

Preisänderungen
vorbehalten

Prices are subject to
change without notice

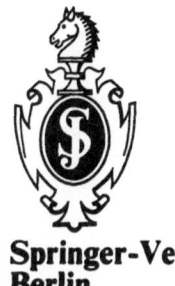

**Springer-Verlag
Berlin
Heidelberg
New York**